Practical Trends in Anesthesia and Intensive Care 2022

Davide Chiumello
Editor

Practical Trends in Anesthesia and Intensive Care 2022

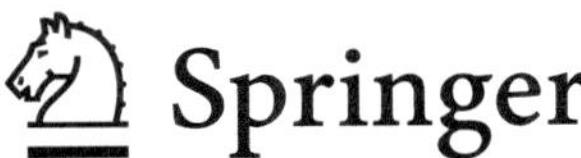 Springer

Editor
Davide Chiumello
SC Anestesia e Rianimazione
Ospedale San Paolo
Milan, Italy

ISBN 978-3-031-43893-6   ISBN 978-3-031-43891-2   (eBook)
https://doi.org/10.1007/978-3-031-43891-2

The translation was done with the help of an artificial intelligence machine translation tool. A subsequent human revision was done primarily in terms of content.

This Springer imprint is published by the registered company Springer Nature Switzerland AG
The registered company address is: Gewerbestrasse 11, 6330 Cham, Switzerland

If disposing of this product, please recycle the paper.

Contents

Part I   Anesthesia

1   TIVA and TCI in Modern Anesthesia 3
Franco Cavaliere and Carlo Cavaliere
  1.1 Indications for the Use of TIVA 4
  1.2 Pharmacokinetics of Intravenous Anesthetics 5
      1.2.1 Peculiarities of Intravenous Anesthetics Versus
             Anesthetic Vapors 5
      1.2.2 Trend of Plasma Concentration After an Intravenous
             Bolus 5
      1.2.3 Distribution in the Organism 6
      1.2.4 Tricompartmental Models 7
  1.3 Manual Adjustment of Anesthetic Infusion 9
  1.4 TCI—Target Controlled Infusion 10
      1.4.1 Effector Site 11
      1.4.2 Anesthetic Half-Life and Recovery of Consciousness 12
      1.4.3 Drug Interactions 13
  1.5 Closed-Loop Anesthesia 13
  1.6 Conclusions: Intravenous Anesthesia as Surfing 14
  References 16

**2   Normothermia in Anesthesia: Impact on Quality and Safety
of Care** 19
Felice Eugenio Agrò and Rita Cataldo
  2.1 Historical Background 19
  2.2 Concepts of Physiology 20
      2.2.1 Thermoregulation of the Body 20
      2.2.2 Factors Affecting Temperature 21
      2.2.3 Changes in Body Temperature 21
      2.2.4 Definition of Fever 22
      2.2.5 Pathophysiology of Fever 22
      2.2.6 Thermal Curves 23
      2.2.7 Hyperthermia 24
      2.2.8 Hypothermia 24

2.3   Preserve the Normothermia   25
2.4   Cardiovascular Effects of Hypothermia   25
2.5   Respiratory Effects of Hypothermia   25
2.6   Coagulation and Hypothermia   25
2.7   Effects of Hypothermia on the Central Nervous System   25
2.8   Effects of Hypothermia on the Immune System   26
2.9   Drugs Effects on Thermoregulation   26
2.10   Hypothermia-Related Complications: 1.4 °C Reduction
       in Core Temperature   26
2.11   Recommendations for Shiver-Free Surgery and Perioperative
       Normothermia   30
Recommended Readings   30

3   **Surgical Site Infections and Antibiotic Prophylaxis in Surgery:
     Update 2023**   33
     Andrea De Gasperi, Marco Merli, Laura Petrò, and Elena Roselli
3.1   Introduction   33
3.2   SSIs—Exogenous or Endogenous Infections?   34
3.3   The "Bundle" Philosophy: The Importance of Aggregated,
       Structured, and Targeted Interventions   36
3.4   The GAIS Bundle   37
3.5   Surgical Antibiotic Prophylaxis (SAP)   39
       3.5.1   SAP has a Precise Rationale Related to   39
       3.5.2   Antibiotic usage in SAP   41
3.6   Assumptions and Indications of Antibiotic Prophylaxis
       in Surgery (SAP)   42
3.7   SAP Schedules   44
3.8   Conclusions   51
References   51

4   **Safety in the Operating Room**   53
     Edoardo De Robertis and Davide Valeri
4.1   Introduction   53
4.2   Medical Error in Anesthesia: Epidemiology and Guidelines   54
4.3   Minimum Standards of Monitoring in Anesthesia   57
4.4   Drug Safety   59
4.5   Use of Checklists, Reports, Surveys   63
References   64

5   **Patient Blood Management**   67
     Francesca Puccini, Lucia M. Bindi, Massimo Esposito,
     and Gianni Biancofiore
5.1   Introduction   67
5.2   Objectives of PBM   68

5.3 PBM: From Theory to Practice 69
    5.3.1 PBM in the Pre-operative Period 71
    5.3.2 PBM in the Intraoperative Period 75
    5.3.3 PBM in the Postoperative Period 78
    5.3.4 PBM: Experiences from Around the World 79
    5.3.5 Strategies for Implementing a PBM Program 79
    5.3.6 PBM: The Problems 81
5.4 Conclusions 81
References 82

6 Monitoring of Sedation and Sleep in Intensive Care Unit 85
Stefano Romagnoli and Francesco Barbani
6.1 Introduction 85
6.2 Guidelines and Monitoring Tools: The Gold Standard 86
6.3 Beyond Clinical Scales: For RASS ≤3—Instrumental
    Monitoring 87
6.4 The pEEG Systems for Monitoring Sedation 90
6.5 Not Only Excessive Sedation: The Phenomenon of Awakenings in
    Patients with Paralysis in ICUs 92
6.6 Summary 92
6.7 Monitoring and the Importance of Sleep 93
6.8 The Concept of Sleep Disruption and Risk Stratification 93
6.9 Preserving the Sleep–Wake Cycle 95
6.10 Conclusions 98
References 98

7 Anesthesia in Robotic Surgery 101
Davide Chiumello and Eleonora Duscio
7.1 Surgical Technique 102
7.2 Pathophysiological Alterations During Robotic Surgery 103
7.3 Hemodynamic Effects 104
7.4 Regional Perfusion, Central Nervous System, Eye
    and Splanchnic Organs 105
7.5 Respiratory Effects 106
7.6 Anesthesia Management 106
    7.6.1 Preoperative Evaluation 106
    7.6.2 Intravenous and Volatile Anesthesia 107
    7.6.3 Neuromuscular Blockade 108
    7.6.4 Positioning 108
    7.6.5 Ventilation Management 109
    7.6.6 Hemodynamic Monitoring 110
    7.6.7 Postoperative Pain Management 111
7.7 Intraoperative Complications 112
7.8 Conclusion 113
References 113

**8   Pre-anesthesia Evaluation and Risk Assessment in Adult Patient
      Candidates for Non-cardiac Surgery** 117
      Rita Cataldo, Sabrina Migliorelli, and Felice Eugenio Agrò
      8.1   Introduction 117
      8.2   Preoperative Anesthesiology Assessment in Patients Undergoing
             Non-cardiac Surgery: A General Overview..................... 118
             8.2.1   Physiological Medical History........................ 118
             8.2.2   Surgical and Anesthesiological Medical History.......... 119
             8.2.3   Which Preoperative Tests to Request?.................. 121
      8.3   Evaluation of the Cardiovascular System in Patients Undergoing
             Non-cardiac Surgery 126
             8.3.1   Functional Capacity Evaluation....................... 126
             8.3.2   Cardiovascular Risk Factors 127
      8.4   Management of Home Drug Therapy 133
             8.4.1   Management of Patients Undergoing Regional
                      Anesthesia While on Anti-thrombotic Medication
                      Treatment...................................... 133
      8.5   Assessment of the Respiratory System 139
      8.6   The Preoperative Approach to the Geriatric/Fragile Patient 140
      8.7   ASA PS Score and International Risk Scores 141
             8.7.1   ASA PS Score 141
             8.7.2   International Risk Scores............................ 141
      8.8   Conclusions 144
      References.. 144

Part II   Critical Care Medicine

9   Purification Techniques 149
      Luigi Tritapepe, Benedetta Cirulli, Stefania Bove, Naike Amato,
      and Aurora Smeriglia
      9.1   Introduction 149
      9.2   Acute Renal Failure...................................... 149
      9.3   Renal Replacement Therapies 151
      9.4   How Does an RRT Work? 153
      9.5   Anticoagulation in CRRT 156
      9.6   When to Start a CRRT?.................................... 158
      9.7   What Is the Optimal Dosage of CRRT?........................ 158
      9.8   Vascular Access 159
      9.9   Depurative Therapy in Liver Failure 160
      9.10   Plasmapheresis.. 160
      9.11   CPFA 161
      9.12   Extracorporeal Removal of CO_2 161
      9.13   Purification Techniques with Special Filters 162
             9.13.1   Polyethyleneimine Filter and Heparin Coating 162

      9.13.2 Adsorbent Resin (Styrene-Divinylbenzene) 163
      9.13.3 Adsorbent Cartridge with Polymyxin B 163
  9.14 Conclusions 164
  Further Reading 164

10 Sepsis from SARS-COV2 Infection (COVID-19): Pathophysiology and Clinic of SARS-COV2 Infection and Sepsis.... 167
Giorgio Tulli
  10.1 The Damage Response Framework (DRF): A New Model to Better Understand the Complexity of Infections.............. 167
      10.1.1 What Are the Clinical and Epidemiological Features of COVID-19 Infection? 168
  10.2 Host-Pathogen-Environment Interactions Underlying Knowledge of Infection 172
  10.3 Viral Sepsis: Early Observations of SARS-COV2 Sepsis 174
  10.4 Viral Infection and Pathogenesis of COVID-19 Infection in Organs 175
      10.4.1 Immune Response to SARS-COV2 and Viral Sepsis 175
      10.4.2 COVID-19 Infection and Abnormal Coagulation 176
  10.5 What Has Viral Sepsis from COVID-19 Infection Taught Us About 177
      10.5.1 What Already Did They Know About Bacterial and Fungal Sepsis?........................... 177
      10.5.2 What Has COVID-19 Sepsis Taught Us? 181
      10.5.3 To Understand the Differences Between SARS-COV2 Infection and Other Systemic Disorders 183
      10.5.4 Pathobiology of COVID-19 185
      10.5.5 Pathobiology of COVID-19 ARDS (C-ARDS) 186
      10.5.6 Pathobiology of Sepsis 187
      10.5.7 Pathobiology of CAR-T Cell-Induced Cytokine Release Syndrome 187
  10.6 Lessons Learned from Bacterial Sepsis Regarding Immunotherapies for COVID-19 Infection 189
  10.7 Immunoparalysis in COVID-19 Sepsis 192
      10.7.1 Monocyte HLA-DR as a Pro-/Anti-inflammatory Marker 193
      10.7.2 Clinical Outcomes in Patients with COVID-19-Immunophenotype In-Depth Studies.................. 194
      10.7.3 Measurements of HLA-DR on Arrival at the Hospital and Various Severities of Patients 194
      10.7.4 Kinetics of HLA-DR Monitoring in Intensive Care Unit Patients.................................... 195
  References..................................... 197

11 Nutrition Therapy in Critically Ill Patients 207
Yaroslava Longhitano, Christian Zanza, Giulia Racca,
and Fabrizio Racca
  11.1   Introduction 207
  11.2   Pathophysiology of Malnutrition in ICU Patients 209
  11.3   Comparisons of Enteral to Parenteral Nutrition
       in Critically Ill Patients 210
  11.4   When to Start Nutrition Therapy 211
  11.5   Refeeding Syndrome Prevention 213
  11.6   What Is the Best Method for Determining Energy
       and Protein Needs in Critically Ill Patients? 214
       11.6.1   Energy Requirement 214
       11.6.2   Protein Requirement 217
       11.6.3   Micronutrients 218
  11.7   Parenteral Nutrition (PN) 218
       11.7.1   PN Venous Access 218
       11.7.2   PN Prescription 219
       11.7.3   Complications 219
  11.8   Enteral Nutrition 220
       11.8.1   Access 220
       11.8.2   Formulations 221
       11.8.3   EN Prescription 224
       11.8.4   Complications 224
  11.9   Conclusions 226
  References 226

12 Patient-Ventilator Interaction in the Patient with ARDS 231
Lucia Mirabella and Cesare Gregoretti
  12.1   Introduction 231
  12.2   Respiratory Physiology and Mechanical Ventilation 231
  12.3   Types of Asynchronies 232
  12.4   Triggering Delay 234
  12.5   Ineffective Effort 235
  12.6   Auto-trigger 236
  12.7   Double Triggering (Double Triggering) 237
  12.8   Reverse-Triggering 237
  12.9   Flow Asynchronies 238
  12.10 Cyclic Asynchronies 238
  12.11 Clinical Implications 239
       12.11.1 Ventilator-Induced Diaphragmatic Dysfunction 239
       12.11.2 Weaning Difficulties 239
       12.11.3 Patient Discomfort and Cognitive Dysfunction 240
       12.11.4 Dyspnea 240
       12.11.5 Monitoring of Asynchronies 240
       12.11.6 Strategies for Improving Patient-Ventilator Interactions 241
  References 245

13 End-of-Life in Intensive Care 249
Giacinto Pizzilli, Alessio Dell'Olio, Maria Della Giovampaola,
and Luciana Mascia
  13.1   Introduction 249
  13.2   Prognostication 250
       13.2.1 Neurological and Neurosurgical Patients. 250
       13.2.2 General ICU. 251
  13.3   Decision-Making Process and Communication. 252
  13.4   End-of-Life Management in the ICU. 255
       13.4.1 Pain Relief and Sedation Management 255
       13.4.2 Respiratory Support. 257
  13.5   Conclusions 257
  References. 258

**14 Point-of-Care Ultrasound (POCUS) in Pediatric Age:
Update** 261
Giovanna Chidini
  14.1   Introduction 261
  14.2   Indications for Chest Ultrasound in Neonatal/Pediatric Age. 262
  14.3   Modalities of Performing Bedside Chest and Cardiac
       Ultrasound in Children. 262
  14.4   Ultrasonographic Features in the Healthy Lung 263
  14.5   Ultrasound in the Diseased Lung. 264
       14.5.1 Pleural Effusion. 264
       14.5.2 Pneumothorax 264
       14.5.3 Consolidation (Atelectasis/Pneumonia). 265
  14.6   Lung Ultrasound Score in the Infant and Child. 265
       14.6.1 LUS POCUS: Bronchiolitis. 267
       14.6.2 LUS POCUS and SARS-COV2 Infection 268
       14.6.3 LUS POCUS: Diagnosis and Follow-Up
              of Neonatal Lung Disease 269
  14.7   Congenital Pulmonary Airway Malformation (CPAM). 272
       14.7.1 Congenital Malformations of the Lung or Chest Wall. 273
  14.8   Chest Trauma and Detection of Signs of Child Abuse. 273
  14.9   Ultrasound of the Diaphragm. 274
       14.9.1 LUS POCUS and Intubation 274
       14.9.2 Point-of-Care Ultrasound: ESPNIC Guidelines. 275
  14.10 Conclusions 277
  References. 277

15 Prehospital and Early Intrahospital Management of Trauma 281
Luca Bolgiaghi, Fabrizio Sammartano, and Davide Chiumello
  15.1   Prehospital Management 281
  15.2   Early Intrahospital Management 289
  15.3   The Activation of the Trauma Team. 291
       15.3.1 Code Red 292
       15.3.2 Code Yellow 292

15.4   First-Level Diagnostics 293
       15.4.1   Extended Focused Assessment Sonography
                for Trauma (E-FAST). 293
       15.4.2   Chest X-Ray. 293
       15.4.3   X-Ray of the Pelvis 294
15.5   Second-Level Diagnostics 294
       15.5.1   X-Ray of the Spine. 294
       15.5.2   X-Rays of the Limbs 295
       15.5.3   Angiography 295
       15.5.4   Nuclear Magnetic Resonance Imaging (RMN) 296
References. 296

Contributors

Felice Eugenio Agrò Fondazione Policlinico Universitario Campus Bio Medico, Rome, Italy

Research Unit of Anesthesia, Intensive Care and Pain Management, Department of Medicine and Surgery, Università Campus Bio-Medico di Roma, Rome, Italy

Naike Amato AO San Camillo-Forlanini, Rome, Italy

Francesco Barbani Department of Anesthesia and Critical Care, Azienda Ospedaliero-Universitaria Careggi, Florence, Italy

SODc Oncology Anesthesia and Intensive Care Unit, Florence, Italy

Gianni Biancofiore Transplant Anesthesia and Critical Care, Pisa University Hospital, Pisa, Italy

Lucia M. Bindi Transplant Anesthesia and Critical Care, Pisa University Hospital, Pisa, Italy

Luca Bolgiaghi Department of Anaesthesia and Resuscitation, ASST Santi Paolo e Carlo, San Paolo University Hospital, Milan, Italy

Stefania Bove AO San Camillo-Forlanini, Rome, Italy

Rita Cataldo Fondazione Policlinico Universitario Campus Bio Medico, Rome, Italy

Research Unit of Anesthesia, Intensive Care and Pain Management, Department of Medicine and Surgery, Università Campus Bio-Medico di Roma, Rome, Italy

Carlo Cavaliere ENT Clinic, University "Sapienza", Rome, Italy

Franco Cavaliere Department of Cardiovascular Sciences, Catholic University of the Sacred Heart, Rome, Italy

Giovanna Chidini Pediatric Intensive Care Unit, Dipartimento Di Emergenza Urgenza- Fondazione IRCCS Cà Granda Ospedale Maggiore Policlinico, Milan, Italy

Davide Chiumello Department of Anesthesia and Resuscitation, ASST Santi Paolo e Carlo, San Paolo University Hospital, Milan, Italy

Department of Health Sciences, University of Milan, Milan, Italy

Benedetta Cirulli AO San Camillo-Forlanini, Rome, Italy

Alessio Dell'Olio Dipartimento di Scienze Mediche e Chirurgiche, Anesthesia and Intensive Care Medicine, Policlinico di Sant'Orsola, Alma Mater Studiorum, Università di Bologna, Bologna, Italy

Maria Della Giovampaola Dipartimento di Scienze Mediche e Chirurgiche, Anesthesia and Intensive Care Medicine, Policlinico di Sant'Orsola, Alma Mater Studiorum, Università di Bologna, Bologna, Italy

Eleonora Duscio Department of Anaesthesia and Intensive Care, ASST Santi Paolo e Carlo, San Paolo University Hospital, Milan, Italy

Massimo Esposito Transplant Anesthesia and Critical Care, Pisa University Hospital, Pisa, Italy

Andrea De Gasperi, MD Anesthesia and Critical Care Service, ASST GOM Niguarda, Milan, Italy

Cesare Gregoretti Department of Surgical, Oncological and Oral Science (Di. Chir.On.S.), University of Palermo, 'Giglio' Foundation, Palermo, Italy

Yaroslava Longhitano Department of Anesthesiology and Intensive Care, Azienda Ospedaliera SS, Antonio e Biagio e Cesare Arrigo, Alessandria, Italy

Luciana Mascia Dipartimento di Scienze Biomediche e Neuromotorie, Anesthesia and Intensive Care Medicine, Alma Mater Studiorum, Università di Bologna, Bologna, Italy

Marco Merli, MD Infectious Diseases Unit - ASST GOM Niguarda, Milan, Italy

Sabrina Migliorelli Graduate School of Anesthesia, Resuscitation, Intensive Care and Pain Management, Fondazione Policlinico Universitario Campus Bio Medico Roma, Rome, Italy

Research Unit of Anesthesia, Intensive Care and Pain Management, Department of Medicine and Surgery, Università Campus Bio-Medico di Roma, Rome, Italy

Lucia Mirabella Department of Medical and Surgical Sciences, University of Foggia, Hospital OO Riuniti di Foggia, Foggia, Italy

Laura Petrò AR 1 - Papa Giovanni 23 Hospital, Bergamo, Italy

Giacinto Pizzilli Dipartimento di Scienze Mediche e Chirurgiche, Anesthesia and Intensive Care Medicine, Policlinico di Sant'Orsola, Alma Mater Studiorum, Università di Bologna, Bologna, Italy

Francesca Puccini Transplant Anesthesia and Critical Care, Pisa University Hospital, Pisa, Italy

Fabrizio Racca Department of Anesthesiology and Intensive Care, Azienda Ospedaliera SS, Antonio e Biagio e Cesare Arrigo, Alessandria, Italy

Giulia Racca Department of Anesthesiology and Intensive Care, Azienda Ospedaliera SS, Antonio e Biagio e Cesare Arrigo, Alessandria, Italy

Edoardo De Robertis Anaesthesia, Analgesia and Intensive Care Section, Department of Medicine and Surgery, University of Perugia, Perugia, Italy

Stefano Romagnoli Department of Health Sciences, University of Florence, Florence, Italy

Department of Anesthesia and Critical Care, Azienda Ospedaliero-Universitaria Careggi, Florence, Italy

Elena Roselli Anesthesia and Critical Care Service, ASST GOM Niguarda, Milan, Italy

Fabrizio Sammartano San Carlo Borromeo Trauma Center, ASST Santi Paolo e Carlo, San Carlo University Hospital, Milan, Italy

Aurora Smeriglia School of Specialization in Anaesthesia and Intensive Care, Sapienza University of Rome, Rome, Italy

Luigi Tritapepe Sapienza University of Rome, Rome, Italy

UOC Anaesthesia and Intensive Care, AO San Camillo-Forlanini-Rome, Rome, Italy

Giorgio Tulli Department of the Florentine Healthcare Trust, Tuscany Region, Florence, Italy

Davide Valeri Anaesthesia, Analgesia and Intensive Care Section, Department of Medicine and Surgery, University of Perugia, Perugia, Italy

Christian Zanza Department of Anesthesiology and Intensive Care, Azienda Ospedaliera SS, Antonio e Biagio e Cesare Arrigo, Alessandria, Italy

Part I

Anesthesia

TIVA and TCI in Modern Anesthesia

1

Franco Cavaliere and Carlo Cavaliere

General anesthesia is characterized by reversible depression of central nervous system functions, with the goal of inducing loss of consciousness, analgesia, amnesia, abolition of neurovegetative responses to stimuli, immobility, and, in some cases, abolition of muscle tone. Over the years, the pharmacological toolbox available to the anesthesiologist has increased considerably. There are a variety of drugs that can be used, some administered by inhalation because they are in the gas or vapor state under ambient conditions, and others administered intravenously. Totally intravenous anesthesia (TIVA: Total IntraVenous Anesthesia) uses only intravenous anesthetics; inhalational anesthesia employs anesthetic vapors; balanced anesthesia, the most widely used, uses both routes. Target-Controlled Infusion (TCI) is a technique for administering intravenous anesthetics that uses advanced infusion pumps, which can autonomously vary the infusion rate to maintain a constant concentration of anesthetic set by the operator in the plasma or effector site; the software with which the pump is equipped continually reevaluates the amount of drug to be infused based on a pharmacokinetic model. Closed-Loop Anesthesia is an anesthesia technique using the TCI method, in which the anesthesiologist does not set the concentration of the anesthetic but the magnitude of the desired effect, e.g., the level of depth of anesthesia as measured by the Bispectral index (BIS). In this mode, the software changes the target plasma concentration based on data from the monitoring system. Table 1.1 shows some important dates in the development of intravenous anesthesia [1].

F. Cavaliere (✉)
Department of Cardiovascular Sciences, Catholic University of the Sacred Heart, Rome, Italy
e-mail: franco.cavaliere@unicatt.it; fcavaliere54@gmail.com

C. Cavaliere
ENT Clinic, University "Sapienza", Rome, Italy

D. Chiumello (ed.), *Practical Trends in Anesthesia and Intensive Care 2022*,
https://doi.org/10.1007/978-3-031-43891-2_1

Table 1.1 Some important dates in the development of intravenous anesthesia

Invention of the syringe, A. Wood, C. G. Pravaz	1853
Intravenous chloral hydrate to produce general anesthesia, P. C. Oré	1872
Synthesis of sodium thiopental, E. H. Volwiler, D. L. Tabern	1934
Development of propofol, JB Glen	1973
Commercialization of propofol, Astra-Zeneca plc	1986
Commercialization of remifentanil, Glaxo Wellcome Inc.	1996

1.1 Indications for the Use of TIVA

The choice of anesthetics and thus the technique, inhaled, intravenous, or balanced, depends on the characteristics of the patient, the type of surgery, and the preferences of the anesthesiologist. The use of TIVA is often motivated by the purpose of avoiding environmental pollution related to the release of anesthetic gases or vapors into the ambient air, although in today's operating rooms air pollution is prevented by the presence of outdoor elimination systems for gases exhaled by the patient. However, the problem of the harmful effects of nitrous oxide on the environment remains. This anesthetic is in fact a more harmful greenhouse gas than carbon dioxide, which can remain in the atmosphere without degrading for many years and which damages the ozone layer in the stratosphere [2].

The main indication for the use of TIVA is the need to avoid inhaled anesthetics. An example is anesthesia in patients at risk of malignant hyperthermia, because anesthetic vapors can trigger this hypermetabolic response of skeletal muscles [3], and in those with long QT syndrome, in whom sevoflurane can trigger ventricular torsion tachycardia [4]. Inhalational anesthetics should also be avoided in patients at high risk for postoperative nausea and vomiting (PONV) because their use is associated with a higher frequency of episodes [5]. In neurosurgery, anesthetic vapors can increase intracranial pressure and interfere with neurophysiologic monitoring.

Another indication for the use of TIVA may arise from the environment where anesthesia or sedation is performed. Indeed, the use of anesthetic vapors requires the availability of the appropriate vaporizer and anesthesia equipment. The unavailability of this equipment may force the anesthesiologist to choose totally intravenous anesthesia. This may occur in surgeries performed outside of operating rooms and in cases where the surgical procedure requires moving the patient still under general anesthesia from one setting to another.

1.2   Pharmacokinetics of Intravenous Anesthetics

1.2.1   Peculiarities of Intravenous Anesthetics Versus Anesthetic Vapors

One of the aspects that differentiate intravenous anesthesia from inhalation anesthesia is the lack of parameters to monitor the concentration of anesthetic in the blood. In inhalational anesthesia, in fact, the use of equipment to measure the concentration of anesthetics in the gases exhaled by the patient is widespread. The end-expiratory value corresponds to the concentration in the pulmonary alveoli and is a good estimate of that in arterial blood. This parameter is universally used to express anesthetic potency, and the end-expiratory concentration sufficient to inhibit the patient's response to surgical incision of the skin in 50% of subjects (MAC, Minimal Alveolar Concentration) is one of the parameters that guide the anesthesiologist. In addition, the use of alarms set to the end-expiratory concentration of anesthetic vapors is very useful in preventing awareness, having demonstrated similar effectiveness to monitoring systems based on electroencephalographic signal analysis [6].

A further difference between intravenous and inhalational anesthesia is that anesthetic vapors result in a global depression of the nervous system, offering the possibility of performing single-drug anesthesia, whereas intravenous anesthetics have more selective actions, particularly on the hypnotic and analgesic components. This makes clinical assessment of the depth of anesthesia and degree of analgesia achieved during TIVA more difficult and increases the risk of an inadequate level of hypnosis and intraoperative awareness episodes [7]. Therefore, the use of anesthesia depth monitoring systems based on electroencephalographic signal analysis is indicated in totally intravenous anesthesia [8].

1.2.2   Trend of Plasma Concentration After an Intravenous Bolus

As with anesthetic vapors, the effects of intravenous anesthetics are closely related to their plasma levels [9]. It is in fact from plasma that they reach the effector site by crossing the blood–brain barrier. A concentration in plasma (or even at the effector site) such that there is no response to surgical incision in 50% of subjects (Cp50) is the equivalent of MAC for intravenous anesthetics.

The concentration achieved after administration of an intravenous bolus depends on the initial dilution of the drug within a central compartment, the volume of which is related to body mass and corresponds to the ratio of the plasma concentration achieved to the dose administered. In this sense, the bolus effect is relatively predictable and dose-dependent. In the literature, intravenous dosages are readily available to achieve for a limited period of time a level of anesthesia sufficient to abolish the patient's response to certain standard stimuli, such as those represented by tracheal intubation or surgical incision.

The difficulty arises from the need to maintain sufficiently stable plasma concentrations to achieve consistent levels of hypnosis or analgesia for a prolonged time. After the initial bolus, in fact, the plasma concentration of the anesthetic gradually decreases both because the drug is distributed within the body and because it is eliminated by the excretory organs. To keep the plasma concentration constant, therefore, it is necessary to infuse the amount of drug needed to balance that which leaves the central compartment. A constant-rate intravenous infusion is unsuitable for this purpose because the amount of anesthetic that leaves the central compartment varies, decreasing progressively over time. During TIVA, therefore, adjustments to the infusion rate are necessary and are set by the anesthesiologist, based on clinical and instrumental monitoring of anesthetic effects, or by the TCI systems software based on a pharmacokinetic model.

1.2.3 Distribution in the Organism

If one follows the plasma concentration of an anesthetic after administration of an intravenous bolus, one can see that its decrease does not have a linear trend corresponding to a constant elimination rate and zero-order kinetics (concentration-independent elimination) (Fig. 1.1a). Instead, the time/concentration graph is represented by a curve showing how the rate at which concentration decreases slows down over time (Fig. 1.2). This occurs because the processes that affect the distribution and elimination of most drugs follow order 1 kinetics, in which the speed of the process varies as the concentration of the drug changes. For example, the diffusion of a drug from one compartment of the body to another occurs with a rate that decreases as the concentration in the first compartment decreases. A process that follows kinetics of order 1 is described by an exponential equation and is represented on a linear graph by a curved line (Fig. 1.1b). If, however, a semi-logarithmic

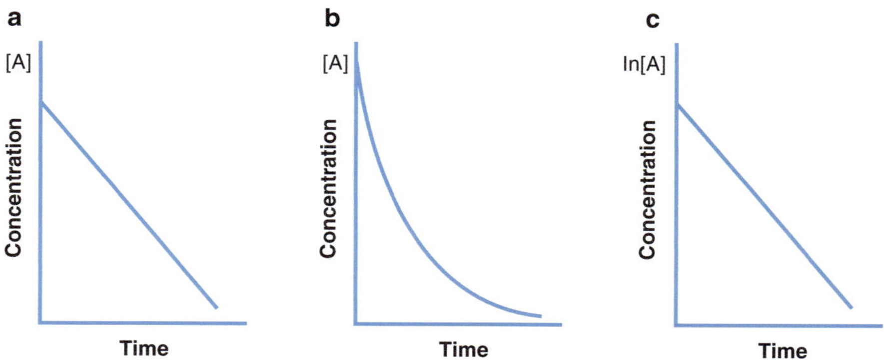

Fig. 1.1 (a) Order 0 kinetics: concentration [A] decreases at a constant rate over time. (b) Order 1 kinetics: concentration [A] decreases at a rate that varies over time and depends on [A] (linear graph). (c) Order 1 kinetics on a semilogarithmic graph

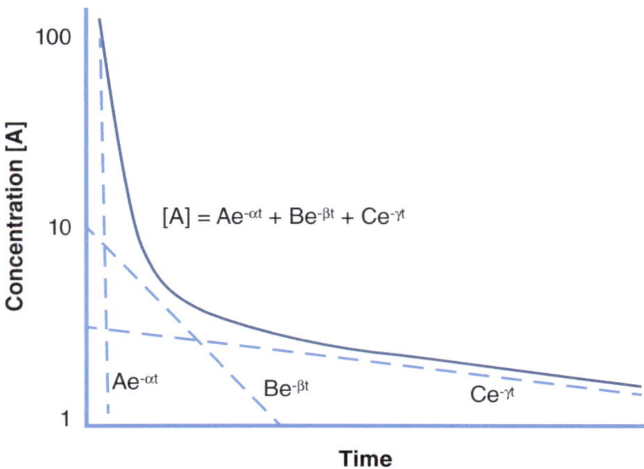

Fig. 1.2 Trend of the plasma concentration of an anesthetic after an intravenous bolus represented on a semilogarithmic plot. The curve can be decomposed into the three components represented by the dashed lines

graph is used, in which the *x*-axis (time) has a linear scale and the *y*-axis (concentration) has a logarithmic scale, the curve becomes a straight line (Fig. 1.1c).

However, the trend in plasma concentration of intravenous anesthetics after an intravenous bolus is more complex than that depicted in Fig. 1.1c and does not assume a linear trend even using a semilogarithmic graph. Figure 1.2 shows the change in concentration of an anesthetic on such a graph. The curve that appears there can be mathematically described by the sum of several exponential functions, represented on the graph by straight lines. In Fig. 1.2, the equation describing the drug concentration trend is given by the sum of three addends and forms the mathematical basis of a tricompartmental pharmacokinetic model.

1.2.4   Tricompartmental Models

The plasma concentration of a drug decreases over time as a result of its distribution within the body and elimination through the excretory organs or metabolism. Distribution in the body exhibits inhomogeneities so that there are better perfused tissues in which the drug diffuses more rapidly and others in which it penetrates more slowly. Each of the three components of the equation shown in Fig. 1.2 describes a process that takes place with kinetics of order 1; these processes have been identified with the diffusion of the drug from the central compartment to a first peripheral compartment (straight line with a greater slope), the slower diffusion of the drug from the central compartment to a second peripheral compartment (straight line with an intermediate slope), and the elimination of the drug through the emunctory organs or metabolism.

Figure 1.3 shows the tricompartmental model that allows a good approximation to describe the processes that influence the pharmacokinetics of intravenous anesthetics. The figure shows a central compartment in which the concentration of the drug is equal to that measurable in plasma and two peripheral compartments, one

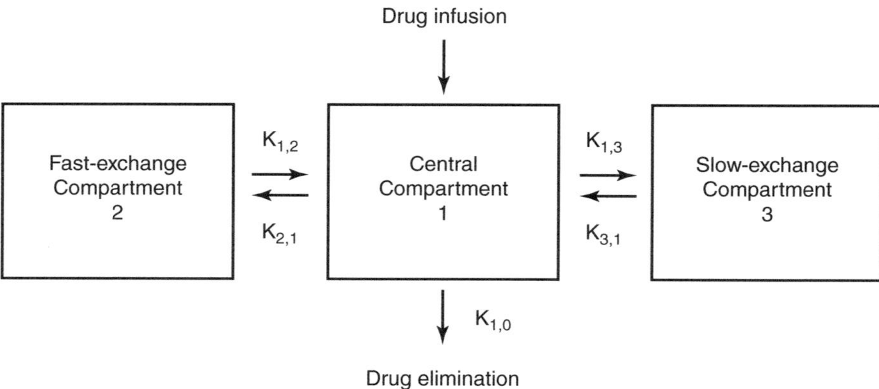

Fig. 1.3 Diagram of tricompartmental model. The drug is administered in the central compartment and from there diffuses to the peripheral compartments and is eliminated through the excretory organs

with rapid and one with slow exchange. These compartments are not real, but only mathematical abstractions. However, the central compartment could be identified with the best-perfused organs; the heart, brain, kidneys, and liver receive about 75% of cardiac output at rest while accounting for about 10% of body weight. The two peripheral compartments balance with the central one at very different rates. The fast-exchange compartment includes tissues that are nevertheless well perfused, mainly muscles. The slow-exchange compartment includes the remaining tissues, such as adipose tissue and bone. The anesthetic administered in the central compartment leaves it by transferring to the two peripheral compartments or through the excretory organs. Diffusion of the drug between the central and peripheral compartments occurs in both directions following the gradient between concentrations. Thus, at the end of an intravenous infusion, the decrease in plasma concentration is slowed by the retrograde diffusion of the anesthetic from the peripheral compartments to the central one.

Figure 1.3 shows the 5 k constants describing the kinetics of drug diffusion and elimination. Each constant is identified by suffix, where $K_{1,2}$ corresponds to the rate of transfer from the central compartment 1 to the fast peripheral compartment 2 and $K_{2,1}$ to the displacement in the opposite direction, $K_{1,3}$ corresponds to the rate of transfer between the central compartment 1 and the slow peripheral compartment, and so on. These constants are derived from the differential equation shown in Fig. 1.2. Table 1.2 presents the mathematical parameters describing the two tricompartmental models most commonly used to perform TCI for propofol; in addition to the k constants, the volumes of the three compartments are given. The differences between the two models highlight the influence of the sample used for database collection and especially the settings chosen by the authors. For example, the volume of the central compartment is a function of body weight in Marsh's model, but not in Schnider's.

Table 1.2 Two tricompartmental models compared

	Marsh [10]	Schnider [11, 12]
$V1$ (L)	$0.228 \times W$	4.27
$V2$ (L)	$0.463 \times W$	$18.9{-}0.391 \times (A - 53)$
$V3$ (L)	$2893 \times W$	238
$k10$ (min^{-1})	0.119	$0.443 + 0.0107 \times (W - 77) - 0.0159 \times (LBM - 59) + 0.0062 \times (H - 177)$
$k12$ (min^{-1})	0.112	$0.302{-}0.0056 \times (A - 53)$
$k13$ (min^{-1})	0.042	0.196
$k21$ (min^{-1})	0.055	$[1.29{-}0.024 \times (A - 53)]/[18.9{-}0.391 \times (A253)]$
$k31$ (min^{-1})	0.0033	0.0035
k_{eo} (min^{-1})	0.26	0.456
TTPE (min)	4.5	1.69

(modified from Absalom AR et al.) [13]

W weight in kg, A age, LBM lean mass in kg, H height in cm

1.3   Manual Adjustment of Anesthetic Infusion

In general, the use of an intravenous anesthetic requires the administration of an initial bolus, the magnitude of which is based on the desired plasma concentration and the theoretical volume of the central compartment. The plasma concentration is that associated with a given effect based on data available in the literature. For example, the recommended starting dose of propofol in an adult younger than 55 years not premedicated with benzodiazepines or opioids is 2–2.5 mg/kg and is reduced to 1–1.5 mg/kg in an adult older than 55 years or ASA class III–IV. Thereafter, the level of anesthesia achieved should be maintained by continuous infusion so as to balance the drug leaving the central compartment by diffusion to the peripheral compartments or elimination through the excretory organs. As shown, this amount varies over time because transfer to the peripheral compartments slows down as the amount of drug contained within them increases. In the case of propofol, the 10/8/6 rule has been proposed whereby propofol is administered at a rate of 10 mg/kg/h in the first 10 min, 8 mg/kg/h in the second 10 min, and 6 mg/kg/h thereafter [14]. Such a scheme results in a relatively constant plasma concentration of about 3.7 mcg/mL for an intervention lasting 80–90 min. Another proposed scheme involves infusion of 1% propofol at a rate of 600 mL/h for induction of anesthesia until adequate depth is reached followed by an infusion rate corresponding to 6 mg/kg/h [15]. Of course, any scheme still requires careful monitoring of clinical and instrumental signs of depth of anesthesia to tailor the dosage to the individual patient, because of individual variability and association with other anesthetics. Furthermore, maintaining a constant plasma concentration does not allow the depth of anesthesia to be changed to match the intensity of the surgical stimulus during the same procedure. In practice, therefore, the anesthesiologist induces anesthesia of adequate depth by administering one or more boluses and then sets up an intravenous infusion based on the pharmacokinetics of the anesthetic, verifying throughout the procedure with clinical and instrumental monitoring the maintenance of adequate depth of anesthesia.

1.4   TCI—Target Controlled Infusion

Target Controlled Infusion (TCI) is a technique in which the drug is administered with a pump controlled by software that, at regular intervals, changes the infusion rate so that the concentration set by the anesthesiologist in plasma or at the effector site is rapidly achieved and then maintained constant over time. The software calculates the drug requirement at regular time intervals, called epochs, using a pharmacokinetic model. The model is generally set by the device manufacturer; if a choice of multiple models is given, the operator must decide which one to use. The software requires entry of one or more patient parameters, such as age, height, and body weight. In practice, the system administers an initial bolus obtained by multiplying the target plasma concentration by the volume of the central compartment; it then administers the amount of drug needed to compensate for the drug leaving the central compartment by diffusion and elimination. TCI also offers the important advantage of being able to change the concentration initially set, such as increasing it if the intensity of the surgical stimulus becomes greater. In this case, the software takes into account the estimated amount of drug in the central compartment, administers as a bolus the amount missing to achieve the desired concentration, then reprograms the infusion rate. In case the target concentration is reduced, the infusion stops until the concentration in the central compartment reaches the set value.

Pharmacokinetic models are developed from data collected on a sample of individuals. They are therefore influenced by the characteristics of the subjects studied, usually healthy individuals, and the variables chosen by the investigator, for example, the decision whether or not to tie the calculation of central compartment volume to the patient's body size. It is therefore necessary to become aware of the limitations of the technique, particularly that actual anesthetic concentrations, which can be measured by analyzing plasma samples, may be significantly different from those estimated by the device. In clinical practice, therefore, it is always necessary to check whether the depth of anesthesia assessed with clinical and instrumental monitoring corresponds to the anesthetic concentration estimated by the TCI device and, if necessary, to vary the concentration set to deepen or superficialize the patient.

The variability of the pharmacokinetic models is easily appreciated by comparing the parameters of two of the most widely used models for propofol TCI, Marsh's and Schnider's (Table 1.2). In the former, the only individual variable is weight, which is involved in the calculation of the volume of the three compartments, while in the latter it is age, sex, body weight, and height that are involved in both the calculation of the volume of the compartments and that of the k constants. The volume of the central compartment predicted by Marsh's model is significantly greater than that predicted by Schnider's model, especially in subjects of larger body size. This difference results in the administration of a larger initial bolus (desired plasma concentration multiplied by the volume of the central compartment) using this model; on the other hand, Schnider's model might be more suitable for induction of anesthesia in elderly or frail subjects, who exhibit increased sensitivity to the action of anesthetic. Minto's model for remifentanil is based on the patient's age and anthropometric parameters weight and height.

1.4.1 Effector Site

The time interval between the administration of an intravenous bolus of anesthetic and the maximum pharmacodynamic effect is called the time to peak effect (TTPE). This interval is independent of the magnitude of the bolus and is characteristic of each drug. Propofol has a value between 1.6 and 3.9 min; Table 1.3 shows the value for some opioids. TTPE represents the time required to reach equilibrium between the plasma concentration of the drug (central compartment) and that at the effector site, where the drug diffuses across the blood–brain membrane. Factors affecting its value include the drug's liposolubility and pKa, which affects the degree of dissociation at blood pH. During TTPE, the concentration in the central compartment decreases after the initial peak due to diffusion phenomena, while the concentration at the effector site increases because the anesthetic diffuses there from the central compartment. Therefore, the concentration at the effector site cannot match the peak maximum plasma concentration obtained immediately after the bolus.

During TCI, the plasma concentration of the anesthetic is kept constant because the infusion rate changes to compensate for diffusion and elimination phenomena. Under these conditions, the diffusion of the anesthetic into the effector site is expressed by an exponential equation characterized by the constant $k_{e,0}$; neither diffusion in the opposite direction, toward the central compartment, nor a volume of the effector site is contemplated in the pharmacokinetic models. The time required for the anesthetic concentration at the effector site to reach half the concentration in the central compartment ($t_{1/2\ ke0}$) expresses a concept similar to that of TTPE. Its value for propofol is 2.77 min, for midazolam 4 min, for remifentanil 1.4 min, for fentanyl 6.9 min, and for morphine 17.7 min. The software in the TCI devices allows the concentration at the effector site to be estimated and allows the operator to set this concentration instead of the plasma concentration. The advantage is a reduction in the latency of the anesthetic's effect, achieved by maintaining a higher plasma

Table 1.3 Time interval in minutes between the administration of an intravenous bolus of some opioids and maximum effect (time to peak effect, TTPE) [16, 17]

	TTPE (min)	pKa	Relative liposolubility
Remifentanil	1.4	7.1	50
Alfentanil	2.6	6.5	90
Fentanyl	3.2	8.4	580
Morphine	19	8.0	1

Values are influenced by the dissociation constant expressed by pKa and the liposolubility of the molecule concentration for the time it takes to reach the desired concentration at the effector site level. Then, when the desired concentration has been reached, the infusion slows or stops for the time required for the two concentrations, in plasma and at the effector site, to equalize.

1.4.2 Anesthetic Half-Life and Recovery of Consciousness

The half-life of a drug ($t_{1/2}$) is equal to the time interval required for the plasma concentration to halve. This parameter is given by the ratio of the volume of distribution (Vd) to the clearance (Cl), which is the volume of plasma that is cleared of the drug in the unit of time. In the formula $t_{1/2} = 0.7 \times Vd/Cl$, 0.7 represents the approximate value of the natural logarithm of 2. The volume of distribution is the ideal space in which the drug would be distributed at a given instant if it had everywhere a concentration equal to the plasma concentration (or to that of the central compartment in the pharmacokinetic model). During the phase in which the drug accumulates in peripheral tissues, the volume of distribution gradually increases and consequently the half-life rises. In practice, the half-life increases because at the end of the infusion not only does the central compartment have to be purified, but also the portion of the drug that has been transferred to the peripheral compartments has to be eliminated. However, the closer we get to achieving equilibrium between the compartments, the more the value of the half-life tends to stabilize.

The concept of context-sensitive half-life thus expresses the variability of drug half-life in relation to the duration of infusion and concerns the period of time from the start of administration to the achievement of equilibrium between pharmacokinetic compartments. In the case of intravenous anesthetics, the relatively short duration of administration (minutes or hours) makes the effects of drug distribution processes in the body particularly important. The context-sensitive half-life of a drug is represented on a graph as a function of infusion duration. For some drugs, such as sodium thiopental or fentanyl, the half-life increases markedly as the infusion is prolonged. For others, such as propofol, the increase is smaller and equilibrium is reached earlier. This is why the concept of context-sensitive half-life is important when conducting anesthesia with propofol, less so during prolonged sedation in the ICU. Remifentanil represents the edge case of a drug with a half-life that rapidly becomes context-insensitive because plasma concentration and half-life stabilize after only 12 min of a constant-rate infusion.

TCI systems offer an estimate of the time required for the patient to wake up by suspending the infusion at that time. The estimate is based on simulation of the plasma concentration decrease curve by zeroing out the external supply and considering only diffusion from the peripheral compartments and elimination through the excretory organs. It is thus possible to calculate the time required for the plasma concentration to fall below the threshold value needed to achieve hypnosis.

1.4.3   Drug Interactions

Intravenous anesthesia generally requires the administration of multiple drugs to achieve adequate levels of hypnosis and analgesia. Classically, a hypnotic and an opioid are combined. One of the advantages of this combination is the ability to reduce the dosages of both. Because of their pharmacokinetic characteristics that make them particularly manageable and their synergism, the drugs most commonly used for this purpose are propofol and remifentanil.

When associated, two drugs can be additive, synergistic, or antagonistic. They are additive when the doses needed by employing them in isolation can be halved by associating them. For example, abolition of the patient's response to surgical incision can be achieved with a TCI of propofol set at a concentration of 11 mcg/mL or with inhalation of sevoflurane at an end-expiratory concentration of 1.8 MAC. The same effect can be achieved by combining a TCI of propofol at 5.5 mcg/mL and inhalation of sevoflurane at an end-expiratory concentration of 0.9 MAC [18]. Two drugs are synergistic when the effect of their combination exceeds the sum of their individual effects. Propofol and remifentanil are an example of synergistic drugs. The patient's response to tracheal intubation can be abolished with a target plasma concentration of propofol of 10 mcg/mL or remifentanil of 10 ng/mL, but by associating the two drugs the required concentrations are 2 mcg/mL and 4 ng/mL [19]. Finally, two drugs are antagonists if their combination at half the dosage results in a lower effect than that of each drug given alone; examples of antagonist drugs are morphine and tramadol.

The synergistic effect between two drugs is graphically represented by a curve that relates the combinations of the two concentrations that achieve the desired effect. The concentrations may be in plasma or, better, at the effector site level, and the desired effect may be, for example, the absence of response to skin incision or tracheal intubation. The curve is a function of the percentage of subjects in whom the effect is achieved. It was shown earlier that the Cp50 of an intravenous anesthetic is the concentration sufficient to obtain the effect in 50% of cases. Synergy between two drugs is thus comprehensively described by a family of curves and is represented by a curvilinear surface within a three-dimensional graph in which the third axis is represented by the percentage of subjects in whom the effect is achieved [19].

1.5   Closed-Loop Anesthesia

Totally intravenous anesthesia is one of the fields of application of new technologies of using autonomous systems in anesthesia [20, 21]. In traditional anesthesia (open-loop), the anesthesiologist completes the circuit starting from the input of clinical parameters and data from monitoring systems, which describe the patient's status, with the effector system, that is, the anesthetic infusion pumps and their speed. The anesthesiologist then assesses the levels of anesthesia and analgesia and sets the drug infusion rate so as to keep the patient's parameters within the optimal range. A

TCI system facilitates the anesthesiologist's task because it independently compensates for the effects of drug delivery.

The closed-loop anesthesia technique autonomously links the monitoring system and the TCI (closed-loop) system. In this case, the anesthesiologist does not set a target anesthetic concentration, but a range of values for one or more measured parameters (e.g., Bispectral Index) and asks the system to keep those parameters within that range. The device software sets and varies the TCI system's target concentration to achieve the goal, changing the concentration as the monitored parameters change.

The potential benefits of a closed-loop system are many. Conceptually, the system optimizes the TCI because it corrects the inaccuracy of a general pharmacokinetic model applied to a particular patient based on the effects that are detected. In practice, numerous studies have shown that the ability of such systems to maintain benchmarks within the set range is superior to that of the human operator and that they often realize significant savings in drug consumption. In addition, the systems prevent over- and underdosing caused by inattention of the human operator or sudden changes in the intensity of the surgical stimulus, and can alert the anesthesiologist if abnormal circumstances occur, such as anesthetic consumption exceeding a limit value.

The limitations and potential risks of a closed-loop anesthesia system are partly related to the anomalies or inadequacy of the signal from the monitoring systems. For example, it is difficult to assess whether the depth of anesthesia is sufficient or excessive based on a single parameter. As a result, the initial one-input, one-output (SISO: Single Input, Single Output) systems have evolved into the multiple input, multiple output (MIMO: Multiple Input, Multiple Output) systems. Certainly, automated systems should not be regarded as devices that replace the anesthesiologist, but as supports that, similar to TCI systems, simplify the anesthesiologist's task [22].

1.6   Conclusions: Intravenous Anesthesia as Surfing

Many years ago, Talmage D. Egan and Steven L. Shafer, two authors who have made important contributions to the development of modern intravenous anesthesia, very effectively described the work performed by the anesthesiologist by resorting to the image of a surfer riding the crest of a wave [23].

The wave represents the curve that links the anesthetic concentration on the x-axis to its effects on the patient on the y-axis. The crest of the wave corresponds to the minimum concentration needed to achieve the required degree of hypnosis and/or analgesia. Increasing the concentration would unnecessarily expose the patient to the side effects of the drug; decreasing it would lead to too shallow anesthesia or insufficient analgesia. The anesthesiologist wants to stay on the crest of the wave to achieve the desired effects of the drug with the least risk of side effects. In addition, staying on the crest of the wave means having a rapid awakening of the patient at the end of the procedure because the decrease in plasma concentration immediately corresponds to a superficialization of the level of anesthesia. From what has been said about the pharmacokinetics of intravenous anesthetics, staying on the crest of the wave is not easy, but to stay there, the anesthesiologist has three useful tools. Pharmacokinetics provides valuable information on reaching the crest of the wave, offering guidance on initial dosing based on patient size, age, and condition. Clinical and instrumental monitoring tells us whether we are actually at the crest of the wave or whether we need to administer additional doses to go up or temporarily stop dosing to go down. TCI systems are the third tool, which makes it easier for us to remain on the crest of the wave because they are very effective in stabilizing the drug concentration in the plasma or at the effector site. In manual adjustment, on the other hand, we have to assess the depth of anesthesia continuously and change the speed of the infusion pumps accordingly.

Alongside these three tools, Egan and Shafer posit a fourth, given by the availability of drugs such as propofol and remifentanil with pharmacokinetics particularly suited to TIVA. In fact, after only 15 min of a constant-rate intravenous infusion with no initial bolus, the plasma concentration of propofol reaches 80% of the concentration it will reach at steady state [24], and remifentanil 100% [25].

Table 1.4 reports some recommendations for safe practice of intravenous anesthesia issued by the Association of Anaesthetists and the Society for Intravenous Anaesthesia [26].

Table 1.4 Recommendations on the practice of intravenous anesthesia [26]

1. All anesthesiologists should be trained and competent on TIVA. Schools of anesthesia should teach, train, and provide hands-on experience for anesthesia and critical care residents

2. When general anesthesia is obtained with propofol, TCI should be used

3. The initial concentration should be set based on the characteristics of the patient, other medications administered, and the clinical situation. Elderly and frail patients may benefit from a lower initial target concentration of propofol and subsequent adjustments

4. Within an anesthesia department, it is preferable to use only one concentration of propofol and always dilute remifentanil to the same standard concentration

5. The infusion set through which TIVA is delivered should have a Luer-lock connector at each end, an anti-siphon valve on the drug delivery line(s), and an anti-reflux valve on any infusion route. The route with the drug should join the others as close as possible to the point of entry into the vein to reduce dead space. The use of TCI-specific sets is recommended

6. Infusion pumps should be programmed only after the syringe containing the drug has been placed

7. The intravenous cannula or central venous catheter through which the infusion is delivered should, when possible, be visible during anesthesia

8. Anesthesiologists should be familiar with the principles, interpretation, and limitations of EEG signal analysis. Direct observation of EEG tracing and muscle activity on electromyography can increase the usefulness of this type of monitoring

9. EEG monitoring is strongly recommended when TIVA is associated with the use of muscle relaxants

10. The standards of TIVA performance and monitoring adopted in the operating room should also be applied when TIVA is used in other environments

References

1. Struys MM, De Smet T, Glen JI, Vereecke HE, Absalom AR, Schnider TW. The history of target-controlled infusion. Anesth Analg. 2016;122(1):56–69.
2. Tian H, Xu R, Canadell JG, et al. A comprehensive quantification of global nitrous oxide sources and sinks. Nature. 2020;586:248–56.
3. Hopkins PM, Girard T, Dalay S, Jenkins B, Thacker A, Patteril M, McGrady E. Malignant hyperthermia 2020: guideline from the Association of Anaesthetists. Anaesthesia. 2021;76(5):655–64.
4. Fazio G, Vernuccio F, Grutta G, King GL. Drugs to be avoided in patients with long QT syndrome: focus on the anaesthesiological management. World J Cardiol. 2013;5(4):87–93.
5. Gan TJ, Belani KG, Bergese S, Chung F, Diemunsch P, Habib AS, Jin Z, Kovac AL, Meyer TA, Urman RD, Apfel CC, Ayad S, Beagley L, Candiotti K, Englesakis M, Hedrick TL, Kranke P, Lee S, Lipman D, Minkowitz HS, Morton J, Philip BK. Fourth consensus guidelines for the management of postoperative nausea and vomiting. Anesth Analg. 2020;131(2):411–48.
6. Association of Anaesthetists of Great Britain and Ireland. Recommendations for standards of monitoring during anesthesia and recovery 2015. Anaesthesia. 2016;71:85–93.
7. Al-Rifai Z, Mulvey D. Principles of total intravenous anaesthesia: practical aspects of using total intravenous anaesthesia. BJA Educ. 2016;16:276–80.
8. https://www.nice.org.uk/guidance/dg6.
9. Tafur LA, Lema E. Total intravenous anesthesia: from pharmaceutics to pharmacokinetics. Colomb J Anestesiol. 2010;38:215–31.
10. Marsh B, White M, Morton N, Kenny GN. Pharmacokinetic model driven infusion of propofol in children. Br J Anaesth. 1991;67:41–8.
11. Schnider TW, Minto CF, Gambus PL, et al. The influence of method of administration and covariates on the pharmacokinetics of propofol in adult volunteers. Anesthesiology. 1998;88:1170–82.
12. Schnider TW, Minto CF, Shafer SL, et al. The influence of age on propofol pharmacodynamics. Anesthesiology. 1999;90:1502–16.
13. Absalom AR, Mani V, De Smet T, Struys MMRF. Pharmacokinetic models for propofol-defining and illuminating the devil in detail. Br J Anaesth. 2009;103:26–37.
14. Roberts FL, Dixon J, Lewis GT, Tackley RM, Prys-Roberts C. Induction and maintenance of propofol anaesthesia. A manual infusion scheme. Anaesthesia. 1988;43(Suppl):14–7.
15. Stokes DN, Hutton P. Rate-dependent induction phenomena with propofol: implications for the relative potency of intravenous anesthetics. Anesth Analg. 1991;72:578–83.
16. Gupta DK, Krejcie TC, Avram MJ. Pharmacokinetics of opioids. In: Evers AS, Maze M, Kharasch ED, editors. Anesthetic pharmacology basic principles and clinical practice. Cambridge University Press; 2011. p. 509–30.
17. https://resources.wfsahq.org/atotw/pharmacology-of-opioids-part-1-anaesthesia-tutorial-of-the-week-64/.
18. Harris RS, Lazar O, Johansen JW, Sebel PS. Interaction of propofol and sevoflurane on loss of consciousness and movement to skin incision during general anesthesia. Anesthesiology. 2006;104(6):1170–5.
19. Mertens MJ, Olofsen E, Engbers FH, Burm AG, Bovill JG, Vuyk J. Propofol reduces perioperative remifentanil requirements in a synergistic manner: response surface modeling of perioperative remifentanil–propofol interactions. Anesthesiology. 2003;99(2):347–59.
20. Ghita M, Neckebroek M, Muresan C, Copot D. Closed-loop control of anesthesia: survey on actual trends, challenges and perspectives. IEEE Access. 2020;8:206264–79.
21. Zaouter C, Joosten A, Rinehart J, Struys MMRF, Hemmerling TM. Autonomous systems in anesthesia: where do we stand in 2020? A narrative review. Anesth Analg. 2020;130:1120–2.
22. Miller TE, Gan TJ. Closed-loop systems in anesthesia: reality or fantasy? Anesth Analg. 2013;117:1039–41.

23. Egan TD, Shafer SL. Target-controlled infusions for intravenous anesthetics: surfing USA not! Anesthesiology. 2003;99:1039–41.
24. Schnider TW. Pharmacokinetic and pharmacodynamic concepts underpinning total intravenous anesthesia. J Cardiothorac Vasc Anesth. 2015;29:S7–S10.
25. Maurtua MA, Pursell A, Damron K, Sonal P. Remifentanil: pharmacokinetics, pharmacodynamics, and current clinical applications. Clin Med Rev Case Rep. 2020;7:304.
26. Nimmo AF, Absalom AR, Bagshaw O, Biswas A, Cook TM, Costello A, Grimes S, Mulvey D, Shinde S, Whitehouse T, Wiles MD. Guidelines for the safe practice of total intravenous anesthesia (TIVA): joint guidelines from the Association of Anaesthetists and the Society for Intravenous Anaesthesia. Anaesthesia. 2019;74:211–24.

Normothermia in Anesthesia: Impact on Quality and Safety of Care

Felice Eugenio Agrò and Rita Cataldo

2.1 Historical Background

In 1850, temperature was recognized as a vital parameter by Wunderlich.

In 1860, special attention was given to thermal rise in the perioperative period and the dreaded malignant hyperthermia syndrome, but it was in those same years that R. W. Pickering asserted that "the most valuable system of cooling a man is to place him under anesthesia."

In 2001 at the Consensus Conference on Perioperative Hypothermia, guidelines and recommendations for temperature management in the perioperative period were established by Società Italiana di Anestesia, Analgesia, Rianimazione eTerapia Intensiva (Italian Society of Anesthesia, Analgesia, Resuscitation and Intensive Therapy, SIAARTI).

In 2007, Agency for Healthcare Research and Quality (AHRQ) identified 20 priority areas of concern and included, with regard to nosocomial infections, perioperative hypothermia as a primary contributing cause deserving of prevention guidelines.

In 2009, the Italian Ministry of Labor, Health and Social Policy included in the "Manual for Safety in the Operating Room: Recommendations and Checklists" body temperature monitoring, by means of a special device for continuous or repeated measurement, in patients exposed to the risk of passive hypothermia (newborns, those of very advanced age) and during procedures accompanied by heat loss.

F. E. Agrò · R. Cataldo (✉)
Fondazione Policlinico Universitario Campus Bio Medico, Rome, Italy

Research Unit of Anesthesia, Intensive Care and Pain Management, Department of Medicine and Surgery, Università Campus Bio-Medico di Roma, Rome, Italy
e-mail: f.agro@unicampus.it; R.Cataldo@policlinicocampus.it

D. Chiumello (ed.), *Practical Trends in Anesthesia and Intensive Care 2022*, https://doi.org/10.1007/978-3-031-43891-2_2

In this operating room safety manual, body temperature monitoring is considered necessary to prevent surgical site infections and to appropriately manage the patient intra- and postoperatively.

2.2   Concepts of Physiology

Body temperature (BT) regulation (THERMOREGULATION) requires the coordination of many body systems: in order for the internal temperature to remain in the normal range, heat gain (THERMOGENESIS) and loss (THERMODISPERSION) must correspond to maintain HOMEOSTASIS.

The HYPOTHALAMUS, located in the pituitary gland in the brain, acts as a thermostat (THERMOREGULATORY CENTER). It senses even slight changes in BT above or below 37 °C and stimulates necessary changes:

- In the nervous and hormonal systems (heat signals).
- In the circulatory system (vasoconstriction or vasodilation).
- In the skin (perspiratio insensibilis).
- In the sweat glands (perspiratio sensibilis).
- In the muscle system (voluntary or involuntary muscle contraction).

The thermoregulatory center is able to sense temperature changes through:

- LOCAL signals, given by blood temperature in the central nervous system (CNS) (hypothalamus, spinal cord), which are an expression of core temperature.
- PERIPHERAL signals, which reach the CNS via the spinal cord conveyed from thermoreceptors residing in various regions of the body, are an expression of EXTERNAL temperature.

2.2.1   Thermoregulation of the Body

The body is unable to endure for long periods in an environment that is extraordinarily cold or excessively hot.

Heat is produced by:

1. Basal metabolic processes
2. Introduction of food
3. Muscle work

To maintain the core temperature at 37 °C, the body employs several mechanisms:

- If temperature is above 37 °C: mechanisms that promote heat transfer such as VASODILATION (to increase blood flow to the skin) or sweating are activated.

– If temperature is below 37 °C: body defenses and heat production start, such as VASOCONSTRICTION to decrease blood flow to the skin and shivering to intensify heat production increasing muscle contractions.

2.2.2 Factors Affecting Temperature

– AGE: In infants: body temperature is unstable, because their thermoregulation mechanisms are immature; in elderly people, axillary BT is usually less than 36 °C.
– ENVIRONMENT: Generally, changes in ambient temperature do not affect the internal BT, but prolonged exposure to extremely hot or cold temperatures can cause some changes. If the internal temperature falls below 25 °C, death (frostbite) can occur. If it rises above 43/44 °C, a state of coma and death (heat stroke or sunstroke) can occur.
– PHYSICAL EXERCISE: BT (body temperature) increases with muscle activity using the metabolism of fats and carbohydrates to produce energy.
– STRESS: It stimulates the sympathetic nervous system (or vegetative or autonomic nervous system) to produce adrenaline and norepinephrine (adrenal medullary hormones); metabolism increases and causes heat production.
– HORMONES: Progesterone secreted during ovulation raises temperature about 0.5 °C above baseline. After menopause, BT is the same for men and women. Thyroid (thyroxine) and adrenal (adrenaline and noradrenaline) hormones increase heat production.

2.2.3 Changes in Body Temperature

A change in body temperature may depend on:

1. Inability of the physiological correction mechanisms to cope with the environmental changes (hypothermia or hyperthermia). These variations may also be called EXTRINSIC (such as frostbite, heat stroke, sunstroke).
2. Altered regulation of thermogenesis and thermodispersion mechanisms.

These changes can also be called variations from an INTRINSIC cause (e.g., intrinsic hypothermia and febrile hyperthermia).

LOW-GRADE-FEVER OR SUBFEBRILE TEMPERATURE is a slight rise in body temperature, between 37 and 38 °C, lasting from days to months.

CAUSES

– Infectious (hepatitis, abscesses, tuberculosis, bacterial endocarditis, etc.)
– Hematological or rheumatological diseases (anemia, rheumatoid arthritis)
– Neoplastic diseases
– Drugs (hormone therapy in women)

FEVER OR PYREXIA is an increase in body temperature above 38 °C.
ETIOLOGY AND CAUSES

- INFECTIVE
- ASEPTIC or due to RESORPTION that occurs after surgery or trauma, related to endogenous decomposition products
- THERMOREGULATORY CENTER disorder due to brain injury
- DEHYDRATION
- HEAT STROKE

SYMPTOMS:

- Increased heart and respiratory rate
- Hot and dry reddened skin
- Poor urinary excretion
- Inappetence
- Increased sense of thirst, dry tongue
- Shining eyes and headache

FEVER
Fever is defined as an increase in core body temperature above normal limits.

According to the World Health Organization, a normal core temperature is defined between 36.5 and 37.5 °C.

2.2.4 Definition of Fever

The definition of fever is arbitrary and depends on the purpose for which it is defined. Some of the literature defines fever as a core temperature >38.0 °C, while others define fever as two consecutive temperature elevations >38.3 °C. Because of the considerable variability of 'normal temperature" in a population of healthy adult subjects, and because the site and method of measurement can influence the measured value, several arbitrary definitions of fever are acceptable depending on the desired sensitivity of the indicator of thermal abnormality to be used. Normal body temperature is generally considered to be 37.0 °C. In healthy individuals, this temperature changes by 0.5–1.0 °C, depending on circadian rhythm and menstrual cycle.

2.2.5 Pathophysiology of Fever

Elevation of core body temperature occurs as a result of increased concentration of prostaglandin E2 (PGE2) in specific brain areas. PGE2, in particular, acts by binding to 4 specific cellular receptors (EP1–EP4) present in the preoptic nuclei of the anterior hypothalamus, which are physiologically deputed to control thermoregulation. As a result of this interaction, an elevation of the equilibrium point of the hypothalamic thermostat ensues. Both heat production and heat loss are then adjusted to this new set point. In the pathogenesis of fever, specific cytokines, known as endogenous pyrogens (inteleukin [IL] 1-beta [IL-1 β], interleukin-6 [IL-6] and tumor necrosis factor-alpha [tumor necrosis factor-α orTNF-α]), play a crucial role. Most exogenous pyrogens, on the other hand (e.g., cell membrane components of some microorganisms) evoke the febrile response stimulating endogenous pyrogens production. For example, endotoxins (lipopolysaccharides from the cell wall of Gram-negative bacteria) act by inducing the production of IL-1 β, which is the signal for PGE2 release in the hypothalamic preoptic region. Pyrogenic cytokines (e.g., TNF-α and IL-1) are in turn implicated in the genesis of many of the metabolic, endocrinologic, and immunologic changes that occur during fever, such as vasodilation; increased hepatic and muscle proteolysis and glycogenolysis; increased basal oxygen consumption; fibroblast proliferation; activation of osteoclasts;production of platelet-activating factors; synthesis of acute-phase proteins; activation of myelopoiesis; synthesis of ACTH and cortisol, insulin, and catecholamines; mobilization and activation of some neutrophil functions; activation of T lymphocytes with increased synthesis of IL-2; and proliferation of B lymphocytes.

2.2.6   Thermal Curves

Depending on the cause, the trend of fever varies over time. This is assessed by constructing the so-called THERMAL CURVE, a graph in which the BT values read throughout the day for the entire febrile period are plotted. In this way the minimum and maximum values, the number of episodes of rise and defervescence, and the length of the acme are noted. Some curves are characteristic:

- LOW-GRADE FEVER: 38 °C is never reached.
- CONTINUOUS FEVER: The acme has fluctuations of less than 1° in the 24 h, so the BT tends to be constant (typical of typhoid).
- REMITTENT FEVER: Daily fluctuations are greater than 1°, but the BT does not return to normal within 24 h.
- INTERMITTENT FEVER: Switching repeatedly in 24 h from a febrile state to a state of apyrexia (typical of malaria).
- ONDULANT FEVER: Gradually increases over several days, reaches a peak, and then slowly decreases over several successive days (by lysis) lasting 1–2 weeks and after an equal period of apyrexia starts again in the same manner (typical of brucellosis or Hodgkin's disease).
- RECURRENT FEVER: 3–4 days of fever that falls abruptly by crisis, alternating with 3–4 days of apyrexia (typical of syphilis).

In the past, the study of thermal curves was very important as a method of diagnosis.

2.2.7 Hyperthermia

- **Increased thermogenesis**
- Considerable muscle exercise
- Thyrotoxicosis (e.g., Basedow-Graves)
- Pheochromocytoma
- Malignant hyperthermia due to halogenated anesthetics
- **Obstacles to thermodispersion**
- Heat stroke (related or not to physical activity)
- Toxicants and drugs (e.g., atropine)
- Autonomic central nervous system (CNS) dysfunction
- Dehydration
- Large burns
- **Hypothalamic disorders**
- Encephalitis or inflammatory processes of the brain
- CNS tumors or trauma or vascular insults
- Central effect of drugs (e.g., phenothiazines) = neuroleptic malignant syndrome

2.2.8 Hypothermia

Several published studies show that the incidence of perioperative hypothermia is still very high. On admission to the intensive care unit, incidental hypothermia is present in 46–66% of patients. Hypothermia, defined as a core temperature below 36 °C, is estimated to occur among 50–90% of surgical patients, even in case of short procedures.

A common mistake is to think that the cause of an accidental perioperative hypothermia is a cold operating room, and that if the room temperature were increased, hypothermia would not occur. Although room temperature plays a role, anesthesia and surgery play the main ones.

General and loco-regional anesthesia alter the patient's thermoregulation. After induction of anesthesia, due to the phenomenon of redistribution, blood flow increases in the peripheral areas of the body (which are usually 2–4 °C lower than the central temperature), cooling and causing the central temperature to decrease.

In addition, anesthesia impairs the body's ability to respond to changes in heat. Normally, the body is able to respond to changes of ±0.2 °C by activating compensatory mechanisms, whereas in anesthesia the response is activated only with changes of ±2 °C.

Hypothermia has been shown to cause:

- Surgical site infection.
- Myocardial ischemia and cardiac disorders.
- Coagulopathies and blood loss.
- Longer awakening/recovery room exit time.
- Prolonged and altered effect of drugs.

2.3 Preserve the Normothermia

During the intraoperative phase, all patients are at risk of a drop in body temperature.

Factors influencing hypothermia incidence include: low ambient temperatures, drugs and anesthetic inhalation agents, infusion of fluids and cold blood products, antiseptic solutions used to prepare the skin site of surgery, for prolonged times of surgery with exposure of large body cavities.

Specifically, anesthetic agents depress metabolism and heat production by 15–30%, inhibit heat-generating protective reflexes (shivering), depress hypothalamic thermoregulatory centers, and increase vasodilation, resulting in heat loss by radiation and conduction.

After induction of anesthesia, heat is redistributed from the core, consisting of the brain, mediastinal, and abdominal organs, to the periphery, and upper and lower limbs; this is the most common cause of hypothermia in the perioperative period.

2.4 Cardiovascular Effects of Hypothermia

From the cardiovascular point of view, hypothermia results in decreased heart rate, depressed systolic output, cardiac contractility, and increased myocardial irritability with increased susceptibility of the patient to arrhythmias.

2.5 Respiratory Effects of Hypothermia

From the respiratory point of view, hypothermia results in depression of the respiratory center and increased blood oxygen solubility.

2.6 Coagulation and Hypothermia

From the coagulative point of view, hypothermia results in decreased coagulation factor activity, thrombocytopenia, and increased risk of cellular agglutination at the microcirculation level due to increased blood viscosity.

2.7 Effects of Hypothermia on the Central Nervous System

The effects of hypothermia on the CNS are a consequence of to the reduction in cerebral blood flow, which is approximately 7% for each degree of temperature in less.

2.8 Effects of Hypothermia on the Immune System

The effects of hypothermia on the immune system increase susceptibility to infections, reduce perfusion and antibiotic penetration, and alter the phagocytic activity of polymorphonucleocytes.

2.9 Drugs Effects on Thermoregulation

Central loco-regional anesthesia results in hypothermia by acting both centrally, on the hypothalamus, and peripherally, on the orthosympathetic system, and blocking the autonomic nervous system fibers in the anesthetic block zones; this results in a redistribution of heat from the center to the periphery.

2.10 Hypothermia-Related Complications: 1.4 °C Reduction in Core Temperature

Decreasing core temperature by about 1.4 °C results in increased oxygen consumption by 35%, increased respiratory rate by 52%, increased carbon dioxide production, and increased clinical risk for patients suffering from heart disease and COPD.

If core temperature drops of 1.4 °C blood pressure increase, as a consequence of increased plasma norepinephrine, this can cause myocardial irritability and greater patient susceptibility to ventricular arrhythmias.

Decrease of about 1.4 °C in core temperature results in increased bleeding of about 200–300 mL in patients undergoing hip replacement under subarachnoid anesthesia causing a 22% increased risk of receiving a blood transfusion, more pain during the postoperative period, and severe postoperative shivering.

To understand the problem, by searching on PubMed *perioperative temperature* we see that there are more than 1800 published papers, including 399 clinical trials and 251 reviews. If we refine the search to *perioperative hypothermia* we find about 1578 published papers, with as many as 114 papers published in the last calendar year alone.

In 2008, the National Institute for Health and Care Excellence (NICE) published a clinical guideline on the prevention and management of perioperative hypothermia, which was revised and updated in 2016.

Also in 2008, NICE published a second document on the management of perioperative hypothermia. These recommendations and the related flowcharts were updated in March 2017.

In 2009, the Italian Ministry of Health issued a manual for safety in the operating room. In the recommendations and checklists, temperature monitoring to maintain normothermia in the patient undergoing anesthesiological–surgical procedures and to prevent surgical site infections is strongly suggested.

In 2010, the American Society of PeriAnesthesia nurses issued guidelines on normothermia.

In 2015, a multidisciplinary study group consisting of German anesthesiologists, surgeons, and nurses issued joint guidelines on the prevention of hypothermia.

In 2016, *The Lancet* published review on perioperative thermoregulation. This article explains in detail the implications of hypothermia on the metabolism of anesthetic and drugs in general.

In 2019, the Italian Society of Anesthesia, Analgesia, Resuscitation and Intensive Therapy (SIAARTI) published new good clinical practices concerning perioperative normothermia, which are now being updated.

The flow chart of the good clinical practices is intended to stress pre-warming, temperature monitoring that should always be documented in the anesthesiology record, during anesthesia, in the recovery room, and until discharge to the ward. The importance of warming in the pediatric patient is also emphasized.

SIAARTI organized an information and awareness campaign regarding perioperative normothermia by conducting an educational tour in various Italian cities with meetings called "normo days" or "shiver-free surgery."

SIAARTI good clinical practices state that incidental perioperative hypothermia alters the metabolism and clinical effects of most drugs used in anesthesia, and contributes to increased incidence of infectious complications, cerebrovascular ischemic events, and hemorrhagic events.

Hypothermia results in increased hospital stay and postoperative mortality; patients and health care workers (including the Emergency Department staff) should be informed about the importance of normothermia, so that preventive measures can always be taken.

The purpose of the good clinical practices published by SIAARTI is to spread and standardize central temperature monitoring in general anesthesia and loco-regional anesthesia in order to enable perioperative normothermia, correcting a major risk factor for perioperative complications, underestimated by many anesthesiology and surgery teams.

Hypothermia increases heath care costs. The costs of just 1 day of prolonging the patient's hospital stay due to a surgical wound infection are about 17 times the cost of a single device suitable for maintaining perioperative normothermia.

PERIOPERATIVE NORMOTHERMIA should be ensured in all surgical procedures lasting longer than 30 min, especially in high-risk subjects (ASA 3 or 4, high BMI, high cardiovascular risk) and always in pediatric surgery.

The SIAARTI document stresses the concept that monitoring and temperature data should always be documented in the anesthesiology record, throughout the duration of anesthesia until discharge from the operating room.

The **SIAARTI good clinical practices** are directed to the entire staff involved in the patient surgical pathway, in the ward, operating block (OB), DEA, and recovery room, and nurses, physicians, and residents.

Accuracy and precision of temperature measurement depend on both the measurement site and the measurement device. The temperature measured peripherally is not accurate, as it is influenced by the ambient temperature and does not reflect the core temperature.

The "gold standard" should be the temperature measured in pulmonary artery by pulmonary artery catheter (PAC). Under general anesthesia, esophageal temperature is currently the clinical standard. More difficult is the monitoring during loco-regional anesthesia, and during the postoperative phase.

It is recommended to monitor core temperature using a heated servo-controlled sensor placed on the front of the patient. The heated servo controlled sensor is accurate, precise and its data are comparable with those from PAC (pulmonary artery catheter).

To counteract redistribution hypothermia, it is essential to consider pre-warming the patient (pre-warming) before the induction of anesthesia for at least 10 min.

To obtain a core temperature higher than or equal to 36 °C, it is recommended to warm patient and fluids as soon as possible before and after entering the operating block:

- Maintain/restore normothermia in ward, before transferring the patient to the operating block (OB).
- Encourage the patient to walk to the OB (when appropriate and if possible).
- Warm the patient and fluids as soon as possible after entering the operating block.
- Always consider pre-warming (10–30 min) to avoid hypothermia from redistribution.
- Monitor BT during surgery and always record the data in the chart.
- Always record BT in the recovery room/post-anesthetic care unit and at discharge from the operating block, providing indications/alerts to the staff.

Shivering at the end of surgery is a major cause of discomfort for patients. It occurs in more than 50% of cases and involves a number of physiological changes including changes in oxygen consumption, lactic acidosis, hypoxemia, and hypercapnia that often increase wound pain.

Always consider:

- Operating block environmental temperature (within the prescribed limits 21–23 °C).
- Active patient warming.
- Warming of infusion and irrigation fluids.

Active warming of the pediatric patient is always recommended, even for surgeries lasting less than 30 min.

If a BT <36 °C occurs:

1. Evaluate implementation of warming (increase forced hot air if possible, or add thermal mats and blankets, based on risk/benefit assessment).
2. Do not discharge the patient from the operating room until the temperature reaches 36 °C (excluding patients to be transferred to the intensive care unit).

To achieve **perioperative normothermia**, it is also recommended to use passive humidification devices, equipped with an electrical resistance inside, which is able to warm the air produced by the patient's exhalation.

1. Core temperature (CT) should always be maintained at or slightly above 36 °C, except in cases of deliberately provoked hypothermia.
2. CT should always be monitored in pediatric patients. In adults, patients who are not at risk for malignant hyperthermia and who are undergoing procedures performed by local anesthesia or loco-regional and general anesthesia for a time not exceeding 30 min may be excluded from temperature monitoring.
3. The site of temperature monitoring can change in consideration of the patient and the surgery. One can opt for tympanic, esophageal, nasopharyngeal, and pulmonary artery measuring. Rectal or bladder probes can be inaccurate in some situations.
4. Anesthetic gases have to always be heated and humidified by means of special filters; low-flow ventilation is also recommended.
5. In case of shivering, it is recommended to increase the concentration of oxygen in the inhaled air, and actively warm the patient.
6. The patient should never be discharged from the recovery room until he or she has reached the state of normothermia, especially if signs of hypothermia are present.

Take-Home Messages
- Do not induce anesthesia if the BT is below 36 °C.
- Use a closed, low-flow system for ventilation.
- Use medical devices of passive humidification with active exhaled gas resistance.
- Always use appropriate noninvasive central temperature monitoring devices and active heating systems according to the surgery.

Reasons for implementing perioperative normothermia are clinical, ethical, economic, and legal:

- **Clinical Reasons**: to prevent hypothermia-related complications in the perioperative period.
- **Ethical Reasons**: to improve patient comfort and outcome.
- **Economic Reasons**: to determine a reduction in costs due to complications.
- **Legal reasons**: to implement good clinical practices to avoid claims.

Perioperative normothermia is vital to:

- Reduce nosocomial infections.
- Improve patient comfort.
- Obtain a reduction in complications-related costs.
- Adhere to the clinical standards and implement good clinical practices in adherence with the Gelli-Bianco law.

2.11 Recommendations for Shiver-Free Surgery and Perioperative Normothermia

- **Central temperature monitoring:** When choosing the device for temperature monitoring, the least invasive and accurate system, such as the heated servo-controlled sensor placed on the patient's forehead, should be preferred, especially in case of loco-reginal anesthesia. The core temperature data should always be documented in the anesthesiology record.
- **Temperature management:** To avoid heat loss and prevent the occurrence of accidental hypothermia, actively warming systems with forced hot air technology and warm infusion and irrigation fluids must be used.
- **Pre-warming:** To prevent hypothermia from redistribution, the good clinical practices suggest pre-warming of the patient before induction of anesthesia for a duration for at least 10 min or ever more, from the ward.
- **Pediatric patients:** Pay very high attention to the youngest patients: warm them up even during interventions of less than 30 min.

Recommended Readings

Borms SF, et al. Bair hugger forced-air warming maintains normothermia more effectively than thermo-lite insulation. J Clin Anesth. 1994;6:303–7. https://doi.org/10.1016/0952-8180(94)90077-9.

Canneti P, et al. SIAARTI clinical best practice: perioperative normothermia. Sapienza Università di Roma; 2017.

Eshraghi Y, et al. An evaluation of a zero-heat-flux cutaneous thermometer in cardiac surgical patients. Anesth Analg. 2014;119:543–9. https://doi.org/10.1213/ANE.0000000000000319.

Fossum S, et al. A comparison study on the effects of prewarming patients in the outpatient surgery setting. J Perianesth Nurs. 2001;16:187–94. https://doi.org/10.1053/jpan.2001.24039.

Frank SM, et al. Perioperative maintenance of normothermia reduces the incidence of morbid cardiac events. A randomized clinical trial. JAMA. 1997;277:1127–34. https://doi.org/10.1001/jama.1997.035403800410296.

Hooper VD, et al. ASPAN's evidence-based clinical practice guideline for the promotion of perioperative normothermia: second edition. J Perianesth Nurs. 2010;25:346–65. https://doi.org/10.1016/j.jopan.2010.10.006.

Karalapillai D, et al. Postoperative hypothermia and patient outcomes after elective cardiac surgery. Anaesthesia. 2011;66:780–4. https://doi.org/10.1111/j.1365-2044.2011.06784.x.

Karalapillai D, et al. Postoperative hypothermia and patient outcomes after major elective non-cardiac surgery. Anaesthesia. 2013;68:605–11. https://doi.org/10.1111/anae.12129.

Kurz A, et al. Perioperative normothermia to reduce the incidence of surgical-wound infection and shorten hospitalization. Study of wound infection and temperature group. N Engl J Med. 1996;334:1209–15. https://doi.org/10.1056/NEJM199605093341901.

Lenhardt R, et al. Mild intraoperative hypothermia prolongs postanesthetic recovery. Anesthesiology. 1997;87:1318–23. https://doi.org/10.1097/00000542-199712000-00009.

Madrid E, et al. Active body surface warming systems for preventing complications caused by inadvertent perioperative hypothermia in adults. Cochrane Database Syst Rev. 2016;2016:CD009016. https://doi.org/10.1002/14651858.CD009016.pub2.

Mahoney CB, et al. Maintaining intraoperative normothermia: a meta-analysis of outcomes with costs. AANA J. 1999;67:155–64.

Ministero della Salute. Manuale per la Sicurezza in sala operatoria: Raccomandazioni e Checklist, a cura di Ministero del Lavoro, della Salute e delle Politiche Sociali, 2009 (ultimo aggiornamento 2013). https://www.salute.gov.it/imgs/C_17_pubblicazioni_1119_allegato.pdf.

NICE Clinical Guidelines. Hypothermia: prevention and management in adults having surgery. No. 65. National Institute for Health and Care Excellence (NICE); 2016.

Schmied H, et al. Mild hypothermia increases blood loss and transfusion requirements during total hip arthroplasty. Lancet. 1996;347:289–92. https://doi.org/10.1016/s0140-6736(96)90466-3.

Sessler DI. Temperature monitoring and perioperative thermoregulation. Anesthesiology. 2008;109:318–38. https://doi.org/10.1097/ALN.0b013e31817f6d76.

Sessler DI. Perioperative thermoregulation and heat balance. Lancet. 2016;387:2655–64. https://doi.org/10.1016/S0140-6736(15)00981-2.

Siew-Fong N, et al. A comparative study of three warming interventions to determine the most effective in maintaining perioperative normothermia. Anesth Analg. 2003;96:171–6. https://doi.org/10.1097/00000539-200301000-00036.

Torossian A. Thermal management during anaesthesia and thermoregulation standards for the prevention of inadvertent perioperative hypothermia. Best Pract Res Clin Anaesthesiol. 2008;22:659–68. https://doi.org/10.1016/j.bpa.2008.07.006.

Winkler M, et al. Aggressive warming reduces blood loss during hip arthroplasty. Anesth Analg. 2000;91:978–84. https://doi.org/10.1097/00000539-200010000-00039.

Young VL, et al. Prevention of perioperative hypothermia in plastic surgery. Aesthet Surg J. 2006;26:551–71. https://doi.org/10.1016/j.asj.2006.08.009.

Surgical Site Infections and Antibiotic Prophylaxis in Surgery: Update 2023

3

Andrea De Gasperi, Marco Merli, Laura Petrò, and Elena Roselli

3.1 Introduction

Surgical site infections (SSIs) are the superficial or deep infections related to a surgical procedure near the incision site and/or affecting organ(s), space(s), site(s), and implanted materials: SSIs occur *within 30 days after surgery* or *up to 90 days in case of prosthetic implantation* [1–4]. According to the Centers for Disease Control and Prevention/National Healthcare Safety Network (CDC/NHSN), SSIs could be classified as follows:

Superficial—SSIs involve only skin and subcutaneous tissue of the incision with at least one of the following: (1) purulent drainage from the superficial incision; (2) organisms isolated from an aseptically obtained culture of fluid or tissue from the superficial incision; (3) among signs or symptoms are pain or tenderness, localized swelling, redness, or heat; superficial incision is deliberately opened by surgeon (responsible for the diagnosis) and is culture-positive or not cultured.

Deep incisional—SSIs occur within 30 days after the operative procedure (no implant left in place) or within 1 year (implant in place) and the infection appears to be related to the operative procedure and involves deep soft tissues (e.g., fascial and muscle layers) of the incision. One of the following should be present: (a) Purulent drainage from the deep incision but not from organ/space component of the surgical

A. De Gasperi (✉) · E. Roselli
Anesthesia and Critical Care Service, ASST GOM Niguarda, Milan, Italy
e-mail: dottdega@gmail.com; elena.roselli@ospedaleniguarda.it

M. Merli
Infectious Diseases Unit - ASST GOM Niguarda, Milan, Italy
e-mail: marco.merli@ospedaleniguarda.it

L. Petrò
AR 1 - Papa Giovanni 23 Hospital, Bergamo, Italy

D. Chiumello (ed.), *Practical Trends in Anesthesia and Intensive Care 2022*,
https://doi.org/10.1007/978-3-031-43891-2_3

"

site. (b) Deep incision spontaneously dehisces or is deliberately opened by a surgeon and is culture-positive or not cultured. (c) The patient has fever (>38 °C) or localized pain or tenderness. (d) An abscess or other evidence of infection involving the deep incision is found on direct examination, during reoperation, or by histopathologic or radiologic examination.

Organ/space SSIs—If infection occurs within 30 days after the operative procedure (no implant left in place) or within 1 year (implant in place), the infection appears to be related to the operative procedure and involves any part of the body, excluding the skin incision, fascia, or muscle layers, that is opened or manipulated during the operative procedure and the patient has: (a) Purulent drainage from a drain that is placed through a stab wound into the organ/space. (b) Organisms isolated from an aseptically obtained culture of fluid or tissue in the organ/space. (c) An abscess or other evidence of infection involving the organ/space that is found on direct examination, during reoperation, or by histopathologic or radiologic examination. (d) Diagnosis of an organ/space SSI by a surgeon.

SSIs are one of the most common postoperative complications/adverse events in the surgical patient, occurring in 3–15% of surgical cases in both EU countries (*European Centre for Disease Prevention and Control, ECDC, 2017—Annual Epidemiological Report for 2015 Healthcare-associated infections: surgical site infections*) and in the USA [1–4]. SSIs included in the *Health Care Associated Infections* (*HCAIs*) and accounting for up to 20% of the cases increase perioperative morbidity and mortality, length of hospitalization, and hospital readmission, sometimes with ICU observation. Importantly, SSIs are considered preventable in close to 50% of cases using evidence-based protocols [1–5].[1] From a public health perspective, SSIs are of such relevance that the WHO defines prevention and interventions aiming at their containment as a real risk management action, while in the USA reimbursements for the treatment may be reduced or even denied [5]. In fact, SSIs containment has long been a primary aim for both scientific societies and institutions, and when achieved, the reduction of SSIs is associated with a relevant improvement in patient safety, global clinical outcomes, and cost containment.[2]

3.2 SSIs—Exogenous or Endogenous Infections?

SSIs are usually classified as *exogenous* infections (caused by nosocomial pathogens), and are part of the HCAIs, given the "nosocomial" origin of the potential reservoir from which infection(s) could be transmitted (health care providers,

---

[1] *For more on this topic, see also Allegranzi B, et al. New WHO recommendations on intraoperative and postoperative measures for surgical site infection prevention: an evidence-based global perspective. Lancet Infect Dis. 2016;16:e288–303. E at 17. Allegranzi B, et al. New WHO recommendations on preoperative measures for surgical site infection prevention: an evidence-based global perspective. Lancet Infect Dis. 2016;16:e276–87.*

[2] *For the interested reader: Umscheid CA, Mitchell MD, Doshi JA et al. Estimating the proportion of healthcare-associated infections that are reasonably preventable and the related mortality and costs. Infect Control Hosp Epidemiol. 2011;32 (2):101–114.*

environments, surfaces, hands, invasive or non-invasive ventilators, instrumentation, surgical and anesthesiologic techniques). It is mandatory the constant reminder for the anesthesiologists of the role of anesthesia equipment, ultrasound (US) probes [6] and non-appropriate conduction (hand hygiene and use of personal protective equipment included) of invasive maneuvers in contributing to this type of infection [7]. Very recent, however, is the hypothesis of the role played by the patient's *microbiome* in SSIs, which may turn SSIs origin from exogenous to *endogenous* [2, 8]. Bacterial genetic analyses have been documenting how a proportion of HCAIs derive from the (altered) microbiome of the patient himself rather than from the hospital environment, making SSIs *endogenous* even in the presence of exogenous-like organisms [2, 3, 8, 9]. In fact, the patient's microbiome prior to contact with the nosocomial environment may become "potentially pathogenic" even in the community environment: in case of inappropriate and/or unnecessary antibiotic therapies in the community setting ("antibiotic pressure") or "stressful" procedures or exposures (surgery, health care environments), microbiota microorganisms may shift from *colonizing commensals* into *infecting* bugs [2, 8]. Skin and nasal microorganisms are the most likely origin of SSIs in clean surgical procedures [2]. Stressful conditions such as disease and injuries—elective surgery or unnecessary antibiotic pressure included—may directly influence and change the gut microbiota, killing commensal organisms but not reducing *Enterococci* and *Staphilococci*. Thus, a proportion of HCAIs (SSIs among them) can be defined as *endogenous* (arising from the altered patient's microbiome) and not necessarily *exogenous* (secondary to "contact" with the nosocomial environment) [2, 8]. Stress conditions are able to alter the host control over the microbiome. The host neutrophils, invaded at remote sites of colonization (nares and gastrointestinal tract) by pathogens (particularly *Staphylococcus aureus*), provide, after re-entering systemic circulation and migrating to traumatized tissues, viable intracellular pathogens: this is the basis of *the Trojan-Horse Hypothesis* [2, 8]. As is for *Candida* infections, procedures capable of "disrupting" or "damaging" anatomical barriers or cells membranes (as occurs during invasive surgical or anesthesiologic maneuvers) cause bacterial translocation from the intestinal canal to surgical sites or to the blood stream [1–3, 8, 9]. "New" possible risk factors, including the (excessive) use of opioids in the perioperative period, volatile anesthetics, overly high perioperative oxygen concentrations, and surgery-related stress conditions should be considered in new SSIs prevention strategies [2, 8]. Such an increased risk of postoperative infections may drive changes in pre-operative preparation strategies, especially for *S. aureus*, including preoperative screening and (nasal) decontamination with mupirocin [2]. According to [2, 8], Methicillin-resistant *S. aureus* bundles (screening, decolonization, contact precautions, and hand hygiene) seem to be highly effective when all components are implemented, in spite of the absence of standard decolonization procedures. Known or suspected reservoir(s) of resistant pathogens should become the target of the surgical antibiotic prophylaxis (SAP) adjustments, aiming at a personalized approach, and not relying upon relevant but not universally standardized guidelines (GLs): one size, once again, does not fit all.

3.3 The "Bundle" Philosophy: The Importance of Aggregated, Structured, and Targeted Interventions

A set of measures and not a single "player" is relevant to contrast SSIs (Box 3.1). In fact, (1) SAP constitutes only one part, even if relevant, of the preventive strategy; (2) a **bundle** refers to *combinations of care-related measures with an evidence-based rationale aiming to achieve a goal of high clinical impact* (e.g., guidelines for sepsis and septic shock from Surviving Sepsis Campaign, CCM 2021) [10]. This set of clinical and organizational interventions addressing the target (the *bundle*) should be extensively and rigorously applied in the different surgical specialties, and strongly supported by institutions, administrations, and trusts; (3) SSIs surveillance, reporting, and results dissemination are important steps to be implemented in the local Continuous Medica Education (CME) programs in both surgical (anesthesiologists, surgeons) and medical (ID specialists, hospitalists) settings; (4) projects able to impact SSIs and developed by the Units could become a relevant part the budget negotiation for the involved Departments, using top-down and bottom-up processes for their implementation (see also [1]). For years the WHO and US Centers for Infectious Disease Control and Prevention (CDC) as well as national and international institutions or scientific societies have been renewing guidelines (GLs) and recommendations for SSIs prevention [1, 11–14]. Guidelines and recommendations are well designed, comprehensive, solid, methodologically appropriate, and frequently updated: real world implementation, despite its evidence, is unfortunately lower than expected, with a negative impact on quality of care [1–3, 15, 16]. A relevant number of clinical and organizational interventions with varying levels

---

Box 3.1 Glossary of "Physical" and "Chemical" Hygiene Measures for SSIs Control
- **Disinfection**: a practice directed at the *destruction of a specific germ or generally of all pathogenic germs* (not necessarily sporigenes) present at a given site. It is generally achieved through the use of *disinfectants*.
- **Sterilization**: a method aimed at *eliminating all living things, pathogenic and non-pathogenic, present on a given solid, liquid, or aeriform substrate*. It is achieved by chemical but mainly physical means (heat, gamma rays, filters).
- **Antisepsis** or bacteriostasis: practice aimed at *neutralizing a microbial load* by blocking reproduction and not necessarily by killing germs.
- **Asepsis**: a procedure designed to prevent contamination by microorganisms of previously sterilized substrates. Asepsis is reserved particularly for items that are part of environments or facilities at high risk of infection to humans such as a surgical compartment may be.
- **Decontamination**: abatement of microbial load by exposing items not previously cleaned to the action of disinfecting or sterilizing agents.

of evidence have been and continue to be available to reduce SSIs [4, 8, 9]. Usually the SSIs *bundle* is based on few interventions (3–5 items) of proven efficacy, aiming at the best patient outcomes. Recently, the ***Global Alliance for Infections in Surgery (GAIS)*** proposed five simple procedures (a bundle) targeting SSIs prevention [13]. Strengths of the GAIS "package" include, among others, easy-to-apply measures whose implementation in the surgical setting should be straightforward. Compliance with these rules, their widest application, and their systematic periodical validations should provide to the surgical patients practices with a significant impact on morbidity and mortality (*good clinical practices*).

3.4   The GAIS Bundle

The measures composing the GAIS *bundle* encompass European, Australian, and American GLs: as alluded to above, antibiotic prophylaxis is one measure, but not the only one, targeting SSIs containment (Fig. 3.1).

Preoperative bath/shower: Patients should be advised to shower or bathe (full body) with soap (antimicrobial or nonantimicrobial) or an antiseptic agent on (at least) the night before surgery to keep the bacterial load as low as possible (*IB–strong recommendation; accepted practice*). According to Berrios Torres et al. the optimal timing of the preoperative shower or bath, the total number of soap or

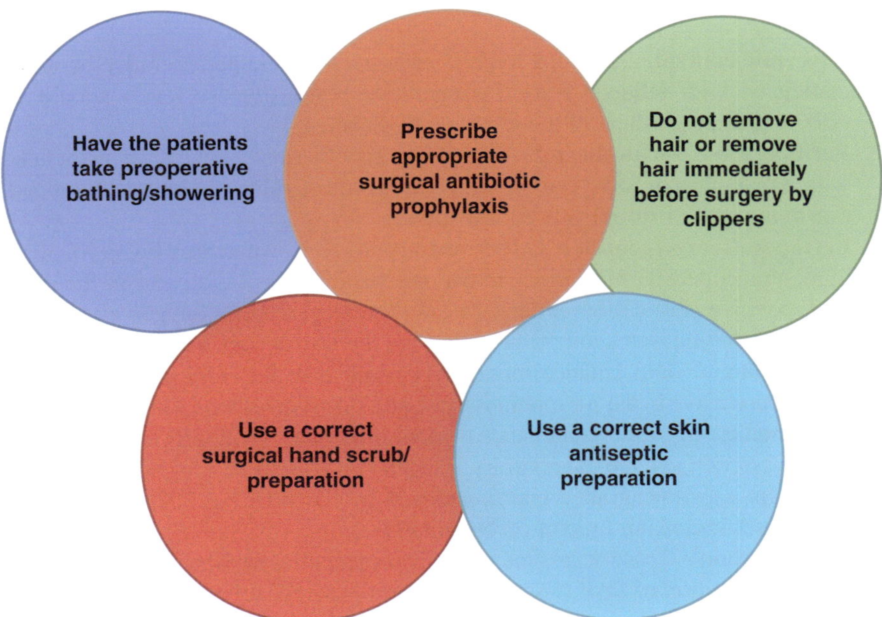

Fig. 3.1 The GAIS scheme (taken from the *Global Alliance for Infections in Surgery* website, www.infectionsinsurgery.org) [13]

antiseptic agent applications, and the use of chlorhexidine gluconate wash cloths for the prevention of SSI are, so far, unresolved issues (*No recommendation*) [5].

Hair removal: In patients undergoing any surgical procedure, hair should not be removed or, if absolutely necessary, should be removed only with a clipper in the operating room immediately before surgery.

Antiseptic skin preparation: Unless contraindicated, perform skin preparation with an alcohol-based antiseptic agent (*IA–strong recommendation; high-quality evidence*). Plastic adhesive drapes with or without antimicrobial properties are not necessary to prevent SSIs (*II–weak recommendation; high- to moderate-quality evidence*) [5].

Intraoperative irrigation of deep or subcutaneous tissues: According to Barrios et al. [5], aqueous iodophor solution for the prevention of SSIs could be an option, while intraperitoneal lavage with aqueous iodophor solution in contaminated or dirty abdominal procedures is not necessary (*II–weak recommendation; moderate-quality*).

Antimicrobial dressings after primary closure: Randomized controlled trials do not show evidence regarding such a dressing in the operating room for the prevention of SSI (*No recommendation/ unresolved issue*) [5].

Surgical hand scrub/preparation: surgical hand preparation should be performed precisely using appropriate soap and adequate hand scrubbing with alcohol-based disinfectants before donning sterile gloves.

Other interventions recognized over the years in helping to contain/reduce SSIs [1, 2, 8] and endorsed by CDC 2017 [1] and NICE 2019 [12] are

1. **Glycemic control**—Avoiding hyperglycemia during the perioperative period is associated with reduced SSIs. Perioperative blood glucose levels should be <200 mg/dL, regardless of the presence of diabetes (I-A).
2. **Perioperative normothermia**—Avoiding hypothermia (<35 °C) is associated with a reduction of SSIs, even if temperature cutoff values are not well defined, due to the lack of sufficiently robust studies.
3. **Perioperative oxygenation** and peripheral perfusion—Increased FiO_2 (40–50%) is recommended during intraoperative mechanical ventilation and in the early postoperative period after extubation to optimize peripheral oxygen availability (DO_2). Other measures to optimize DO_2 are the appropriate perioperative circulating volume (fluid balance moderately positive in the intraoperative period, mildly restrictive in the postoperative period), invasive or noninvasive cardiovascular monitoring, and maintenance of normothermia. NICE GLs suggest to aim at SaO_2 >95% [12]. On the contrary, elevated FiO_2 (80%) during surgery to prevent SSIs was downgraded and abandoned by the WHO in 2020, after recent re-analyses indicating little or no benefit [8].
4. **SAP duration**—Trials across many surgical specialties have clearly documented that long duration of SAP (>24 h) does not prevent SSIs, but may increase antibiotic resistance, *Clostridium Difficile* infections, and, even if rarely, acute kidney injury: short antibiotics (ATB) courses are then to be implemented, representing a further chance for a wise antibiotic stewardship [8] (see below).

Adhering to the antiseptic measures, while implementing the interventions related to hemodynamics and metabolism, and appropriately applying SAP at local level (timing, duration, local microbiological ecology, periodical revision) should contribute to the reduction of surgical site infections: anesthesiologists are given a relevant chance to contribute to safety and quality of surgical care, underlining once again their role as perioperative physicians.

3.5   Surgical Antibiotic Prophylaxis (SAP) [1–3, 11–14]

SAP refers to the use of antibiotics for the prevention of SSIs. SAP, the administration of an anti-infective drug *before bacterial contamination of the surgical field*, aims at avoiding the potential subsequent development of infection at the surgical site. SAP is not intended to "sterilize" tissues, but to reduce the microbial load at the surgical site to a level affordable by "normal" host defenses [1–3, 11–14]. SAP constitutes a pillar of prevention and is one of the most relevant, and, if well applied, clinically and economically valuable measures to prevent surgical wounds infection [2]: the routine addition of SAP—started in the 1960s and mandatory since the 1980s—resulted in a 50–60% reduction in the incidence of SSIs in most surgical procedures. The routine administration of prophylactic antibiotics is standard in cases of artificial implant/prosthesis as part of the procedure, bone grafting procedures, and other surgeries with extensive dissections or expected high blood loss. SAP constitutes one of the most common indications for antibiotic use in many hospitals (indication close to 40%). It does not include possible preoperative decolonization, particularly nasal decolonization with mupirocin in **MSSA** (*Methicillin Susceptible Staphylococcus aureus*) or **MRSA** (*Methicillin Resistant Staph Aureus*) carriers, this latter being a cutting-edge item, with pros and cons. NICE GLs support its use for patients at risk of *S. aureus* infection*s,* together with chlorhexidine bath from 2 days before to post operative day (POD) 3 [12]. SAP does not include treatment of known, pre-existing infections. Should this be the case, the perioperative antibiotic indication must be guided by antibiotic *stewardship* and should include type of surgery, site of infection, knowledge of local microbial ecology, and drug choice: a treatment and not a prophylaxis, by definition [17]. Appropriate prophylaxis should reduce both the incidence of superficial and deep surgical site infections (at the site of surgery) and systemic infections: sepsis or septic shock and the need for an intensive treatment are the possible feared evolutions.

3.5.1   SAP has a Precise Rationale Related to [1, 11–14, 17]

- Type of intervention (*clean, clean-contaminated, contaminated, dirty*) (Table 3.1)
- Use of prosthetic material/foreign body implantation
- Operative risk associated with comorbidities, almost always defined using the American Society of Anesthesiologists (ASA) score, but more recently also employing National Surgical Quality Improvement Program (which includes ASA) or similar scores (SURPAS) [19]

Table 3.1 Classification of surgical wounds (modified from Talbot) [18]

Classification of surgical wounds	Criteria
Clean	Uninfected operative wounds in which • No inflammation is encountered • Respiratory, gastrointestinal, genital, or urinary tracts are not entered • No break in aseptic technique • Primarily closed and, if necessary, drained with closed drainage • Operative incisional wounds after nonpenetrating (blunt) trauma included in this category if they meet the criteria
Clean-contaminated	Operative wounds in which • Respiratory, gastrointestinal, genital (including female and male reproductive tracts), or urinary tracts entered under controlled conditions and without unusual contamination • Operations involving the biliary tract, appendix, vagina, and oropharynx included in this category • Evidence of infection or major break in technique encountered
Contaminated	• Major breaks in sterile technique (e.g., open cardiac massage) • Gross spillage from the gastrointestinal tract • Incision of acute, non-purulent inflammation (including necrotic tissue without evidence of purulent discharge) • Open, fresh, or accidental wounds
Dirty (or infected)	• Existing clinical infection or perforated viscera, old traumatic wounds with retained devitalized tissue • Organisms causing postoperative infection present before surgery • Antibiotic treatment required

• "Timing" and "dosing" (schedule), which must be *timely and appropriate*

The indication for SAP is well supported in numerous GLs (perhaps too many, and often repetitively) in every surgical specialty and for groups of surgeries [1, 11–14, 17].

The administration of antibiotics (ATB) in community aquired pneumonia (CAP) has precise rules related to the type of surgery, choice of drug, and type of patient (vide infra), e.g., obese or the very elderly. Main points are time of administration (*timing*), doses (*dosing/scheduling*) and *redosing if indicated, and* pharmacokinetic (pK) characteristic of the molecule. Reasons for "*redosing*" include intraoperative bleeding—"critical" if greater than 1500 ml, or in case of massive transfusion (usually considered administration of PRCs > 6 units) or in case of prolongation of surgery due to technical difficulties. Unfortunately, compliance with these GLs is "worldwide" low even if a trend toward improvement is now present in the literature [15, 20]. *Timing* and *scheduling* aim at achieving effective plasma and tissue concentrations at the start of and during surgery to lower the risk of infection during the period of maximum exposure: short-term prophylaxis and appropriate doses are cornerstones of SAP. The administration of any antibiotic after skin incision greatly reduces its efficacy. For this reason, the NICE guidelines (GLs) [12] emphasize standardizing the timing of prophylactic dose administration at induction of anesthesia, providing for its anticipation in surgeries where tourniquet use is planned and when vancomycin is used. If timing of antibiotic administration varies, optimum way in which to have the highest concentration in the tissues at the start of and during surgery is to start antibiotics at least 30 min but no more than 60 min before the skin incision.

3.5.2 Antibiotic usage in SAP

For this review we have used the most recent GLs (Medical Letter 2016 [11], NICE 2020 [12], GAIS [13], SA 2020 [14], CDC 2019 [1], UPTODATE 2023 (accessed March 2023) [21]. Some of the main points dealing with the mode of administration include:

- **Beta Lactams**—To be administered within 5–60 min *before* skin incision.
- **Gentamicin** (if and when indicated)—3 mg/kg bw (NICE suggests 2 mg/kg) within 120 min before surgical incision. To be administered intravenously over 15 min in 100 mL saline solution.
- **Metronidazole** and **clindamycin**—To be administered over 20 min.
- **Vancomycin**—1 g in at least 60 min and 1.5 g in at least 90 min (adults). Vancomycin should be started 15–120 min before skin incision to provide adequate concentration at the time of incision and to allow any potential infusion-related toxicity prior to induction.

The use of "common" antibiotic molecules (e.g., *cefazolin*) is based on balance between cost, safety, PK profile, and antimicrobial activity. The anti-infective drugs chosen for SAP should protect against the most likely infectious risk(s) associated with the intervention: this strategy is closely correlated to the need to avoid antibiotics to be used in case of complicated infections sustained by multidrug-resistant (MDR) microorganisms: main aims are to contain bacterial resistance, while effectively counteracting the most probable SSIs. In fact, there is no scientific support to use broad-spectrum antibiotics to reduce the incidence of postoperative SSIs compared to narrower-spectrum, more common antimicrobial agents: possible benefits might be present only in patients with known MDR colonization and only in specific settings. Crucial in this regard are antibiotic *stewardship*, local SSIs epidemiology, and local microbiological ecology [17].

Unfortunately, too common seems to be the non-complete adherence to these indications [1, 15, 16, 20]: according to a 2015 Australian review (National Antimicrobial Prescribing Survey, NAPS) [20] the proportion of inappropriate SAP indications was around 40%, reduced to 27% in the most recent review (2019), but still to be improved [16]. Critical points are the choice of class of antibiotics (inappropriate) and the duration of administration, not infrequently prolonged well beyond 24 h after the intervention [1]. The negative implications are not only economic but also associated with increased bacterial resistance, overinfection (fungal infections are possible), and changes in the microbiota [2, 8], not to mention possible adverse reactions. Interestingly, a recent US report dealing with the efficacy of current standard surgical prophylaxis regimens underlined

1. Close to 40–50% of SSIs are sustained by germs resistant to standard antibiotics for the procedure.
2. Such a trend may result in an increase in infections associated with surgery [22].

The widespread use of antibiotics to treat community infections or some questionable prophylaxis schemes in case of cancer chemotherapy [22] has resulted in the emergence of resistant strains at the level of the "community microbiome" [2, 8], a condition that now poses a complex set of challenges for prophylaxis against surgical site infection, potentially turning into "endogenous" [2, 8]. Such a setting makes relevant the chance of using in selected cases an individualized approach and not necessarily the "standard" [2]: antibiotic stewardship should play a strategic role using data coming from "local" SSIs epidemiology [1–3, 17]. Each hospital should build locally adapted SAP guidelines starting from the robust and evidence-based national and international schemes [17]. In fact, the strength of an SAP should rely upon the "quali-quantitative" knowledge of "immediate" local post-surgical infectious complications (first 92 postoperative hours). Ideal, even if complex, would be to track SSIs at POD 30. Such a set of information should include incidence of SSIs by type of surgery, site, severity, microbiology, and the presence of MDR: of the utmost importance is the 2017 ECDC document, addressing the relevance of surgery if performed using an "open" or minimally invasive approach [23]. Structuring such an intervention guided by the Hospital Strategic Management and HCAI local committee allows the fine-tuning of the local SSIs GLs, making a "dynamic" adaptation to the local epidemiology and creating a sort of *context-sensitive SAP*, i.e., SAP based on evidence-based national or international guidelines, adapted and revised (possibly at least every 2 years) with data coming from the local SSIs epidemiology.

3.6 Assumptions and Indications of Antibiotic Prophylaxis in Surgery (SAP) [21]

SAP has a strong indication in any surgical procedure that, referring to the surgical wound classification (***clean; clean-contaminated; contaminated; dirty***), is classified as **clean-contaminated, contaminated, or dirty** (see Table 3.1). SAP has no indication in clean procedures, unless special conditions/risk factors are present and related to the local setting. Worth underlining are the following notes of microbiology underlying the rationale for the choice of antibiotics [18, 21–23]:

- The predominant organisms causing SSIs after clean procedures are present in the skin flora, including *Streptococcal* species, *Staphylococcus aureus,* and *coagulase-negative Staphylococci (CoNS)* (frequently *Staphylococcus epidermidis*).

- In clean contaminated procedures the predominant organisms include *Enterococcus* spp. and Gram-negative bugs in addition to skin flora.
- When the surgical procedure involves the viscera, pathogens reflect the endogenous flora of the viscera or of the mucosal surface; such infections are typically polymicrobial. Hence the importance of the microbiome and its modifications (see above) [2, 8].
- The causative pathogens associated with SSIs have changed over time. In the USA between 1986 and 2003, the percentage of SSIs caused by gram-negative bacilli decreased from 56 to 33%. *S. aureus* was the most common pathogen (22%). Between 2006 and 2007, the increase in the incidence of infections sustained with *S. aureus* (30%) was associated with a substantial increase in *MRSA* (about half of the isolates), with obvious increases in hospital stay, morbidity, mortality, and costs. Surveys performed in the last 10 years show a reversal of this trend and a reduction in MRSA infections [21, 22]. The differences in the EU (see specific table reported by ECDC) are interesting to note [23].
- Fungal infections, and particularly *Candida albicans infections* are on the rise among SSIs. Overly liberal and unnecessary use of prophylactic and empiric antibiotics, coupled with the increasing comorbidities of the surgical candidates and the increasing number of immunocompromised/immunomodulated patients undergoing surgical procedures, probably plays a role in this trend.
- Among exogenous sources of infection, there is a role played by organisms from the environment or from health care workers (healthy carriers).
- Although rare, SSIs have been associated with so-called unusual pathogens, found on dressing material or ultrasound probes, or in disinfection solutions.

Key points to optimize SAP are [1, 11–14, 18, 21–23]:

1. Appropriate indication of the surgical procedure.
2. Risk of postoperative infection and possible systemic consequences: prophylaxis in the absence of evidence of reducing postoperative infections should be critically reviewed (useless).
3. Appropriate timing, dosage (and redosage if and when necessary), scheduling.
4. Patient's risk factors, including (but not limited to) state of immunosuppression, immunomodulation, use of prosthetic material, allergies, obesity, liver and kidney dysfunction, malnutrition, diabetes, and oncological pathology. These issues are discussed by Decker et al. [3].
5. Preoperative presence of infections or preoperative MDR colonization deserves a different, individualized approach. MDR colonization should by no means automatically lead to the use of "special" antibiotic prophylaxis, to be considered instead for the treatment of infections for which ID *stewardship* is mandatory [17], and a solid consensus is eagerly awaited.
6. The risk of bacterial endocarditis in the presence of specific cardiological conditions;
7. In case of prosthetic surgery or implanted devices, SAP has an indication also in cases of clean surgery: screening *for MSSA/MRSA* is strongly suggested: the

presence of *MRSA* colonization (targeted screening) is an indication for decolonization.

8. Splenectomized patients deserve special attention and consideration. GLs are available to prevent and treat infections in patients with dysfunctional (or absent) splenic function. Relevant points among others are (1) pneumococcal immunization; (2) haemophilus influenza type B vaccination; (3) meningococcal group C conjugate vaccination; (4) yearly influenza immunization; and (5) lifelong prophylactic antibiotics (oral phenoxymethylpenicillin or erythromycin) (under discussion).

9. In case of manifest/known allergy to betalactams, NICE [12] suggests the use of **gentamicin** 2 mg/kg 5–15 min in 100–250 mL saline solution or **gentamicin** 3 mg/kg in 5–15 min in 100–250 mL saline solution **plus** Metronidazole 500 mg ev in intestinal surgery.

3.7 SAP Schedules [11–14, 18, 20, 21, 24]

The interested reader is asked to refer to the specific references for further insights in SAP related to surgical procedures. In Table 3.2 (from Talbot, Chap. 313 in Mandell, Douglas, and *Bennett's Principles and Practice of Infectious Diseases*, 2-Volume Set, ninth Edition Elsevier 2021) the recommended doses of antibiotics and redosing intervals [18] are given.

1. **Surgery of the gastrointestinal tract**—In gastrointestinal (GI) tract surgery in case of clean-contaminated procedures and in case of entry into the hollow viscera, **cefazolin** still constitutes the antibiotic of choice. These procedures include both minimally invasive endoscopic or radiologic interventional procedures (percutaneous gastrostomy, percutaneous endoscopic gastrostomy/radiologically inserted gastrostomy (PEG/RIG)) and bariatric surgery as well as oncologic procedures with minimally invasive (videolaparoscopic or robotic) or "open" approaches (major gastric, major pancreatic oncologic surgery). In procedures such as selective vagotomy and antireflux procedures, by definition "clean," antimicrobial prophylaxis is deemed necessary only in the presence of the risk factors listed below.

   - Decrease in gastric pH
   - Gastroduodenal perforation
   - Diminished gastrointestinal motility
   - Obstruction (esophageal/gastric/enteric)
   - Obesity
   - ASA status ≥ 3

   The relevance of appropriate SAP is underscored by the following figures: the incidence of SSIs in patients **not** receiving antimicrobial prophylaxis was 6% after vagotomy and drainage, 13% after gastric ulcer procedures, 7–17% after gastric cancer procedures, 8% for duodenocephalopancreasectomy (DCP), and up to 26% after PEG/RIG insertion.

Table 3.2 The recommended doses of antibiotics and redosing intervals for more commonly used antibiotics for SAP

ANTIMICROBIAL	RECOMMENDED DOSE FOR ADULTS	RECOMMENDED REDOSING INTERVAL (FROM INITIATION OF PREOPERATIVE DOSE) (h)[a]
Intravenous Agents		
Ampicillin-sulbactam	3 g (ampicillin 2 g/sulbactam 1 g)	2
Ampicillin	2 g	2
Aztreonam	2 g	4
Cefazolin	2 g; 3 g for persons with weight ≥120 kg	4
Cefotaxime	1 g	3
Cefoxitin	2 g	2
Cefotetan	2 g	6
Ceftriaxone	2 g	NA
Ciprofloxacin	400 mg	NA
Clindamycin	900 mg	6
Ertapenem	1 g	NA
Fluconazole	400 mg	NA
Gentamicin	5 mg/kg	NA
Levofloxacin	500 mg	NA
Metronidazole	500 mg	NA
Moxifloxacin	400 mg	NA
Piperacillin-tazobactam	3.375 g	2
Vancomycin	15 mg/kg	NA
Oral Agents for Colorectal Procedures (in Conjunction With Mechanical Bowel Preparation)		
Erythromycin base	1 g	NA
Metronidazole	2 g	NA
Neomycin	1–2 g	NA

[a]Based on typical case length; for prolonged cases, antibiotics noted as "NA" (not applicable) may require redosing.
Modified from Bratzler DW, Dellinger EP, Olsen KM, et al. Clinical practice guidelines for antimicrobial prophylaxis in surgery. Am J Health Syst Pharm. 2013;70:195–283.

(From Talbot, Chap. 313 in Mandell, Douglas, and Bennett's *Principles and Practice of Infectious Diseases*, 2-Volume Set, ninth Edition Elsevier 2021)

The most common organisms sustaining SSI after gastroduodenal procedures are coliforms (*Escherichia coli*, *Proteus* spp., *Klebsiella* spp.), *Staphylococci, Streptococci, Enterococci* spp., and occasionally *Bacteroides.*

For small bowel surgery without obstruction antimicrobial prophylaxis with **cefazolin** is still recommended. Coverage for anaerobes should be used in case of obstructive pathology and includes: **cefazolin + metronidazole** 500 mg ev over 20 min (NICE) or **ampicillin/sulbactam** or **cefoxitin**.

The incidence of SSIs for small bowel procedures (UK data, 2010) was between 3 and 7%, depending on the risk categories. The microorganisms isolated included gram-negative enteric bugs (aerobes and anaerobes) and gram-positive species such as *Streptococci, Staphylococci, and Enterococci* spp. Knowledge of local epidemiology is, as underlined above, paramount.

Cefazolin	2 g ev to be repeated after 4 h if needed
	3 g ev in case of BW >120 kg
Redosing needed in case of surgery lasting >4 h (interval between doses equal to one to two half-lives of the drug)	
Alternatives to Cefazolin	
Cefuroxime	2 g (additional dose of 1 g after 3 h if needed)
Cefoxitin	2 g (additional dose of 1 g after 3 h if needed)

The NICE GLs [12] suggest adding **Vancomycin** 1 g (1.5 g in case of actual BW >80 kg) in case of high risk of MRSA (history of MRSA colonization or infection *or* an ongoing prolonged stay in health care environments with high prevalence of MRSA, *or* residence in the last 12 months, in a correctional institution).

2. **Biliary tract and pancreatic surgery**—in patients undergoing open biliary tract procedures **cefazolin** is the drug of choice. Alternatives include other **beta-lactams, cefoxitin, cefuroxime, and ampicillin/sulbactam**. The appropriateness of SAP in cases of elective laparoscopic cholecystectomy in low-risk subjects is still a matter of debate and the choice is left to local expertise according to local epidemiology.

   Routine antimicrobial prophylaxis is not warranted for patients undergoing endoscopic retrograde cholangiopancreatography (ERCP), even in patients with biliary tract stones or distal bile duct stenosis. Antimicrobial prophylaxis *is warranted for ERCP* in patients with cholangitis, biliary obstruction, and incomplete drainage: association with metronidazole is proposed in selected cases [12, 21]. **Ampicillin/sulbactam** (3 g up to 120 kg) could be an alternative to **cefazolin**. The use of broad-spectrum antibiotics has a rationale in cases of ongoing infectious disease and/or with stigmata recalling sepsis or even septic shock (a therapy and not a prophylaxis).

   The organisms responsible for biliary tract infections include *E. coli, Klebsiella* spp., and *Enterococci*; less frequently *Streptococci or Staphylococci* and occasionally anaerobes (also *Clostridioides*) are reported. Increased antimicrobial resistance has been observed among pathogens causing intra-abdominal infections and resistant *E. coli* (extended-spectrum betalactamase producer, ESBL) accounting for up to 40%. Again, local epidemiology has to guide internal GLs.

3. **Pancreatic procedures**—In general, the guidelines for biliary tract surgery can also be applied to pancreatic procedures. The risk of SSIs is increased in the context of endoscopic or percutaneous biliary or pancreatic drainage procedures performed before pancreatic surgery [22]. Therefore, antimicrobial prophylaxis before pancreatic procedure should be extended to cover microorganisms recovered from biliary drains. The possible contamination of the sample obtained during the endoscopic procedures should be considered.

4. **Splenectomy**—The standard schedule includes **cefazolin 2 g** ev and **vancomycin** in case of high risk of MRSA. Post-splenectomy vaccination for meningococcal, pneumococcal, and *H. influenzae* is required in all cases (NICE GL; see above) [12]. In case of elective splenectomy, vaccination is recommended at least 2 weeks before surgery.

5. **Procedures related to hernia repair**—Antimicrobial prophylaxis for patients undergoing hernioplasty with or without use of prosthesis relies on **cefazolin**. In selected cases without the use of prosthetic material, SAP can be avoided. The most common organisms isolated from SSIs after hernia repair are gram-positive aerobic MO (*Streptococci, Staphylococci, and Enterococci*). In cases in which hollow viscera perforation is expected (or suspected) NICE [12] suggests the use of **Metronidazole** 500 mg ev + **Gentamicin** 2 mg/kg.

6. **Appendectomy**—Complicated appendicitis is usually defined as "perforated, abscessualized or peritonitis-associated appendicitis." Antimicrobial prophylaxis is warranted in the context of uncomplicated appendicitis: **cefazolin 2 g ev + metronidazole 500 mg ev is the choice**, but **cefuroxime or cefoxitin** is an appropriate alternative. In case of peritonitis the antibiotic treatment should be continued treatment for 3 (to 5) days, particularly if inadequate *source control is suspected* [13, 17]. The most common organisms isolated from SSIs after appendectomy are anaerobic gram-negative enteric microorganisms (MOs) (*Bacteroides fragilis*) and/or aerobes (*E. coli*). Aerobic and anaerobic *Streptococci, Staphylococci,* and *Enterococci have* also been reported. NICE suggests the use of vancomycin in case of high MRSA risk [12].

7. **Colorectal procedures** [11–14, 18, 21, 24–26]—Intravenous antimicrobial prophylaxis for colorectal procedures, able to reduce SSIs and mortality, includes as mainstays **cefazolin and metronidazole**: this association covers both aerobic and anaerobic gram-negative enteric bacilli. Alternatives include second-generation cephalosporins (cefoxitin 2 g + intraoperative dose of 1 g after about 2 h, or cefuroxime). According to NICE [12] and UPTODATE [21], cefazolin plus metronidazole is the solution of choice due to increased resistance of *E. coli* to second-generation cephalosporins, the occurrence of *Clostridioides difficile* infections, and the emergence of resistance or MDR infections (particularly carbapenemase-resistant Enterobacteriaceae). According to Talbot [18], alternative approaches include EV antibiotics and oral (often nonabsorbable) antibiotics or combination therapy. A recent

Cochrane review [25] may help clarify the issue of optimal antimicrobial prophylaxis for colorectal surgery. Analysis of 260 studies with more than 43,000 patients found a significant reduction in post-surgical infections with the use of oral and EV prophylaxis compared with EV prophylaxis or oral prophylaxis alone. Still debated is bowel preparation (MBP) in colorectal surgery associated or not with oral antibiotics [25]: conflicting results are reported in the literature particularly in case of anastomotic leaking. A retrospective analysis found that MBP in combination with oral antimicrobials resulted in significantly lower rates of SSI than MBP without oral antimicrobials. In contrast, a larger study reported by Talbot [18] as part of the National Surgical Quality Improvement Program found that MBP with oral antibiotics was associated with significantly lower incidence of anastomotic leaking, SSI, and postoperative ileus. The 2013 US surgical prophylaxis GLs recommended the use of MBP combined with oral antimicrobials and EV for most colorectal procedures [26].

8. **Urologic procedures** [11–14, 18, 21, 24]—For open or laparoscopic surgeries (including robotic surgery) involving prostate, bladder, or ureter, **cefazolin** 2 g + **gentamicin** 3 mg/kg is the appropriate choice. **Metronidazole** 500 mg ev should be associated in case of risk factors for anaerobes and in case of intestinal perforation. In case of true allergy to betalactams, **gentamycin** 3 mg/kg + **metronidazole 500 mg** should be considered. In case of patients carrying MRSA, **vancomycin** is advised. For prostate transurethral resection procedures, the first choice is **gentamicin 2–3 mg/kg bw** in 100–250 Saline within 5–15 min (cefazolin in case of contraindication to gentamicin) [12]. In case of prostate biopsy **amoxicillin clavulanate** (2.2 g) in preferred to **cefazolin 2 g ev** [12, 21].

   Pre-existing or suspected infections deserve treatment with appropriate antibiotics. For patients at risk of endocarditis, treatment is warranted: please refer to the NICE GL [12].

9. **Gynecologic and obstetric surgery**—SAP for gynecologic surgery does not differ from abdominal surgery, with **cefazolin and metronidazole** for oncologic and non-oncologic procedures. For *cesarean section* NICE proposes **cefazolin** 2 g alone; **cefazolin and metronidazole** or **amoxicillin/clavulanate** (2 g) is suggested in case of vaginal delivery and presence of anal sphincter damage [12].

10. **Cardiac surgery** [11–14, 18, 21, 24]—Scheduled procedures in cardiac surgery include coronary artery bypass (CABG), valve replacement procedures, and placement of implantable devices. SSIs include mediastinitis and sternal wound infection (range 0.35–8.49%). A large number of the infections are superficial. Risk factors include pre-existing obstructive pulmonary disease, heart failure, vascular grafts with internal mammary artery, number of grafts, and nasal colonization by *S. aureus*. Common MOs are *S. aureus* and *CoNS* (*coagulase-negative staphylococci*); less common are Gram-negative MOs (*Enterobacteriaceae, Pseudomonas* and *Acinetobacter*, associated, according to some, with saphenous vein grafts. Cephalosporins (first- and second-generation) are the antimicrobial agents of choice for the prevention of SSIs in

cardiac surgical procedures, **cefazolin** perhaps more performant than cefuroxime. **Vancomycin** prophylaxis is warranted for patients colonized by MRSA and/or at high risk of MRSA infection. Alternatives for patients with known beta-lactam allergy are **vancomycin** or **clindamycin**. Still under debate is the use of third-generation cephalosporins, aminoglycosides, or aztreonam, in the presence of risk factors, to cover Gram-negative bugs. The optimal duration of antimicrobial prophylaxis after cardiothoracic procedures is controversial, but always limited to 24 h. No advantage has been demonstrated to extend the duration of antimicrobial prophylaxis until removal of central catheters, epicardial wires, drains, etc.

11. **Implanted devices**—Antimicrobial prophylaxis is indicated for implantation/ replacement of permanent pacemakers, implantable cardioverter defibrillators, and cardiac resynchronization devices. The antibiotic of choice is **cefazolin.** Risk factors for SSIs include fever in the 24 h prior to implantation, temporary pacing prior to definitive implantation, and hematoma.

    The optimal approach to antimicrobial prophylaxis in the setting of ventricular assist devices (VADs) is still not well defined. Data on infection rates are limited, and no published studies demonstrate, so far, the effectiveness of preoperative antimicrobial therapy. Most infections are bacterial, sustained mainly by *Staphylococcus* spp., although fungal infections have also been observed (9%).

12. **Thoracic surgery**. In case of known infections, current antibiotic therapy is continued and will be modified based on the material recovered and cultured during surgery. In the case of elective surgery (lobar resections, pneumonectomies, pleural decortications) and in the absence of any infectious disease, NICE proposes **cefazolin** 2 g with redosing every 8 h for the first 24 h [12]; in fact, infections after thoracic procedures are <2%, and even less in the case of video-assisted thoracoscopic surgery. Pulmonary infections may complicate the first postoperative period and are sustained by gram-positive (*Streptococcus* and *Staphylococcus* spp.) and gram-negative MOs (*Haemophilus influenzae, Enterobacter cloacae, Klebsiella pneumoniae, Acinetobacter, Pseudomonas aeruginosa*, and *Moraxella catarrhalis*). Suspected anaerobes infections (empyema/abscesses) require a combination with **metronidazole** 500 to be repeated twice in the first 24 h. Third-generation betalactams, aminoglycosides, and aztreonam should be considered only in case of positive cultures (protected distal bronchial aspirate, bronchoalveolar lavage, blood cultures) and with an appropriate and wise use of antimicrobials. **Vancomycin** prophylaxis is warranted for patients known to be colonized with MRSA, while **vancomycin** and **clindamycin** are the alternatives in case of beta lactam allergy.

    The presence of *Candida* on the aspirate is for the majority of cases colonization and does not require treatment. Antiinfective stewardship is mandatory in such settings.

13. **Prophylaxis of bacterial endocarditis (BE)** [27, 28].

    According to the most recent review of this issue [27], whose last release dates back to 2007 [28], antibiotic prophylaxis for the prevention of bacterial endocarditis should be limited to high-risk patients, as the benefits for a wider use have not been documented. Use should be considered in patients undergoing procedures that may result in bacteremia (*2C*). In a recent US review, however, extreme care and monitoring is recommended to avoid underestimating the risk [29]: "the fall in antibiotic prophylaxis prescribing in those at high risk is of concern and, coupled with the borderline increase in Infective Endocarditis incidence among those at moderate risk, warrants further investigation."

High-risk conditions of BE are [27]:

- Presence of cardiac prosthetic valve
- Transcatheter implantation of prosthetic valves (TAVI)
- Cardiac valve repair with devices, including annuloplasty, rings, or clips
- Left ventricular assist devices or implantable heart
- Previous, relapse, or recurrent Infectious Endocarditis
- Unrepaired cyanotic congenital heart disease, including palliative shunts and conduits
- Completely repaired congenital heart defect with prosthetic material or device, whether placed by surgery or by transcatheter procedures during the first 6 months after the procedure
- Heart transplant recipients who develop valvulopathy

In such settings, prophylaxis is recommended [27, 28] in case of procedures involving manipulations on

- periapical region of the teeth and gum tissue
- perforation of the oral mucosa
- routine dental cleaning
- incision or biopsy of the respiratory mucosa
- procedures on infected skin, skin structure, or musculoskeletal tissue
- surgery to place prosthetic heart valves or intravascular or intracardiac prosthetic materials

In contrast, recommendations are **against** antibiotic prophylaxis in other forms of valvulopathy, in the presence of patent foramen ovale or mitral prolapse.

For SAP GLs for orthopedic surgery, see the recent SIOT 2022 release [30]; for neurosurgery and head and neck surgery, refer to SNLG 2008–2011 [31]. We also suggest the most recent review by Pinchera et al. [29] for an update on the management of surgical site infections.

Even though scarce evidence is currently available regarding antibacterial prophylaxis and multidrug-resistant microorganisms colonization, the latest ESCMID EUCIC recommendations consider screening patient candidates for colorectal surgery and liver transplantation for extended-spectrum beta-lactamase producing *Enterocbacterales* (ESBL-E) and to subsequently adapt perioperative prophylaxis. Nonetheless, it is yet to be defined which drug would be more appropriate as prophylaxis in ESBL colonized subjects, since the wide use of carbapenems could potentially favor the diffusion of carbapenem-resistant *Enterobacterales* (CRE), which are already widely diffused in areas of high ESBL prevalence. Solid organ transplant, especially liver transplant, is currently the only setting where preoperative CRE and carbapenem-resistant *Acinetobacter baumannii* screening is recommended, though with low certainty of evidence. Adaptation of prophylaxis is nonetheless not supported by clinical studies or by guidelines even in this context, but further studies are ongoing to examine this relevant issue.

3.8   Conclusions

SSIs are still a relevant postoperative problem and a cause of increased morbidity, mortality, and social costs worldwide. SSIs prevention and containment, as underlined by the WHO, is a real risk management operation and institutions and scientific societies are strongly committed to empower every possible effort to support health care workers to reach this goal. Strict adherence to the SSI bundle and its rigorous implementation adapted to local epidemiology seem to be the game changer. Well-designed studies are needed to overcome the gap so far present between guidelines and clinical practices.

References

1. Berrios Torres SI, Craig A, Bratzler DW, et al. Centers for disease control and prevention guideline for the prevention of surgical site infection. JAMA Surg. 2017;152:784–91.
2. Long DR, Alverdy JC, Vavilala MS. Emerging paradigms in the prevention of surgical site infection: the patient microbiome and antimicrobial resistance. Anesthesiology. 2022;137:252–62. https://doi.org/10.1097/ALN.0000000000004267.
3. Decker BK, Nagrebetsky A, Lipsett PA, Wiener-Kronish JP, O'Grady NP. Controversies in perioperative antimicrobial prophylaxis. Anesthesiology. 2020;132:586–97.
4. Surgical Site Infection Event (SSI)—NHSN—CDC. 2022.
5. Badia JM, Casey AL, Petrosillo N, Hudson PM, Mitchell SA, Crosby C. Impact of surgical site infection on healthcare costs and patient outcomes: a systematic review in six European countries. J Hosp Infect. 2017;96:1–15.
6. Loftus RW, Campos JH. Anaesthetists' role in perioperative infection control: what is the action plan? Br J Anaesth. 2019;123:531–4.
7. Géry A, Mouet A, Gravey F, Fines-Guyon M, Guerin F, Ethuin F, Borgey F, Lubrano J, Le Hello S. Investigation of *Serratia marcescens* surgical site infection outbreak associated with peroperative ultrasonography probe. J Hosp Infect. 2021;111:184–8.
8. Wenzel RP. Surgical site infections and the microbiome: an updated perspective. Infect Control Hosp Epidemiol. 2019;40:590–6.
9. Alverdy JC, Hyman N, Gilbert J. Re-examining causes of surgical site infections following elective surgery in the era of asepsis. Lancet Infect Dis. 2020;20:e38–43.
10. Evans L, et al. Surviving sepsis campaign: international guidelines for management of sepsis and septic shock 2021. Crit Care Med. 2021;49(11):e1063–143. https://doi.org/10.1097/CCM.0000000000005337.
11. The Medical Letter. Antibiotic prophylaxis in surgery. Italian ed. 2016.
12. NICE. NG 125—Surgical site infections: prevention and treatment, vol. 11. National Institute for Health Care and Excellence; 2019. p. 4.

13. Sartelli M, Labricciosa FM, Coccolini F, et al. It is time to define an organizational model for the prevention and management of infections along the surgical pathway: a worldwide cross-sectional survey. World J Emerg Surg. 2022;17:17. https://doi.org/10.1186/s13017-022-00420.
14. SAAGAR. Surgical antimicrobial prophylaxis prescribing guideline. Version 3-12.7.21. South Australia Health System.
15. Ierano C, et al. Surgical antimicrobial prophylaxis. Aust Prescr. 2017;40:225–9. https://doi.org/10.18773/austprescr.2017.073.
16. Dias P, Patel A, Rook W, Edwards MR, Pearse RM, Abbott TEF. Contemporary use of antimicrobial prophylaxis for surgical patients: an observational cohort study. Eur J Anaesthesiol. 2021;38:1–7.
17. Sartelli M, Pagani L, Iannazzo S, Moro ML, Viale P, Pan A, et al. A proposal for a comprehensive approach to infections across the surgical pathway. World J Emerg Surg. 2020;15:13.
18. Talbot RT. Surgical site infections and antimicrobial prophylaxis. In: Mandell GL, editor. Mandell, Douglas and Bennett's principles and practice of infectious diseases. Elsevier; 2018.
19. Brienza N, Biancofiore G, Cavaliere F, Corcione A, De Gasperi A, et al. Clinical guidelines for perioperative hemodynamic management of noncardiac surgical adult patients. Minerva Anesthesiol. 2019;85(12):1315–33.
20. Australian Commission on Safety and Quality in Health Care. Antimicrobial prescribing practice in Australian hospitals: results of the 2015 national antimicrobial prescribing survey. Sydney: ACSQHC; 2016. https://www.safetyandquality.gov.au/wp-content/uploads/2017/01/Antimicrobial-prescribing-practice-in-Australian-hospitals-Results-of-the2015-National-Antimicrobial-Prescribing-Survey.pdf
21. Anderson DJ, Sexton MPH. Antimicrobial prophylaxis for prevention of surgical site infection in adults. UpToDate; 2019.
22. Teillant A, Gandra S, Barter D, et al. Potential burden of antibiotic resistance on surgery and cancer chemotherapy antibiotic prophylaxis in the USA: a literature review and modelling study. Lancet Infect Dis. 2015;15:1429–37.
23. ECDC. Annual Epidemiological Report for 2015 Healthcare-associated infections: surgical site infections. 2017.
24. Bassetti M. Infection therapy and prophylaxis. 2nd ed. Mediprint.
25. Nelson RL, Gladman E, Barbateskovic M. Antimicrobial prophylaxis for colorectal surgery. Cochrane Database Syst Rev. 2014;5:CD001181.
26. Deierhoi RJ, Dawes LG, Vick C, et al. Choice of intravenous antibiotic prophylaxis for colorectal surgery does matter. J Am Coll Surg. 2013;217:763–9.
27. Sexton DJ, Chu VH. Antimicrobial prophylaxis for the prevention of bacterial endocarditis. UpToDate; 2022.
28. Wilson W, Taubert KA, Gewitz M, Lockhart PB, Baddour LM, Levison M, Bolger A, et al. Prevention of infective endocarditis: guidelines from the American Heart Association Rheumatic Fever, Endocarditis, and Kawasaki Disease Committee, Council on Cardiovascular Disease in the Young, and the Council on Clinical Cardiology, Council on cardiovascular Surgery and Anesthesia, and the quality of care and outcomes research interdisciplinary working group. Circulation. 2007;116(15):1736.
29. Pinchera B, Buonomo AR, Schiano Moriello N, Scotto R, Villari R, Gentile I. Update on the management of surgical site infections. Antibiotics. 2022;11:1608. https://doi.org/10.3390/antibiotics11111608. www.mdpi
30. SIOT. Guideline prevention of infections in orthopedic surgery guideline published in the National Guideline System Rome, 2021.
31. SNLG 17 Perioperative antibiotic prophylaxis in adults GUIDELINE—2008–2011.

Safety in the Operating Room

4

Edoardo De Robertis and Davide Valeri

4.1 Introduction

Patient safety in the care process is a challenge for all health care systems, and results in prevention of medical error, a tangible sign of the quality of service provided by professionals, leading to important clinical as well as organizational-economic repercussions.

Today the management of health care systems has as its primary target the improvement of the quality and safety of health care services that fall within the Essential Levels of Care. This is one of the pivotal elements of integrated clinical governance, which, by placing the needs of the patient at the center, sees a comprehensive management of health care services, within the framework of planning and service management policies based on clinical choices that enhance the role and responsibility of physicians and other health care professionals.

Surgery, due to volumes of activity and the inherent complexity of all related procedures, requires planned and shared actions and behaviors aimed at preventing the occurrence of peri-operative accidents and ensuring the successful outcome of operations. It was with this purpose that the *Manual for Safety in the Operating Room: Recommendations and Checklist,* drawn up by the General Direction of Health Planning of the Ministry of Health, was born; it includes the Recommendations and checklist developed by the World Health Organization as part of the *Safe Surgery Saves Lives* program, adapted to the national context (https://www.salute. gov.it/imgs/C_17_pubblicazioni_1119_allegato.pdf).

E. De Robertis (✉) · D. Valeri
Anaesthesia, Analgesia and Intensive Care Section, Department of Medicine and Surgery, University of Perugia, Perugia, Italy
e-mail: edoardo.derobertis@unipg.it

D. Chiumello (ed.), *Practical Trends in Anesthesia and Intensive Care 2022,* https://doi.org/10.1007/978-3-031-43891-2_4

Because of its high complexity, the clinical practice of anesthesiology, including anesthesia, pain medicine, intensive care, and critical emergency medicine, is one of the settings in which it is necessary to ensure high levels of safety. Increasing attention is being paid internationally to issues related to safety in the operating room, since peri-operative adverse events constitute a significant percentage both in Italy and in other European and non-European countries.

In this regard it is essential to develop an appropriate training strategy for every health professional involved in peri-operative activities, with the goal of enhancing both technical and cognitive-behavioral skills.

The World Health Organization (WHO) states that *unsafe care* represents one of the top ten causes of death and disability worldwide to date. Despite a large number of national and international initiatives focused on reducing preventable risks, patient safety still remains a large-scale problem [1].

Anesthesiologist plays a crucial role in ensuring the safety and quality of patient care. This role is not limited to peri-operative time, but extends to intensive care, acute and chronic pain management, and intra- and extrahospital emergency medicine, all settings in which the patient is exposed to high risks [2]. A British study found that anesthesiologists are involved in the care process of about 60% of hospital patients; therefore in several settings the anesthesiologist is called to share skills and experience to ensure patient safety.

4.2 Medical Error in Anesthesia: Epidemiology and Guidelines

Clinical risk management in health care represents the set of various actions put in play to improve the quality of health care delivery and ensure patient safety; among other things, this process is based on learning from error. Only integrated risk management can lead to changes in clinical practice, promoting the growth of a health culture that is more attentive and close to the patient and providers, contributing indirectly to a decrease in the cost of services, and, finally, encouraging the allocation of resources on interventions aimed at developing safe and efficient health care organizations and facilities.

Every year millions of patients suffer complications as a result of preventable errors; it is estimated that in high-income countries about one in 10 (9.2%) patients are involved in adverse events during their hospital stay; about half of these turn out to be related to preventable errors. More than half (56.3%) of these patients experience little or no disability, but 7.4% of these events turn out to be fatal [1]. Recent studies have pointed out that adverse events related to medical error are mainly related to surgical procedures and wrong medication administration [3].

A 2018 monthly report carried out by the US Department of Health [4] found that 25% of hospital patients admitted for acute events under Medicare were encountering adverse events during their stay; about half (12%) of these adverse events were accompanied by prolonged hospital stay, permanent damage, life-saving interventions, or death. The most common cause of adverse event was related to drug therapy (43%); the remainder were related to patient care (23%), surgical procedures and interventions (22%), and infectious complications (11%). Physicians involved in this survey pointed out that 43% of adverse events were preventable and consequent to inadequate care compared to expected standards. In terms of health care expenditures, about a quarter (23%) of the patients involved in these adverse events, both preventable and non-preventable, required additional treatments resulting in increased medical costs, estimated to be in the range of hundreds of millions of dollars for the only month analyzed by the US report.

It is no coincidence that the World Health Organization (WHO), after addressing the issue of surgical risk, has focused its third *Global Patient Safety Challenge in 2017* on the issue of safe medication (*Medication without harm*) [5], setting as a goal to reduce over the next 5 years the harm caused by unsafe practices and avoidable medical errors by 50% through the development of less fragile health care systems worldwide. For this purpose three areas of priority action were identified: high-risk situations, poly-pharmacotherapy, and transition of care. It is evident how anesthesiologists can make a substantial impact in each of these three areas.

Every year around 230 million people worldwide undergo anesthesia for major surgery: peri-operative complications with permanent damage are observed in 1 in every 170–500 patients, while anesthesia-related deaths in Europe, Australia, and the United States occur in less than 1 in every 100,000 patients [3]. In recent years we have certainly seen a reduction in anesthesia-related mortality, thanks to advances in available drugs and equipment, improved training, and the availability of recovery rooms and appropriate airway management devices. However, these undoubted advances should not induce a false sense of security, as in parallel specialists have to deal with increasingly elderly and frail patients, new surgical procedures, and more complex care processes, all of which combine to increase the risks of error in anesthesiology practice.

In recent years, the major scientific societies of Anesthesia and Intensive Care, both national and supranational, have collaborated to provide specialists and hospital facilities with minimum standards and protocols aimed at implementing patient safety and quality of anesthesiology practice. These standards aim to address different aspects of the anesthesiologist's work: from the organization of services to the management of the equipment provided, from the choice of the best monitoring to the correct administration of drugs, from the safest anesthesiological conduct to the process of detecting medical errors.

A major step forward in this regard was taken with the 2010 Declaration of Helsinki, in which the European Board of Anaesthesiology (EBA) and the European Society of Anaesthesiology (ESA), now the European Society of Anaesthesiology and Intensive Care (ESAIC), collaborated to draft a document in which they defined the goals necessary to improve patient safety, by providing protocols to be adopted in daily clinical practice by specialists and health care organizations [3].

The Statement was built from pre-existing recommendations and guidelines, and presents a European consensus view of what needs to be done to improve patient safety. All institutions providing anesthesiologic care are urged to adopt the minimum monitoring standards recommended by the EBA and to provide protocols and

Table 4.1 Main requirements of the Declaration of Helsinki for institutions providing anesthesia care

1. Adhere to the minimum monitoring standards recommended by the EBA in operating rooms and recovery rooms
2. Provide protocols and services to manage: Preoperative preparation, equipment and drug control, syringe labeling, difficult intubations, malignant hyperthermia, anaphylaxis, local anesthetic toxicity, massive hemorrhage, infection control, postoperative care
3. Adhere to recognized anesthesiological standards in the management of patient sedation
4. Support the WHO *Safe Surgery Saves Lives* initiative and related checklist
5. Produce annual reports of measures taken and results achieved in improving patient safety
6. Collect the necessary data to produce annual reports on patient morbidity and mortality
7. Contribute to national safe practice audits and incident reporting

services to better manage the following phases of anesthesiologic practice: preoperative preparation, drug and medical equipment control, syringe labeling, difficult intubation, malignant hyperthermia, anaphylaxis, local anesthetic toxicity, massive hemorrhage, infection control, and postoperative care (Table 4.1).

A shared document is then provided to European anesthesiologists that can be presented to political and health authorities for the purpose of encouraging the introduction of necessary safety measures at both local and national level. Since its endorsement, most European anesthesia societies have subscribed to the Declaration of Helsinki, and in the following years about three-quarters of national societies around the world have transposed and adopted its principles.

In order to understand how much the Declaration of Helsinki has influenced our daily clinical practice, in 2018 the ESA(IC) carried out a survey [6] involving hundreds of European specialists; the questionnaire revealed, for example, an established and widespread adoption of the minimum levels of monitoring, as well as of the *Safe Surgery Checklist* proposed by the *WHO*; protocols for preoperative assessment and airway management are also widely used, while there is still a lack of annual reporting regarding safety measures, morbidity, and mortality. However, this survey testifies how this Europe-wide shared statement still holds true today, serving as a guide on what is practical and appropriate to do to improve patient safety during perio-perative care.

In the wake of these developments, in 2016 the WHO in collaboration with the World Federation of Societies of Anesthesiologists (WFSA), a non-profit organization representing anesthesiologists from 150 countries, produced an important document [7] that revises and redefines international standards for safe practice of anesthesia (these standards were first published in 1992, followed by revisions and updates); this document serves as a guide and assistance to professional organizations, hospitals, and governmental bodies, going on to address, with recommendations of varying degrees, numerous aspects of anesthesiological practice (work organization, staff training, facilities and equipment, pharmacotherapy, monitoring, conduct of anesthesia). It should be emphasized that these international standards represent minimum standards: the goal of anesthesiology care providers should be to continuously provide the highest possible standards, exceeding those proposed by the guidelines if possible.

4.3   Minimum Standards of Monitoring in Anesthesia

To ensure patient safety, it is essential to adopt a certain standard of monitoring during anesthesia, as well as specified both by the recommendations of the European Board of Anaesthesiology (EBA) [8] and by the minimum standards defined by the WHO and WFSA [7].

The risk of human error is drastically reduced through the use of proper monitoring equipment; in fact, this provides the anesthesiologist the possibility to note the consequences of any errors, or warn him early if the patient's clinical condition is deteriorating for other reasons.

The minimum monitoring standards [7, 8] (Table 4.2) that have been defined over the years should be adhered to regardless of the type and duration of anesthesia, and regardless of the setting in which one works.

First the anesthesiologist has the responsibility to check the equipment before it is used, setting the appropriate alarm levels (which should be audible throughout the operating room). At this stage, the anesthesiologist must ensure that he or she is familiar with all the equipment that is provided and that he or she plans to use. He or she should also make sure that an adequate oxygen source is available, check the

Table 4.2 Monitoring standards according to the WHO-WFSA International Standards for a Safe Practice of Anaesthesia (2017)

	Strongly recommended	Recommended	Suggested
Intra-operative	– Clinical observation by a health care provider adequately trained in anesthesia – Audible signals and alarms throughout the duration – Continuous pulse oximetry – Non-invasive intermittent blood pressure monitoring – Capnography (if intubated patient)	– Donitoring of the fraction of inspired oxygen – Device to prevent delivery of a hypoxic gas mixture – Deconnection alarms (in case of mechanical ventilation) – Use of continuous ECG – Intermittent temperature monitoring – Peripheral monitoring of myoresolution (if used myorelaxant)	– Continuous measurement of inhaled and exhaled gas volumes – Continuous measurement of inhaled and exhaled concentrations of inhalation anesthetics – Continuous blood pressure measurement (in selected cases) – Continuous temperature monitoring (in selected cases) – Monitoring of urinary output (in selected cases) – EEG analysis (in selected cases)

(continued)

Table 4.2 (continued)

	Strongly recommended	Recommended	Suggested
Postoperative	– Clinical observation – Continuous pulse oximetry – Non-invasive intermittent blood pressure monitoring – Assessment of pain intensity with appropriate scale	– Intermittent temperature monitoring	– Monitoring urinary output (in selected cases)

ventilator and vapor delivery systems, and check the infusion lines and their accesses, which should be secure and preferably visible.

During anesthesia, the physiological state of the patient and the depth of anesthesia require continuous evaluation: in this regard, a fundamental prerequisite for patient safety is the continuous presence in the surgical setting of a properly trained and experienced anesthesiologist [5], who should first make use of appropriate clinical observation (e.g., mucosal color, pupillary diameter, pulse, precordial auscultation, responses to the surgical stimulus, chest wall or reservoir movements, etc.).

Minimal monitoring of the patient undergoing anesthesia, however, cannot be separated from the presence of certain equipment, such as pulse oximeter, non-invasive blood pressure monitoring, electrocardiogram, capnograph, gas mixture analyzer delivered to the patient, and airway pressure monitoring. Neuromuscular monitoring (if muscle relaxant medication is used) and patient temperature monitoring are also strongly recommended. It's up to the anesthesiologist to decide whether a particular patient, depending on comorbidities or operative risks, will require additional monitoring (e.g., invasive blood pressure, cardiac output, processed electroencephalography, anesthesia depth monitoring, hematobiochemical tests).

On the other hand, in the case of procedures under loco-regional anesthesia or sedation, according to the EBA and WHO guidelines, proper patient monitoring includes the indispensable presence of the following devices: pulse oximeter, non-invasive blood pressure monitoring, electrocardiogram, and capnography (the latter in the case of moderate or deep sedation).

The above minimum standards of monitoring must be maintained until the patient fully recovers from anesthesia; if the recovery room is not immediately adjacent to the operating room, or if the patient's condition is deemed critical, adequate monitoring of vital parameters must be ensured during patient transfer (transport remains under anesthesiologist's responsibility).

Once the transfer to the recovery room has taken place, it will be the anesthesiologist's job to make sure that the patient is placed in the care of an appropriately trained health care professional. In this setting, it is a good idea to have the following supplies readily available at all times: an oxygen source, suction equipment, ventilation devices, and resuscitation medications.

In the postoperative period, the minimum recommended monitoring is pulse oximeter and intermittent blood pressure monitoring. Clinical observation, in addition to assessing the patient's oxygenation and hemodynamic stability, should pay attention to the evaluation of postoperative pain.

A recent survey [6] addressed to European anesthesiologists showed satisfactory adherence to minimum standards of monitoring in the peri-operative period; pulse oximetry, capnography, electrocardiogram, and blood pressure measurement are used by almost all respondents. It is also encouraging to note the good uptake of recommended but not mandatory monitoring such as that of temperature (monitored by 89.7% of respondents), neuromuscular block (87.4%), and bispectral edge (86.5%).

A separate issue that should be discussed is the management of sedation, on which the joint ESA and EBA working group focused, arriving at the publication in 2018 of the new guidelines for procedural sedation and analgesia. Although about 80% of European anesthesiologists claim to follow in daily practice the sedation standards described by national or local guidelines, there is still a lack of procedural uniformity in certain settings, especially in the management of sedation practiced by other professionals. The Declaration of Helsinki itself stresses the need for all institutions practicing sedation to adopt recognized anesthesiological standards.

4.4 Drug Safety

One of the most interesting and topical issues in the complex field of safety in clinical practice is certainly the prevention of errors in the preparation and administration of drug therapy. This type of error can occur at different stages of the therapeutic process and involves both human and organizational factors.

Experimental studies have shown a 6.5% error rate during syringe preparation by anesthesiologists [9]. The frequency of errors in drug administration in anesthesia is reasonably estimated to be about 1 in every 200 anesthesia procedures, and the most frequent causes of error are administration of incorrect doses (in 20% of cases) and drug substitution (in another 20% of cases), i.e., administration of a different drug than what was believed [10].

Recent surveys have shown that the most common errors in clinical practice are: drug swapping for similar names or packaging, syringe swapping, infusion route error, inadequate or absent labeling, incorrect dilution or dosages, and contamination of the preparation to be administered [11]. Medication administration errors are more frequent and in fact more dangerous when carried out in pediatric patients [12]. It is worth noting that 70–80% of errors are related to human factors, such as operator fatigue or inattention.

Recent national and European guidelines seek to create a safe drug pathway in the highest risk areas (operating rooms, intensive care unit, and emergency area), identifying key points for error prevention in an integrated, multidisciplinary view [7, 11, 13].

In fact, the three recommendations most supported by the evidence are: syringe labeling, use of internationally validated color code, and use of pre-filled syringes.

First and foremost, it is always a good practice for the preparation of medications to be done by the person administering them, avoiding distractions or interruptions during the procedure. It is good practice to perform double-checking at each step, especially when handling high-risk drugs. A useful expedient aimed at preventing unplanned administration of anesthetic drugs in recovery rooms or inpatient wards is to properly "wash" the intravenous cannulas at the end of each use.

A second crucial step in error prevention is proper syringe labeling. All drugs prepared for routine use in anesthesia, intensive care, emergency medicine, and pain medicine should be clearly labeled and dated; syringe labeling should be done only after filling the syringe. It is also a good practice to label infusion lines at both ends, preferably near their connections, to make them easier to check and limit connection errors.

The use of labels with internationally validated color codes is strongly suggested. To date, all societies and regulatory agencies recognize and share the use of color codes responding to ISO 26825:2008 for recognition of different classes of anesthesia drugs; the introduction of these specific color codes has resulted in a 66% reduction in errors due to syringe exchange.

In the absence of availability of preprinted labels, it is possible to identify the drug using handwritten labels or indelible markers, although these exceptions may certainly be accompanied by increased inconsistency and confusion in clinical practice.

Any drug or fluid that cannot be identified during clinical practice should be considered unsafe and therefore discarded. In emergency situations the EBA considers infusing aspirated drugs in unlabeled and unidentifiable syringes a viable solution, as long as these remain in the hands of the person actually injecting the drug.

A further step forward for patient safety is the use, whenever possible, of pre-filled syringes; this practice has several advantages, such as: increased safety by removing the risk of human error in preparation and labeling, dosage standardization, increased sterility, ready availability, and less needle use. In addition, in time-dependent settings such as those of anesthesiology and resuscitation practice, the use of pre-filled syringes, especially for acute cardio-circulatory treatments, reduces the time of preparation and thus drug administration [14]. It has been shown that the use of ready-to-use formulations would reduce the vulnerability of the system by about 30% compared to self-filling, especially when the specialist is forced to perform actions simultaneously or in rapid temporal sequence. Suffice it to say that while the use of an operator-filled syringe requires 20 steps, the use of a pre-filled syringe requires 12 steps, and thus there is a 40% reduction in the number of operations to be performed. This is a substantial reduction in time, which can optimize work, but also reduce the time between detection of a pharmacological need and ability to administer, which is particularly important in emergency conditions. For example, the time between deciding to use an emergency drug (e.g., adrenaline or noradrenaline) and administering it, using a pre-filled syringe versus a syringe prepared for the purpose by the operator, is reduced by about 106 s.

Again, variations in drug concentration are much greater if the syringe is prepared at the patient's bedside than when the preparation is done by the pharmacy or industry. From a strictly organizational point of view, although pre-filled syringes may initially seem more expensive, their use leads in the medium term to reduced costs due to less wasted drug, and reduced cost for storage, transportation and disposal of ampoules, syringes, and needles [15].

Any contamination should be avoided in the preparation of drugs; the anesthesiologist should be aware of the infectious risk associated with his or her practice, and in the administration of drugs should operate with aseptic techniques designed to reduce postoperative infectious complications [16]. To minimize the risk of cross-infection between patients, the contents of each vial should be administered only to one patient. In addition, preparations not used for the individual patient should be disposed of appropriately at the end of each anesthesia procedure.

In order to reduce error in the preparation of medications, arrangements must also be made in the organization and management of work plans. The purchase of drugs with clearly identifiable packaging should be encouraged, and drugs should be divided into their respective cabinets and/or drawers respecting their division by pharmacological classes, taking into consideration that any error in the administration of drugs of the same class will certainly be less harmful than an error in administration between drugs of different classes. In addition, local anesthetics should be stored separately from other drugs, while high-risk drugs (e.g., potassium) should be stored in locked locations.

Vials should be kept in their original packaging until they are actually needed for preparation. Additional care should be taken when handling vials of similar shapes or colors, or with labels that are difficult to read.

In recent years, various models of logistics management and drug procurement have been designed in order to increase the safety and traceability of the drug pathway; examples are the so-called smart cabinets, which with controlled access open according to the operator's requests, or the "Kanban model," which bases the supply of the department on the logic of restoring what has been consumed, cutting down stock and occupied space, or the use of "Radio Frequency Identifier" (RFiD) technology, which associates drugs and patient by providing quick feedback on the medical record.

It's now clear how the safe drug pathway consists of a complex set of tasks to be performed and requires the intervention of different professionals who must be properly sensitized and trained. An effective collaborative relationship between the anesthesiologist and the hospital pharmacist becomes important, involving greater range in the choice of therapeutic pathways, still respecting the respective professional competencies. For example, in a rational and shared perspective, we should not consider only drug cost savings as a factor of expenditures control, but we should evaluate the clinical, economic, and organizational benefits of introducing specific health care devices or interventions.

It is necessary to standardize and simplify the drug pathway in an integrated and rational vision especially in the highest-risk areas (operating rooms, intensive care unit), and in this sense the effort of national and international Societies in producing appropriate guidelines should be understood: an example is the recent Società Italiana Anestesia, Analgesia, Rianimazione e Terapia Intensiva (SIAARTI) document regarding Good Clinical Practices on *Safety of Drug Management in the Operating Room, Intensive Care, Pain Therapy and Emergency,* published in 2019 [11]. It is based on data collected from a National Survey conducted in 2018 and from the review of the 2012 Societal Guidelines on syringe labeling; it offers different levels of recommendations to all the involved actors in the therapeutic process (Table 4.3).

On the other hand, the same SIAARTI survey [11] highlighted how clinical practices related to medical administration are still not homogeneous and not optimized. For example, it appears that only half of Italian specialists work in operating units that adopt a standardized protocol for drug preparation; labeling is not a standardized practice for 35.5% of the sample; and indelible marker or writing on a patch is still too often used. Pre-filled syringes are available only in a few settings (18.4%), just as only 33% of specialists have pre-diluted medications. Drug storage also appears to be non-standardized, even in the specific area of local anesthetics.

The SIAARTI Survey also shows that 64.8% of anesthesiologists have an operational scheme for locating and managing emergency medications (e.g., dantrolene, sugammadex, or lipid emulsions), but 6% admit to ignoring protocols in use at their unit, a percentage that rises to 51% in pain management and 41.9% in critical and emergency medicine.

And while it is true that a large majority of respondents (65%) are unaware of dedicated drug labeling guidelines and only 11.9% are aware of national guidelines, it is clear how much further acceleration is needed in terms of implementation and dissemination of good clinical practices.

Table 4.3 SIAARTI recommendations for safe medication management (from Buone Pratiche Cliniche (Good Clinical Practices) 2019)

Warning	Never use infusions prepared with unlabeled drugs and syringes
Strongly recommended	Always clearly label syringes and infusions containing drugs
Strongly recommended	Use ISO 26825:2008 (E) standard colors for labeling
Recommended	The preparation of drugs must be done by those who administer them
Recommended	Load the syringe before labeling it
Strongly recommended	Dispose of unused preparations immediately at the end of the procedure
Rrecommended	Prepare drugs immediately before possible use
Auspicable	Where available, use ready-to-use formulations
Suggested	Logical organization of work plans with clear separation of drugs by class

4.5   Use of Checklists, Reports, Surveys

A key to improving safety in the care pathway consists in reducing the gap between what we know needs to be done and what is actually done in clinical practice [1]. Reducing this gap requires a systematic approach, enhancing not only learning platforms but also systems for monitoring and evaluating clinical practice in relation to patient safety in anesthesiology.

To reduce the risk of peri-operative error, checklists (generally modified, according to local needs, from the WHO Surgical Safety Checklist) have been in use for years now. In a simple and intuitive way they help to carry out safety checks during crucial phases of the anesthesiological and surgical process (usually before induction of anesthesia, before surgical incision, and before leaving the operating room). The Declaration of Helsinki itself pushes institutions to support the WHO's *Safe Surgery Saves Lives* initiative and to adopt its checklist. All over Europe there is now widespread use of such checklists, which are used by about 78% of anesthesiologists, although their use appears to be in some settings still fragmentary. This is because the mere introduction of a checklist does not guarantee its effective implementation, but must be accompanied by an appropriate division of roles and responsibilities within the team, maintaining structured communication even when the team faces emergency situations.

In order to adequately promote a culture of safety and improve the care pathway, all anesthesiologists should fill in local and national reports about errors and incidents that occurred in clinical practice (*incident reporting*); this process allow them to reanalyze periodically their actions and understand how to prevent or manage any future errors. On the other hand, unrecognized or unreported adverse events contribute to inadequate interpretation of the problem in the clinical setting. Suffice it to mention that only 39.6% of Italian anesthesiologists say they fill out Incident Reporting forms in case of incidents deemed 'serious,' while as many as 30.5% do not follow this directive. At the European level, the overall picture does not differ much: although nearly 80% of hospitals provide incident reporting systems, adherence among specialists is still low, while the use of morbidity/mortality reporting systems or participation in national audits is even more limited. Underlying this deficiency, specialists complain of problems in data collection and organization, lack of a responsible figure in compiling such reports, and lack of time.

Again, the Declaration of Helsinki incentivizes the various institutions to collect data for the production of annual reports on patient morbidity and mortality, to provide resources to complete local or national audits, and to make annual reports about the measures put in place each year to improve patient safety at their place of employment.

In this sense, we can understand the usefulness of periodic surveys aimed at verifying the state of the art regarding certain clinical practices and the transposition of current guidelines nationally and internationally.

For example, it is with this purpose that SIAARTI decided to proceed by first conducting a National Survey [11], a prerequisite for the development of specific recommendations aimed at defining Good Clinical Practices for the anesthesiologist.

Adequate dissemination of proper anesthesiologic practices in relation to patient safety goes through a complex process of awareness, training, and continuous education. Over time this will result not only in better care for the patient and a reduction of health care expenditures, but also in greater safety and satisfaction for the anesthesiologist.

Highlights
- The issue of safety in anesthesia is a priority. This priority depends on the critical and emergency conditions in which we often operate and on the characteristics of patients who are increasingly complex and often fragile.
- The need to work at a high pace and under conditions where speed of action is required for critical patient issues means putting in place operating modes (protocols, procedures) to avoid error.
- Proper labeling and use of pre-filled syringes offer the possibility of limiting errors with limited costs.
- There is a need to enhance training, optimize procedures, and consider safety benefits when decisions are made about the introduction of new medical devices or interventions.
- It is important that anesthesiologists are always well aware of the recommendations promulgated by scientific societies. Their consideration stimulates greater cognition of the problems and prompts the implementation of behaviors/methods designed to reduce errors due to drug preparation or administration. For the latter, it is important that the responsibilities of every nurse, physician, or hospital facility are clearly understood. Each health care centre must put in place adequate systems of prevention, organization, and staff training.
- There should be constant and accurate tracking and documentation of all steps and procedures followed in the drug pathway, from its arrival at the hospital to its preparation and finally administration.
- Close collaboration between hospital pharmacy and clinicians is essential, and it certainly contributes to increased safety in drug administration. While respecting each other's professional expertise, a shared choice of treatment pathways is now more desirable than before.

References

1. NHS, Patient Safety Learning, Mind the implementation gap—the persistence of avoidable harm in the NHS. www.patientsafetylearning.org. Accessed 7 Apr 2022.
2. Martin C, De Robertis E, De Hert S. The anesthesiologist: the unsung hero of peri-operative intensive care. Eur J Anaesthesiol. 2019;36(6):387–9.
3. Mellin-Olsen J, Staender S, Whitaker DK, et al. The Helsinki Declaration on patient safety in anaesthesiology. Eur J Anaesthesiol. 2010;27:592–7.

4. U.S. Department of Health and Human Services Office of Inspector General. Adverse events in hospitals: a quarter of Medicare patients experienced harm in October 2018. May 2022, OEI-06-18-00400.
5. WHO Global Patient Safety Challenge: Medication without harm. WHO/HIS/SDS/2017.6. www.who.int/patientsafety/medication-safety/en/.
6. Wu HHL, Lewis SR, Čikkelová M, Wacker J, Smith AF. Patient safety and the role of the Helsinki Declaration on patient safety in anaesthesiology: a European survey. Eur J Anaesthesiol. 2019;36(12):946–54.
7. Gelb AW, Morriss WW, Johnson W, et al. World Health Organization–World Federation of Societies of Anaesthesiology international standards for a safe practice of anesthesia. Can J Anesth. 2018;65:698–708.
8. European Board of Anaesthesiology. EBA recommendations for minimal monitoring during anesthesia and recovery. 2012.
9. Garnerin P, Pellet-Meier B, Chopard P, Perneger T, Bonnabry P. Measuring human-error probabilities in drug preparation: a pilot simulation study. Eur J Clin Pharmacol. 2007;63(8):769–76.
10. Dhawan I, Tewari A, Sehgal S, Sinha AC. Medication errors in anesthesia: unacceptable or unavoidable? Braz J Anesthesiol. 2017;67(2):184–92.
11. SIAARTI Good Clinical Practices. Safety of medication management in the operating room, ICU, pain therapy, and emergency. 2019. www.siaarti.it/standardclinici.
12. Lobaugh LMY, Martin LD, Schleelein LE, Tyler DC, Litman RS. Medication errors in pediatric anesthesia: a report from the wake up safe quality improvement initiative. Anesth Analg. 2017;125(3):936–42.
13. Whitaker D, et al. European Section and Board of Anaesthesiology of the UEMS. The European Board of Anaesthesiology recommendations for safe medication practice: first update. Eur J Anaesthesiol. 2017;34(1):4–7.
14. Adapa RM, Mani V, Murray LJ, Degnan BA, Hercules A, Cadman B, Williams CE, Gupta AK, Wheeler DW. Errors during the preparation of drug infusions: a randomized controlled trial. Br J Anaesth. 2012;109(5):729–34.
15. Benhamou D, Piriou V, De Vaumas C, Albaladejo P, Malinovsky JM, Doz M, Lafuma A, Bouaziz H. Ready-to-use pre-filled syringes of atropine for anaesthesia care in French hospitals—a budget impact analysis. Anaesth Crit Care Pain Med. 2017;36(2):115–21.
16. Gargiulo DA, Mitchell SJ, Sheridan J, Short TG, Swift S, Torrie J, Webster CS, Merry AF. Microbiological contamination of drugs during their Administration for Anesthesia in the operating room. Anesthesiology. 2016;124(4):785–94.

Patient Blood Management

Francesca Puccini, Lucia M. Bindi, Massimo Esposito, and Gianni Biancofiore

5.1 Introduction

The term Patient Blood Management (PBM) was first used in 2005 by an Australian hematologist, Professor James Isbister, on the insight that the focus of transfusion in medicine should be shifted from products from the blood bank to patients [1]. PBM, in a nutshell, is a multidisciplinary, multimodal strategy that, by placing patient health and safety at its core, aims to improve clinical outcomes. This approach significantly reduces the use of blood products by addressing all modifiable transfusion risk factors even before transfusion use needs to be considered [2–5]. Therefore, compared to tradition, PBM represents an innovative approach to the management of the "blood resource" that results in the simultaneous adoption of all techniques, interventions, and strategies that are usable in that individual case whose overall outcome is derived from the summation of the results of the interventions themselves. Therefore, PBM works only through the simultaneous application in the same individual of the entire "package' of interventions. Thus, it is a multiprofessional, multidisciplinary, multimodal, and patient-centered approach to the optimal management of anemia and hemostasis (especially in surgery) that aims to contain allogeneic transfusion requirements by emphasizing the appropriate use of blood components and, where applicable, plasma-derived drugs. It is important to stress the concept that PBM is not focused on a specific pathology or procedure or on a specific discipline or field of medicine, but aims to manage the blood resource in the individual patient who, therefore, acquires a central and priority role. Therefore, PBM goes beyond the concept of appropriate use of blood products and plasma products as it aims to prevent or significantly reduce their use by managing

F. Puccini · L. M. Bindi · M. Esposito · G. Biancofiore (✉)
Transplant Anesthesia and Critical Care, Pisa University Hospital, Pisa, Italy
e-mail: giandomenico.biancofiore@unipi.it

D. Chiumello (ed.), *Practical Trends in Anesthesia and Intensive Care 2022*,
https://doi.org/10.1007/978-3-031-43891-2_5

all modifiable risk factors that may involve transfusion in a timely manner. All of this is clearly spelled out in the Society for the Advancement of Blood Management's definition of PBM, which states that Patient Blood Management should be understood to mean the timely application of evidence-based medical and surgical principles conceived and designed for the maintenance of hemoglobin concentration, optimization of hemostasis, and minimization of blood loss for the purpose of improving patient outcomes [2]. The PBM principles are also used in the implementation of PBM. Implementation of PBM principles requires that:

1. The dogma that the same strategy can be applied indiscriminately to all different types of patients be set aside.
2. Red blood cell transfusion is no longer used as the sole and primary solution for correcting low Hb levels.
3. PBM strategies are implemented through the collaboration of members of a multidisciplinary team working based on four guiding principles [2, 3]: management of anemia, optimization of possible coagulopathy, use of techniques that aim to save blood, and communication with the patient.

In this review, current knowledge on the implementation methods, applications, and outcomes of PBM in surgical and perioperative settings will be summarized.

5.2 Objectives of PBM

PBM has three main objectives:

1. Improving erythrocyte mass including through treatments aimed at stimulating erythropoiesis and treating possible iron and vitamin deficiency.
2. Minimizing blood loss as much as possible, such as by optimizing specific surgical and anesthesiological techniques.
3. Harnessing and optimizing anemia tolerance by promoting maximal pulmonary and cardiac function and the use of restrictive transfusion thresholds [2]. Over the years, a number of researchers and clinicians have attempted to combine the individual elements of these three PBM goals in order to promote optimal management of patients in different clinical settings. Certainly, one of the most important areas of application of PBM is the surgical patient in the perioperative period [4, 5]. Indeed, while some of the risks and complications historically associated with blood transfusions (e.g., transmission of pathogens) have been largely reduced by advances in the field of transfusion medicine [6, 7], in surgical patients, anemia and perioperative transfusions still remain associated with increased morbidity and mortality. Therefore, the systematic application of PBM in the perioperative period appears to be a very attractive tool for improving clinical outcomes and results after surgery [8, 9]. However, in order not to create dangerous misunderstandings, it is important to emphasize that PBM does not absolutely *proscribe* blood transfusion: instead, it is a mode of management of

the anemic patient in which the use of transfusion is no longer considered as the only possible and applicable approach. This mode of considering transfusion therapy requires the caregiver, in collaboration with the patient, to carefully assess the risks and benefits of transfusion, taking into consideration the available evidence about its benefits but also the potential harms. Therefore, transfusion is viewed as the result of clinical reasoning and not as the mere application of a transfusion trigger. Accordingly, PBM emphasizes (a) education and improvement of knowledge about the risks, effects, and benefits of blood transfusion; (b) the adoption of the best available evidence in combination with expert opinion and experience as a guide for behaviors and the clinical approach to the individual patient; and (c) the use of technology, which provides real-time guidance to help clinicians in their diagnostic and therapeutic choices also with a view to improving appropriateness and limiting variability within clinical practice [1–5, 8, 9].

5.3 PBM: From Theory to Practice

As mentioned above, PBM aims to improve patient outcomes and transfusion safety by preventing both unnecessary transfusions and the need for transfusions themselves through preventive optimization of various parameters by having the most up-to-date knowledge as a reference and employing specific techniques and behaviors.

Traditionally, red blood cell transfusion has always been the treatment of choice for anemia partly due to the fact that it is an established therapeutic procedure with now more than 100 years of history behind it. A number of factors have contributed to the widespread and often inappropriate use of blood bank products: the only seemingly "harmless" nature of blood transfusion, its perceived easy availability, its relative low cost, the simplicity with which it can be prescribed, and the ability to immediately observe its efficacy (in terms of increased Hb levels). In contrast, evidence highlighting possible harmful effects related to the use of transfusions of both red blood cell concentrates and the other blood components has been increasing over the years. In fact, several studies have shown that transfused patients may more frequently manifest clinical problems and worse outcomes, including an increased risk of mortality and complications such as stroke, renal damage, thromboembolic events, infections, respiratory failure, and prolonged hospitalization [9]. Also deserving of emphasis is the fact that PBM greatly encourages the patient's active involvement in his or her care process through discussions between the patient and the caregivers about the various alternative options to transfusion that can be adopted in his or her specific case in view of his or her clinical condition and actual needs. Ultimately then, PBM aims to ensure that all patients to whom it is proposed are provided with a personalized transfusion pathway that takes into account their peculiar needs, medical and/or surgical, and their physiological and clinical characteristics.

From everything reported so far we can derive the general founding principles of a hospital PBM program:

(a) *Anemia management.* This principle defines the implementation of a diagnostic-therapeutic pathway that identifies anemic patients early on for whom nutritional and pharmaceutical treatments will be adopted to support erythropoiesis (if the anemia is not primarily genetic or related to cancer pathology). During anemia treatment, physiological tolerance of anemia may be improved through interventions or treatments that minimize oxygen consumption and/or increase oxygen transport.

(b) *Optimization of any altered hemostatic function.* This involves knowledge of the current status of the individual patient's hemostasis. Of course, drugs characterized by some influence on coagulation competence that may be taken by patients as part of therapy for concomitant (usually cardiologic) conditions should be taken into account [2].

(c) *Perioperative use of blood-saving techniques, instruments, and drugs.* It will be necessary to ensure the adoption of techniques and the availability of instrumentation that can minimize perioperative blood loss. Surgeons and anesthesiologists will therefore have to strive for early detection and immediate treatment of any blood loss. In addition, intra- and postoperative blood salvage techniques should be considered, and attention should be paid to the volume and frequency of blood draws for diagnostic purposes so as to minimize or eliminate this source of iatrogenic anemia.

(d) *Continuous communication with the patient about the treatments that are intended to be adopted for his or her specific case.* There is a need to effectively communicate to patients the risks and benefits of the various interventions that may be adopted on a case-by-case basis and to decide with them on a shared course of action.

The goals and principles of PBM listed so far are pursued by following a now classic and well-identified strategy, that of the so-called *three pillars of PBM* (Table 5.1):

- **First pillar of PBM: optimizing hematopoiesis**
- **Second pillar of PBM: minimization of blood loss**
- **Third pillar of PBM: optimization of anemia tolerance**

The most significant actions and strategies under the 3 pillars of PBM will be described below following the pattern of PRE-, INTRA-, and POST-operative according to the perspective of Perioperative Medicine, which now forms the basis of the planning of the clinical activities of the Resuscitative Anesthesiologist.

Table 5.1 The three pillars of PBM

Period	PILLAR 1 Optimization of erythropoiesis	PILAST 2 Containment of blood loss	PILAST 3 Optimization of anemia tolerance
PRE-OP	• Detect anemia • Identify and treat the cause of anemia	• Identifying and managing hemorrhagic risk • Containment of iatrogenic bleeding • Planning and preparation of the procedure • Predeposit (very selected cases)	• Assess/optimize the patient's physiological reserve • Adopt restrictive transfusion thresholds
INTRA-operative	• Intervention planning after optimization of erythropoiesis	• Less invasive surgical technique • Meticulous hemostasis • Blood-sparing surgical techniques • Anesthesiologic blood-sparing techniques • Algorithms for diagnosis and management of coagulopathy	• Optimize hemodynamics • Optimize ventilation and oxygenation • Restrictive transfusion thresholds
POST-operative	• Stimulate erythropoiesis if necessary • Detect and manage drug interference that may promote/accentuate anemia	• Management of hemostasis • Maintenance of homeothermy • Infection prophylaxis/treatment	• Optimize anemia tolerance • Maximize oxygen supply • Minimize oxygen consumption • Restrictive transfusion thresholds

5.3.1 PBM in the Pre-operative Period

5.3.1.1 Preoperative Anemia

Anemia is a common observation of the period before surgery in patients who are candidates for major surgery. In fact, the reported incidence of this condition ranges from 8%, in patients undergoing radical prostatectomy, to 64% in gynecologic surgery [6]. The prevalence of iron deficiency (defined as ferritin levels <30 ng/mL or <100 ng/mL with transferrin saturation <20% or C-reactive protein >5 mg/L) is high in anemic patients and about 62% of them have absolute deficiency [6]. Interestingly, even patients defined as nonanemic can be characterized by a high prevalence of iron deficiency, which can be as high as 60% of cases in gynecologic surgery and 44% of subjects undergoing surgery for colorectal cancer [6]. Even in cardiac surgery, iron deficiency is common, with about 50% of anemic patients and 20% of nonanemic patients showing absolute deficiency of this essential element [3].

Several studies support the benefits of preoperative treatment of anemia. For example, in orthopedic surgery, treatment with intravenous iron combined with subcutaneous erythropoietin 1–3 days before surgery resulted in (a) a reduction from 37 to 24% in the need for erythrocyte transfusion; (b) a containment of the incidence of nosocomial infections (from 12 to 8%); and (c) a reduction in hospital stay (from 11.7 to 10.7 days) [7]. In addition, in the specific population of hip fracture patients, this treatment resulted in a decrease in mortality from 9.4 to 4.8% [7]. However, the reduction in infection rates reported in this experience is in contrast to an increase in infectious complications related to intravenous iron treatment described in a previous meta-analysis [10]. However, it should be noted that in this meta-analysis only 11 of the 75 included studies had been performed in the surgical setting. In addition, a study of 605,000 surgical patients verified a 21% reduction in postoperative infections [11]. A similar finding (−9%) is also reported in a recent meta-analysis [12]. Furthermore, in a prospective randomized study in patients with preoperative iron deficiency anemia undergoing gastrointestinal surgery, intravenous iron treatment conducted about 10 days before surgery was shown to reduce erythrocyte transfusions with also a decrease in the duration of hospitalization (from 9 to 6 days) [13]. Finally, a recent prospective, randomized, double-blind study in anemic or iron-deficient patients who were candidates for cardiac surgery showed that a combined treatment of intravenous iron, subcutaneous erythropoietin, vitamin B12, and folic acid per os administered 1 day before surgery was able to reduce the number of erythrocyte transfusions from a median of 1 unit to 0 with no difference in clinical outcomes [14]. Of note, there are currently no studies available that focus on the treatment of iron deficiency specifically before gynecologic surgery [1]. However, it is likely that even in this type of surgery, preoperative treatment of anemia and iron deficiency may prove useful and beneficial. An important factor is the timing with which preoperative anemia is diagnosed. Indeed, although its late treatment may have some success, early correction (2–3 weeks before surgery) is recommended. Such an approach has been strongly recommended by a group of experts [15]. From the above, the importance of carefully planning the timing of surgery strongly emerges. Therefore, from the perspective of PBM, it is important for each hospital to prepare a dedicated diagnostic treatment plan in which timelines and task assignments are clear. An algorithm regarding preoperative sideropenic anemia must also be established where the tests to be performed and the treatments made available to patients are defined [1]. In this regard, an interesting algorithm is shown in Table 5.2.

The treatment of individuals with preoperative iron deficiency anemia can be complex because the diagnosis of this condition is not always straightforward since its causes are often combined [16]. Another factor that requires attention by treating physicians and personalization of the treatment approach is that oral iron

Table 5.2 Scheme of possible treatment of sideropenic anemia

Hb	Condition					Treatment
	Ferritin		TSAT	CCl	CRP	
Hb <130 g/L	<100 ng/mL	o	<20%	≥50 mL/min		Iron IV: 20 mg/kg Vit B12 SC Folic acid 5 mg PO
Hb <130 g/L	≥100 ng/mL	e	≥20%	<50 mL/min		Epoetin alpha SC 600 U/kg Iron IV: 20 mg/kg Vit B12 SC Folic acid 5 mg PO
Hb <130 g/L		e	≥20%		>5 mg/L	Epoetin alpha SC 600 U/kg Iron IV: 20 mg/kg Vit B12 SC Folic acid 5 mg PO
Hb >130 g/L	<100 ng/mL	o	<20%			Iron IV: 20 mg/kg

(Modified from Spahn D, Muñoz M, Klein AA et al. Patient Blood Management. Effectiveness and Future Potential. Anesthesiology 2020;133:212–22)

TSAT transferrin saturation, *CCL* creatinine clearance, *CRP* C-reactive protein, *IV* intravenous, *SC* subcutaneous, *PO* per os

administration, which remains the first-line treatment, still has well-documented problems. Those of greatest clinical significance are the poor tolerance to the drug resulting in dose-dependent gastrointestinal side effects and the prolonged times that are required to adequately replenish iron stores [17]. Therefore, IV infusion of iron is nowadays the preferred route of administration especially when time for optimization of martial reserves is limited due to the need to proceed with celerity to surgery, for example, in subjects with cancer diseases. From this point of view, it may be useful to mention how it has been shown that a positive response to therapy can be detected as early as when treatment is started at least 5 days before surgery, while maximal efficacy is believed to last 2–4 weeks after infusion. Also worth mentioning is how, historically, iron parenteral preparations may be associated with a certain rate of adverse effects, including anaphylaxis especially when dextran-containing preparations are used. In contrast, more modern preparations have a significantly improved tolerability and safety profile with an overall anaphylaxis rate comparable to that of penicillin IV [17]. Relative to erythropoiesis-stimulating agents, it should be highlighted that the National Institute for Health and Care Excellence (NICE) guidelines caution against their liberal and routine use unless patients refuse blood transfusion or have a rare or non-rapidly supplied blood type. This caution stems not only (or not so much) from economic reasons since they are expensive drugs, but from the observation that their use has been linked to an increased risk of thromboembolic events and tumor growth through promotion of angiogenesis. In practice, according to the most recent recommendations [1]:

- Erythropoietin should not be used routinely but based on a case-by-case analysis of its risks and benefits

- Individuals with severe cerebrovascular disease and/or history of recent severe thromboembolic events should not be treated with erythropoietin
- In patients with anemia of renal etiology or inflammatory anemia, combined treatment with intravenous iron and erythropoietin is recommended
- Net of the above, the lower the preoperative hemoglobin level and the shorter the time to surgery, the more freely erythropoietin can be used

5.3.1.2 A Special Surgical Population: Anticoagulated and/or Antiplatelet Patients

Also in the PBM setting, an important aspect to consider when preparing a patient for surgery is the management of any anticoagulant (vitamin K antagonist drugs and direct oral anticoagulants) or antiplatelet therapy, especially with dual platelet inhibition. Relative to the first group of subjects, a standardized timing of drug discontinuation has been proposed that is based on their pharmacokinetic properties and the expected bleeding risk for the specific surgical procedure for which they are candidates [18]. In addition, drug discontinuation times should take into account other situations characterizing the patient and be longer in individuals with renal or hepatic impairment or those taking other drugs with the ability to interfere with the metabolism of anticoagulants at the same time [19, 20]. To this end, measurement of plasma levels of the drugs in question can help in guiding patient management [21]. Initially, such an attitude was proposed mainly for cases operated in emergency. However, because plasma levels of rivaroxaban above 100 ng/mL have been found to be associated with significant intraoperative blood loss, measurement of plasma levels of this drug may also be indicated in patients operated on electively, particularly in patients at risk of having higher plasma levels than expected and based on the drug's dosage such as those with impaired renal function, very advanced age, concomitant treatment with amiodarone, and in those in whom the time of last drug intake is unknown [19]. In case plasma levels of the drug are indeed greater than 100 ng/mL, it may be justified to postpone surgery if there is a high risk of bleeding [19]. Administration of a "bridging" anticoagulant treatment during discontinuation of the main anticoagulant drug is not recommended for most cases because bridging with heparin has been shown to fail to prevent thromboembolic complications and results in increased perioperative bleeding [22]. Relative to the perioperative management of patients with coronary stents and undergoing dual antiplatelet therapy, the American College of Cardiology/American Heart Association guidelines recommend postponing any elective noncardiac surgery by 30 days after bare metal stent implantation and optimally by 6 months after medicated stent implantation. If surgery requires discontinuation of P2Y12 platelet inhibitor-based medications, it is recommended to continue aspirin and resume P2Y12 platelet inhibitor as soon as possible after the surgery itself. In individuals with a medicated stent, any surgery requiring discontinuation of the platelet P2Y12 inhibitor may be performed between 3 and 6 months after stent implantation if the risk of further delaying surgery is greater than the expected risk of stent thrombosis [23]. In this regard, an observational study found a high incidence of major cardiac adverse events (20%) with a maximum incidence in the first 42 days after stent placement despite the fact that 69% of patients had taken aspirin up to 3 days before surgery [24]. Since most of the events were myocardial infarctions without ST-segment elevation, they may have been caused by an imbalance between oxygen demand and availability. Therefore, treatment of preoperative anemia might be particularly important in this category of patients.

5.3.2 PBM in the Intraoperative Period

Surgical and anesthesiological techniques having as their goal the containment of blood loss have markedly improved in the last decade both from a "conceptual" point of view and in terms of their effectiveness and efficiency also thanks to the progressive development of technology and specific knowledge. In particular, a surgically minimally invasive approach, resulting in decreased transfusion requirements, is synergistic with the goals of PBM. This principle is now well established for various types of surgeries that until a few years ago were performed exclusively by *open* modality and are now routinely conducted by both robot-assisted and "traditional" laparoscopy [25]. However, net of the modality by which any surgery is performed, blood loss always plays a key role in the principles of PBM. Another very important point is regarding the use of restrictive transfusion triggers for erythrocyte transfusion [12, 15]. For most patients, hemoglobin values above 70 g/L are adequate [26]. This value rises to 75 g/e for high-risk patients undergoing cardiac surgery [27]. Recovery of blood from the surgical field, its processing by dedicated instrumentation (cell-saver), and its reinfusion are also an important part of PBM programs, and in a recent meta-analysis, this technique was shown to be associated with a reduction in allogeneic erythrocyte transfusions and infection rates, length of hospital stay, and mortality [28]. A Cochrane review also found that the use of blood salvage can reduce the rate of allogeneic red blood cell concentrate transfusions by up to 38% with an average unit savings of 0.68 units per patient [29]. These numbers are even higher in the case of orthopedic surgery where the reduction in transfusions can be as high as 55%. Intraoperative blood salvage has also proven useful in vascular, cardiac, and obstetric surgeries where, therefore, its use, particularly in cases of severe hemorrhage, should definitely be considered [29]. Along with precise and, when possible, minimally invasive surgical technique, the use of appropriate transfusion triggers, and cell-saving techniques, the reduction of transfusion requirements during surgery is aided by the anesthesiologist's maintenance of temperature, acid-base, and hydro-electrolyte balance parameters within ranges of normality throughout the operative period. Therefore, careful positioning of the patient on the operating table, adequate hemodynamic monitoring, strict control of body temperature through the use of fluid warmers, air heaters, heated mattresses, and careful thermal isolation of the patient from the ambient air are all useful measures to prevent dysfunction of hemostasis and subsequent coagulopathy. Attention should also be paid to maintaining a normal acid–base balance and calcemia since acidosis and hypocalcemia significantly adversely affect coagulation [17, 30]. Fluid administration should be judicious and goal-directed using cardiac output monitoring. Careful volemic resuscitation will go a long way toward avoiding dilution coagulopathy while maintaining tissue perfusion within optimal levels. The use of vasopressors should, when possible, be avoided during active hemorrhage as well as volemic overload. It follows from the above that, in patients at significant risk of hemorrhage, instrumental monitoring should be performed as completely as possible [17, 30].

5.3.2.1 Monitoring and Treatment of Intraoperative Coagulopathy

Detection of possible intraoperative coagulopathy is greatly facilitated by hemostasis monitoring performed with viscoelastic tests (thromboelastography, thromboelastometry) that, in combination with laboratory testing, can be used following specific algorithms [30, 31]. Ideally, such algorithms should focus on individualized treatment of specific hemostatic defects detected through dedicated monitoring [32–36]. Therefore, recent years have seen a significant increase in the use of the thrombooestograph (TEG®, Haemonetics, Braintree, MA, USA) and the rotational thromboelastometer (ROTEM®, Tem International, Basel, Switzerland). Indeed, these instruments provide a rapid description of hemostatic function by detecting with good accuracy both cellular and humoral deficits. Finally, the data obtained from these instruments provide a reliable guide for the targeted and patient-specific administration of fresh frozen plasma, platelets, cryoprecipitate, coagulation factor and fibronogen concentrates, and antifibrinolytic drugs, thus reducing inappropriateness and thus waste [30, 31].

As with any diagnostic test, coagulation monitoring with the viscoelastic method has some problems. For example, it cannot detect both hereditary and drug-induced platelet dysfunction. In addition, the method itself has low sensitivity for detecting the activity, or lack thereof, of von Willebrand factor. Finally, the activity of factor XIII, which is primarily responsible for stabilizing the fibrinogen lattice, is not adequately evidenced [31].

One type of patient in whom the use of viscoelastic tests is of particular interest is cirrhotic subjects [37]. However, even in this part of the population, data from viscoelastic tests must be considered in light of the inherent limitations of this technology [38].

One might wonder whether the results from TEG® and ROTEM® are interchangeable. In this regard, it should be noted that although the two instruments share basic operating principles, the results obtained may not be directly comparable probably due to the use of different activators [39]. Therefore, data from the two instrumentations to date cannot be considered overlapping.

A detailed description of the targeted and individualized management of intraoperative coagulopathy using algorithms guided by viscoelastic testing is beyond the scope of this review and therefore is deferred to individual and personal study. However, it is useful here to mention how the utility and efficacy of such an approach has been shown in cardiac surgery [40], in major obstetric hemorrhage [41], in that of the cirrhotic cirrhotic patient [42] as well as in that of the trauma patient [43].

Importantly, these studies not only demonstrate a significant reduction in the need for allogeneic transfusions but also a shorter ICU stay and reduced mortality [43]. Finally, of particular relevance is the early use of tranexamic acid in various acute bleeding conditions such as trauma, postpartum, in cardiac surgery [1], and in the cirrhotic patient [42]. Tranexamic acid can also be used for preventive purposes in most types of surgery, and nearly 200 meta-analyses describe its efficacy in reducing blood loss and erythrocyte transfusions without evidence of increased thromboembolic complications. However, the use of this drug should be limited to individuals who experience significant blood loss during surgery [1].

One of the cornerstones of PBM is the appropriate use of blood bank products with a strong focus on limiting their use. From this point of view, since fibrinogen is a critical protein in the hemostatic process, it is strongly suggested that, in bleeding patients, its blood level be maintained at a level greater than or equal to 1.5 g/L [43, 44]. It should be noted, however, that fresh frozen plasma (FFP) is not a good source of fibrinogen because its concentration within FFP units depends on that of the respective donor and therefore, in addition to not being predictable, can vary from unit to unit (from 1.0 to 3.0 g/L with an average of about 2.0 g/L) [44]. In addition, some treatments aimed at pathogen inactivation can also reduce the average fibrinogen concentration even to lower levels [32]. Consequently, administration of FFP alone often cannot increase patients' total fibrinogen also because, when administered in a certain amount, it can cause dilution. Another source of fibrinogen is cryoprecipitate. However, this is a product that is no longer available in many countries because of transfusion safety issues. Therefore, the use of pharmaceutical products based on fibrinogen concentrate is growing significantly. However, it should be mentioned that no clear signal regarding this product can yet be traced in the literature. For example, a recent systematic review that included 21 randomized controlled trials conducted between 2009 and 2018 on the use of fibrinogen concentrate in the perioperative period revealed great variability in the design of the studies, thus making it complicated to draw definitive conclusions about the efficacy of this drug [33]. However, in a nutshell, this review has shown that in approximately 60% of the studies in which fibrinogen concentrate was used for the treatment of clinically relevant bleeding, a decrease in bleeding tendency along with a reduction in transfusion requirements was shown compared with comparative treatment. It was also noted that in studies in which fibrinogen concentrate did not prove superior to the comparator, most treated patients had an initial fibrinogen level above 1.8–2 g/L. Therefore, it is not surprising that in studies where patients treated with fibrinogen concentrate had normal levels of this protein, no difference in the incidence of bleeding or use of blood products is shown. Consequently, the efficacy of fibrinogen concentrate products is shown in patients with active bleeding who also have significant hypofibrinogenemia. Finally, as a data point related to the safety of the drug, the cumulative evaluation of the more than 700 patients who had received fibrinogen concentrate did not show an increased perioperative rate of thrombosis compared with the comparison groups [33].

5.3.3 PBM in the Postoperative Period

During the postoperative period, the maintenance of restrictive transfusion thresholds and the use of individualized *goal-directed* algorithms for coagulation management remain of great importance [26]. Regarding coronary patients, several authors agree that the transfusion trigger remains that of a hemoglobin value below 80 g/L [34]. Even in the postoperative period, it is critical to maintain a high level of clinical vigilance regarding the possibility of bleeding and, when this occurs, to act quickly to control it. In addition, still too often too little attention is paid to the fact that anemia can persist, but also worsen, after surgery and that even at this stage it can be successfully treated with the administration of intravenous iron and, possibly, subcutaneous erythropoietin [1]. In this regard, there is evidence that postoperative treatment of sideropenic anemia with intravenous iron can improve hemoglobin levels in a few weeks and reduce erythrocyte transfusions, postoperative infections, and length of hospital stay [1]. A recent meta-analysis highlighted how erythropoietin treatment of patients with severe trauma is associated with a 37% reduction in mortality (RR 0.63 [0.40–0.79]; $P < 0.0001$) without adverse thromboembolic events or other side effects despite the lack of a significant reduction in erythrocyte transfusion [35]. Therefore, it is important to set transfusion goals based on the patient's comorbidities and that they are adhered to and taken into consideration throughout the patient's course. In this regard, it is noteworthy how, for the maintenance of a given Hb level, today it is recommended to transfuse even a single unit of concentrated red blood cells at a time as opposed to what was thought until a few years ago when the culture reigned that required transfusions of at least 2 units of blood even in nonbleeding patients [36]. It is understood that after each transfusion of concentrated red blood cells, an evaluation of the effectiveness of the transfusion should be performed with hemoglobin monitoring in order to proceed with further transfusions only in cases of proven necessity.

An often underestimated factor in the postoperative period is that of blood draws for diagnostic purposes. Indeed, it has been estimated that in patients admitted to the ICU, on average, about 300 mL of blood is drawn per week [45]. Inevitably, this contributes to the development of anemia and the subsequent need for erythrocyte transfusions. Therefore, it is necessary to limit the number of blood draws for diagnostic purposes by perhaps using small sampling volumes [46]. Finally, in the context of perioperative management of patients with coronary stents and undergoing dual platelet inhibition, an important consideration is when to restart medications to avoid thrombotic events. For patients treated with oral anticoagulants or dual antiplatelet inhibition before surgery, medications should be resumed 1–3 days after surgery depending on the risk of postoperative bleeding without resorting to the loading dose for P2Y12-inhibitor drugs (e.g., clopidogrel) [18, 23].

Relative to hemodynamic management, even in the postoperative setting of patients at increased hemorrhagic risk, the adoption of all possible strategies aimed at optimizing oxygen availability, cardiac output, and factors affecting oxygenation is strongly recommended. In this regard, a series of maneuvers based on physiological anemia tolerance can be put into practice. Indeed, tissue oxygenation can generally be optimized by acting on the respiratory side, increasing ventilation and the inspired fraction of oxygen, and also by manipulating hemodynamic function with fluids and the use of vaso/cardio-active drugs. On the other hand, oxygen consumption can be reduced by ensuring adequate control of perioperative analgesia [3]. Clearly, all of these interventions must be conducted in an individualized manner depending on the type of surgery but especially taking into consideration the patient's age and any comorbidities they may have.

5.3.4   PBM: Experiences from Around the World

Implementation of the package of interventions included in PBM has been shown to reduce the extent of allogeneic blood product transfusions and substantially improve patient outcomes in various international experiences [1]. In practice, it is reported to reduce (a) erythrocyte transfusions by 39%; (b) hospital length of stay by 0.45 days; (c) major complications by 20%; (d) incidence of acute kidney injury by 26%; (e) incidence of infections by 9%; (f) thromboembolic complications by 25%; and finally (g) mortality by 11% (Fig. 5.1) [47, 48]. According to some recent experience, the application of PBM could also result in significant economic savings [49, 50]. It should be noted that these savings refer only to the direct costs related to decreased consumption of blood products and therefore underestimate the real costs related to the entire transfusion process. In addition, they do they take into account the savings related to the reduction of transfusion-related complications [50].

5.3.5   Strategies for Implementing a PBM Program

The management of transfusion resources according to the principles of PBM is increasingly recognized as valid, and therefore its implementation is being rolled out in various hospitals [48]. Generally, an implementation strategy of PBM principles is suggested that goes by successive steps that can be summarized as follows.

1. The first step in implementing a PBM program in one's care setting is to analyze the local situation in terms of the prevalence of preoperative anemia and perioperative transfusion triggers in use regarding erythrocytes, FFP, and platelets. Knowledge of these data is essential to convince the hospital management that "something needs to be done." In addition, such analyses also allow estimation of potential clinical benefits and associated cost savings.
2. The second step is to introduce restrictive transfusion triggers after sharing them among anesthesiologists, surgeons, intensivists, blood center physicians, and hematologists.
3. The third step is the introduction of a coagulation monitoring and treatment algorithm, again, through a joint effort of all relevant specialties.
4. The fourth step is early detection and treatment of iron deficiency anemia. The implementation of this last step could also be quite challenging because it will

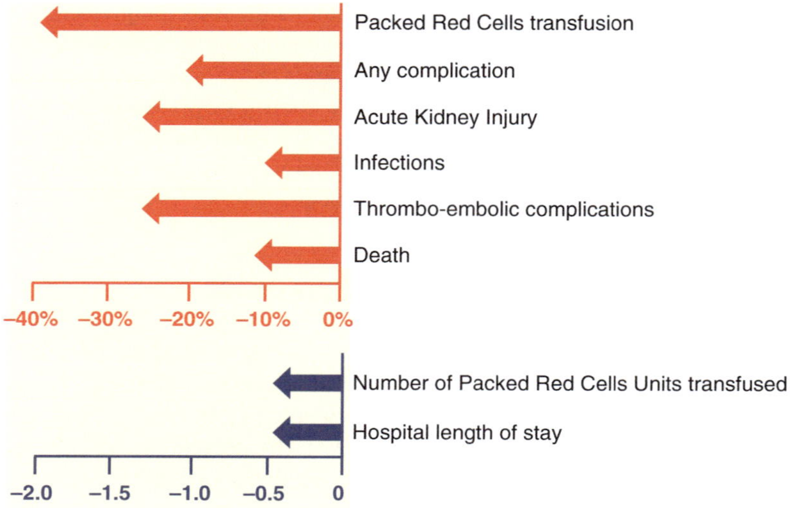

Fig. 5.1 Positive effects of implementing a PBM program (modified from Althoff FC, Neb H, Herrmann E, et al. Multimodal patient blood management program based on a three-pillar strategy: A systematic review and meta-analysis. Ann Surg 2019;269:794–804)

involve various categories of specialists within the hospital. Of course, surgeons will have to schedule well in advance (2–3 weeks) surgeries for which significant blood loss (greater than or equal to 500 mL) is expected in order to be able to refer patients to the appropriate specialists (see chapter 5.3.1). In this regard, computerized tracking using dedicated software can be very helpful.

The decision of the departments from where to start the PBM program depends on several different specific characteristics of the hospital in question. Generally, orthopedic, colorectal, and cardiac surgery are the settings to start with given the high prevalence of preoperative anemia and the potential for blood loss [1]. Once you have started, it is important to monitor the PBM program through a collection of the data that characterize it. In fact, documenting the results as they are obtained is critical for acquiring additional staff and expanding the experience to other departments. Once the PBM program has reached a certain level of priority within the hospital, it will be useful to create an ad hoc PBM committee where all the directors of the facilities involved in the program are involved. This committee will have the function of coordinating all the activities included in the hospital PBM pathway and updating the protocols as and when they are achieved [1]. Finally, another key element is the development and maintenance of continuing education accompanied by some form of monitoring with feedback from all professionals involved [49, 51].

5.3.6 PBM: The Problems

In view of its benefits, there is increasing awareness of the need to integrate the pillars of PBM into the routine approach to the surgical patient. In the United States, PBM has been successfully introduced in some centers while in Australia it has become standard of care. PBM initiatives in Europe have been variable and generally inconsistent reflecting the difficulties that can be encountered in its implementation. In fact, there are many barriers that limit its dissemination but in particular a lack of information, a lack of interdisciplinary involvement, and a shortage of resources seem to be the obstacles that limit the translation of PBM principles into practice. Therefore, nationwide initiatives are needed to expand the number of clinicians sufficiently informed about this approach. It is very useful for the drive and commitment of scientific societies and opinion leaders from the various specialties involved [51] to be added to such strategic actions, especially those that are educational in nature. Finally, a very recent meta-analysis that seems to be cooling some enthusiasm about PBM should be noted here [52]. The meta-analysis in question covered 393 randomized controlled trials that had enrolled a total of 54,917 patients. The use of PBM strategies resulted in reduced exposure to red blood cell transfusion (RR 0.60) but without a significant effect on in-hospital or 30-day mortality. Thus, the most important finding of this review is that although PBM reduced red blood cell transfusions by one-third, it had no major clinical effects even in cohorts of patients at medium or high risk of bleeding. Therefore, further studies conducted with high-quality methodology are needed to better clarify the clinical effects of PBM and to more accurately define the indications for PBM interventions.

5.4 Conclusions

Before a decision is made to transfuse any blood bank product to a patient, all the benefits, risks, and issues should be assessed from a perspective that is personalized for the individual patient in the context of his or her particular physiological and/or disease conditions. In the surgical patient, PBM represents a strategy that tends to simplify the complex decision-making process related to the use of transfusion resources. PBM is based on a personalized approach to the individual patient throughout the perioperative period. A very important factor is that the principles of PBM help to structure interventions and decisions related to anemia and blood transfusion, representing a shift in the transfusion paradigm actually, moving it to a more thoughtful approach recognizing the risks and maximizing the use of alternatives to blood transfusion. All three pillars of PBM are equally important and must therefore all be implemented and structured within the perioperative pathway of surgical patients. Although it is not simple and straightforward, it is now increasingly clear that a PBM program offers a real possibility for the adopting hospital to reduce transfusion needs and transfusion-related risks. As for the influence of PBM to act concretely on clinical outcomes, further investigation conducted with methodologically sound studies is needed.

References

1. Spahn D, Muñoz M, Klein AA, et al. Patient blood management: effectiveness and future potential. Anesthesiology. 2020;133:212–22.
2. Society for the Advancement of Blood Management (SABM). http://www.sabm.org. Accessed 6 Jan 2018.
3. Meybohm P, Richards T, Isbister J, et al. Patient blood management bundles to facilitate implementation. Transf Med Rev. 2017;31:62–71.
4. Muñoz M, Acheson AG, Auerbach M, et al. International consensus statement on the perioperative management of anaemia and iron deficiency. Anaesthesia. 2017;72:233–47.
5. Muñoz M, Franchini M, Liumbruno GM. The postoperative management of anaemia: more efforts are needed. Blood Transfus. 2018;16:324–5.
6. Munoz M, Laso-Morales MJ, Gómez-Ramírez S, et al. Preoperative haemoglobin levels and iron status in a large multicenter cohort of patients undergoing major elective surgery. Anaesthesia. 2017;72:826–34.
7. Munoz M, Gómez-Ramírez S, Cuenca J, et al. Very-short-term perioperative intravenous iron administration and postoperative outcome in major orthopedic surgery: a pooled analysis of observational data from 2547 patients. Transfusion. 2014;54:289–99.
8. Spahn DR, Theusinger OM, Hofmann A. Patient blood management is a win–win: a wake-up call. Br J Anaesth. 2012;108:889–92.
9. Franchini M, Marano G, Mengoli C, et al. Red blood cell transfusion policy: a critical literature review. Blood Transfus. 2017;15:307–17.
10. Litton E, Xiao J, Ho KM. Safety and efficacy of intravenous iron therapy in reducing requirement for allogeneic blood transfusion: systematic review and meta-analysis of randomized clinical trials. BMJ. 2013;347:f4822.
11. Leahy MF, Hofmann A, Towler S, et al. Improved outcomes and reduced costs associated with a health-system-wide patient blood management program: a retrospective observational study in four major adult tertiary-care hospitals. Transfusion. 2017;57:1347–58.
12. Althoff FC, Neb H, Herrmann E, et al. Multimodal patient blood management program based on a three-pillar strategy: a systematic review and meta-analysis. Ann Surg. 2019;269:794–804.
13. Froessler B, Palm P, Weber I, et al. The important role for intravenous iron in perioperative patient blood management in major abdominal surgery: a randomized controlled trial. Ann Surg. 2016;264:41–6.
14. Spahn DR, Schoenrath F, Spahn GH, et al. Effect of ultra-short-term treatment of patients with iron deficiency or anaemia undergoing cardiac surgery: a prospective randomized trial. Lancet. 2019;393:2201–12.
15. Mueller MM, Van Remoortel H, Meybohm P, et al. Patient blood management: recommendations from the 2018 Frankfurt Consensus Conference. JAMA. 2019;321:983–97.
16. Kotzé A, Harris A, Baker C, et al. British Committee for Standards in Haematology guidelines on the identification and management of pre-operative anaemia. Br J Haematol. 2015;171:322–31.
17. Butcher A, Richards T. Cornerstones of patient blood management in surgery. Transf Med. 2018;28:150–7.
18. Kristensen SD, Knuuti J, Saraste A, et al. 2014 ESC/ESA guidelines on non-cardiac surgery: cardiovascular assessment and management: the joint task force on non-cardiac surgery: cardiovascular assessment and management of the European Society of Cardiology (ESC) and the European Society of Anaesthesiology (ESA). Eur Heart J. 2014;35:2383–431.
19. Kaserer A, Schedler A, Jetter A, et al. Risk factors for higher-than-expected residual rivaroxaban plasma concentrations in real-life patients. Thromb Haemost. 2018;118:808–17.
20. Chang SH, Chou IJ, Yeh YH, et al. Association between use of non-vitamin K oral anticoagulants with and without concurrent medications and risk of major bleeding in nonvalvular atrial fibrillation. JAMA. 2017;318:1250–9.

21. Godier A, Dincq AS, Martin AC, et al. Predictors of pre-procedural concentrations of direct oral anticoagulants: a prospective multicenter study. Eur Heart J. 2017;38:2431–9.
22. Raval AN, Cigarroa JE, Chung MK, et al. Management of patients on non-vitamin K antagonist oral anticoagulants in the acute care and periprocedural setting: a scientific statement from the American Heart Association. Circulation. 2017;135:e604–33.
23. Levine GN, Bates ER, Bittl JA, et al. 2016 ACC/AHA guideline focused update on duration of dual antiplatelet therapy in patients with coronary artery disease. Circulation. 2016;134:e123–55.
24. Wąsowicz M, Syed S, Wijeysundera DN, et al. Effectiveness of platelet inhibition on major adverse cardiac events in non-cardiac surgery after percutaneous coronary intervention: a prospective cohort study. Br J Anaesth. 2016;116:493–500.
25. Preisser F, Pompe RS, Salomon G, Rosenbaum C, et al. Impact of the estimated blood loss during radical prostatectomy on functional outcomes. Urol Oncol. 2019;37(298):e11–7.
26. Hébert PC, Carson JL. Transfusion threshold of 7 g per deciliter-the new normal. N Engl J Med. 2014;371:1459–61.
27. Mazer CD, Whitlock RP, Fergusson DA, et al. Six-month outcomes after restrictive or liberal transfusion for cardiac surgery. N Engl J Med. 2018;379(13):1224–33.
28. Meybohm P, Choorapoikayil S, Wessels A, et al. Washed cell salvage in surgical patients: a review and meta-analysis of prospective randomized trials under PRISMA. Medicine (Baltimore). 2016;95:e4490.
29. Klein A, Bingham RM, Brohi K, et al. AAGBI guidelines: the use of blood components and their alternatives 2016. Anaesthesia. 2016;71:829–42.
30. http://pbm.centronazionalesangue.it/MC-API/Risorse/Raccomandazioni%20Patient%20Blood%20Management.pdf. Accessed Feb 2022.
31. Liumbruno GM, Vaglio S, Grazzini G, Spahn DR, Biancofiore G. Patient blood management: a fresh look at a fresh approach to blood transfusion. Minerva Anesthesiol. 2015;81:1127–37.
32. Theusinger OM, Goslings D, Studt JD, et al. Quarantine *versus* pathogen-reduced plasma-coagulation factor content and rotational thromboelastometry coagulation. Transfusion. 2017;57:637–45.
33. Cushing MM, Haas T. Fibrinogen concentrate for perioperative bleeding: what can we learn from the clinical trials? Transfusion. 2019;59:3295–7.
34. Wang Y, Shi X, Du R, Chen Y, Zhang Q. Impact of red blood cell transfusion on acute coronary syndrome: a meta-analysis. Intern Emerg Med. 2018;13:231–41.
35. French CJ, Glassford NJ, Gantner D, et al. Erythropoiesis-stimulating agents in critically ill trauma patients: a systematic review and meta-analysis. Ann Surg. 2017;265:54–62.
36. Carless P, Henry D, Moxey A, et al. Cell salvage for minimizing perioperative allogeneic blood transfusion. Cochrane Database Syst Rev. 2010;4:CD001888.
37. Montalvá E, Rodríguez-Perálvarez M, Blasi A, Bonanad S, Gavín O, Hierro L, et al. Consensus statement on hemostatic management, anticoagulation, and antiplatelet therapy in liver transplantation. Transplantation. 2022;106:1123–31.
38. Lisman T. Interpreting hemostatic profiles assessed with viscoelastic tests in patients with cirrhosis. J Clin Gastroenterol. 2020;54:389–90.
39. Chitlur M, Sorensen B, Rivard GE, et al. Standardization of thromboelastography: a report from the TEG-ROTEM working group. Haemophilia. 2011;17:532–7.
40. Weber CF, Görlinger K, Meininger D, et al. Point-of-care testing: a prospective, randomized clinical trial of efficacy in coagulopathic cardiac surgery patients. Anesthesiology. 2012;117:531–47.
41. Mallaiah S, Barclay P, Harrod I, Chevannes C, Bhalla A. Introduction of an algorithm for ROTEM-guided fibrinogen concentrate administration in major obstetric haemorrhage. Anaesthesia. 2015;70:166–75.
42. Biancofiore G, Blasi A, De Boer MT, et al. Perioperative hemostatic management in the cirrhotic patient: a position paper on behalf of the Liver Intensive Care Group of Europe (LICAGE). Minerva Anesthesiol. 2019;85:782–98.

43. Spahn DR, Bouillon B, Cerny V, et al. The European guideline on management of major bleeding and coagulopathy following trauma: fifth edition. Crit Care. 2019;23:98.
44. Levy JH, Goodnough LT. How I use fibrinogen replacement therapy in acquired bleeding. Blood. 2015;125:1387–93.
45. Vincent JL, Baron JF, Reinhart K, Gattinoni L, et al. ABC (anemia and blood transfusion in critical care) investigators: anemia and blood transfusion in critically ill patients. JAMA. 2002;288:1499–507.
46. Fischer DP, Zacharowski KD, Meybohm P. Savoring every drop—vampire or mosquito? Crit Care. 2014;18:306.
47. Spahn DR. Patient blood management: what else? Ann Surg. 2019;269:805–7.
48. Spahn DR. Patient blood management: the new standard. Transfusion. 2017;57:1325–7.
49. Kaserer A, Rössler J, Braun J, et al. Impact of a patient blood management monitoring and feedback program on allogeneic blood transfusions and related costs. Anaesthesia. 2019;74:1534–41.
50. Mehra T, Seifert B, Bravo-Reiter S, et al. Implementation of a patient blood management monitoring and feedback program significantly reduces transfusions and costs. Transfusion. 2015;55:2807–15.
51. https://www.nice.org.uk/guidance/ng24. Accessed Feb 2022.
52. Roman MA, Abbasciano RG, Pathak S, et al. Patient blood management interventions do not lead to important clinical benefits or cost-effectiveness for major surgery: a network meta-analysis. Br J Anaesth. 2021;126:149–56.

Monitoring of Sedation and Sleep in Intensive Care Unit

6

Stefano Romagnoli and Francesco Barbani

6.1 Introduction

After a profound, albeit incomplete, evolution in the field of anesthesia monitoring and management in the operating room through the use of new instruments for the analysis of frontal brain electrical activity (processed electroencephalography [pEEG]), the concept of neurological monitoring of critical patients is being looked at from new clinical and diagnostic–therapeutic perspectives.

In recent years, there has been a rise in the number of studies and investigations aimed at optimizing and improving new, modern outcomes that are radically different from the historical goals of utmost importance such as length of stay in the intensive care unit (ICU), duration of mechanical ventilation, and incidence of renal failure, mortality. These new outcomes address the preservation and integrity of the central nervous system in its most complex joints and functions: delirium, dysfunction, and neurocognitive decline. Now, we consider the brain at risk of biological and functional damage not only in the field of neuro-traumatology, neurosurgery, and neuro-ICU but in radically different fields such as general resuscitation, sepsis and septic shock, cardiac surgery, and cardiac arrest, emphasizing the importance of early identification of the patients at higher risk (e.g., frail patients, elderly patients, and patients with an impaired neuro-cognitive status).

S. Romagnoli (✉)
Department of Health Sciences, University of Florence, Florence, Italy

Department of Anesthesia and Critical Care, Azienda Ospedaliero-Universitaria Careggi, Florence, Italy
e-mail: stefano.romagnoli@unifi.it

F. Barbani
Department of Anesthesia and Critical Care, Azienda Ospedaliero-Universitaria Careggi, Florence, Italy

SODc Oncology Anesthesia and Intensive Care Unit, Florence, Italy

D. Chiumello (ed.), *Practical Trends in Anesthesia and Intensive Care 2022*, https://doi.org/10.1007/978-3-031-43891-2_6

6.2   Guidelines and Monitoring Tools: The Gold Standard

Many guidelines, recommendations, and position papers have been published in the recent years [1–4]. These important documents seek to guide clinicians in managing sedation in a way that safeguards these difficult neurological outcomes as much as possible. The major international guidelines, including the American, Spanish, German, and English guidelines, recommend achieving a minimum level of sedation as soon as possible with the goal of having a patient easily awakened, in full comfort, and with optimal pain control [1–3]. The American PADIS [1] guidelines recommend maintaining light sedation versus deep sedation in a critically ill patient on mechanical ventilation based on the analysis of numerous randomized controlled trials. A group of researchers in critical care medicine have advanced the concept of eCASH (early comfort using analgesia, minimal sedation, and maximal human care) [3]. These researchers emphasized the importance of optimal pain management and the careful use of sedation medications to achieve a neurological state in a patient that was characterized by the three Cs: comfortable, calm, and cooperative. Similarly, the American Society of Critical Care Medicine (SCCM) and ICU Liberation through their ABCDEF bundle emphasized the importance of having an awake, "cognitively engaged," and physically active patient through the combination of careful monitoring of neurological status and pain, early identification of delirium, early mobilization, careful choice of specific sedative molecules, and involvement of family members [5]. Improved survival, shorter coma periods, fewer delirium incidents, shorter duration of mechanical ventilation, fewer ICU readmissions, and higher likelihood of discharge are the goals achieved by studies based on the ABCDEF bundle [5]. A recent study showed that the depth of sedation correlates with increased risk of mortality, increased incidence of delirium, delayed extubation time, and longer ICU and hospital stay [6].

Current guidelines and recommendations for the management and monitoring of sedation recommend the use of validated clinical scales: Richmond Agitation Sedation Scale (RASS; Table 6.1), Sedation Agitation Scale (SAS), and Ramsay. The most widely used clinical scale is the RASS, which provides a set of 10 items that can be divided into sedative states identified by negative values from −1 to −5 and states of wakefulness or agitation identified by positive values from +1 to +4; the zero alert/calm level divides the two domains. The sedative state considered optimal is that of mild sedation, in cases where sedation is considered useful and necessary. Mild sedation can be identified at −2 (Table 6.1).

There are numerous clinical conditions, such as severe respiratory failure with patient–ventilator asynchrony, patients receiving neuromuscular blockers, epileptic states that are difficult to control, surgical conditions requiring absolute immobility, and some conditions of severe head trauma with endocranial hypertension, in which exclusive clinical monitoring is not feasible because states of moderate-to-profound sedation (RASS <−3) are absolutely necessary [3]. We have unfortunately recently witnessed how a respiratory virus pandemic can force clinicians to keep patients deeply sedated and paralyzed, sometimes on extracorporeal respiratory assistance. All of these conditions listed above prevent the use of a clinical rating scale for

Table 6.1 Richmond Agitation Sedation Scale (RASS)

Score	Definition	Description
+4	Combative	Clearly combative, violent, and of imminent danger to himself and staff
+3	Very agitated	Aggressive; obvious risk of catheter or tube removal
+2	Agitated	Frequent non-purposeful movements and maladaptation to mechanical ventilation
+1	Restless	Anxious but without aggressive and vigorous movements
0	Alert and calm	Includes moments of physiological sleep
−1	Drowsy	Not fully awake, opens eyes to verbal stimulus, and maintains eye contact for >10 s
−2	Mildly sedated	Brief awakenings to verbal stimulus, eye contact for <10 s
−3	Moderately sedated	Movement or opening of the eyes to verbal stimulus (without eye contact)
−4	Deep sedation	Non-response to verbal stimulus, movement or eye opening to physical stimulation
−5	Unarousable	No response to tactile/painful stimulation

obvious reasons involving the administration of analgo-sedative doses that keep a patient at a very low RASS score.

In particular, the American guidelines suggest that if sedation is absolutely necessary, which suggests careful and conditional use of sedation, the patient's condition in terms of the depth of sedation should be frequently assessed and reassessed throughout the day using scales that are reliable and validated [1]. Indeed, these guidelines emphasize that if the patient is admitted to the ICU, by virtue of his or her condition (hemodynamic instability, altered tissue perfusion, impaired function of the systems suitable for drug metabolism, organ failure, altered hepato-renal function, change in distribution volumes, etc.), the pharmacokinetics and pharmacodynamics of numerous molecules, including sedatives, may be different from what we would expect in the same patient under other clinical conditions [7].

6.3 Beyond Clinical Scales: For RASS ≤3—Instrumental Monitoring

When deep sedation is necessary, we must realize that we are exposing the patient to additional risks related precisely to the use of sedation. Among the potential problems associated with deep sedation, we can identify the following: decreased contact with the external environment, family members, and clinicians (predisposition to the development of delirium); depression of respiratory function; inactivity of respiratory muscles and, in particular, the diaphragm; hemodynamic instability; myocardial depression; altered gastrointestinal function with an increased tendency to develop ileus; risk of micro-inhalations; increased risk of pneumonia;, thrombophlebitis; pressure ulcers; delirium; ICU-acquired weakness; hospitalization; immunosuppression; prolonged mechanical ventilation with increased difficulty in weaning; long ICU and hospital stay; development of permanent cognitive deficits; development of chronic psychological illness; and significant increase in costs [1, 3].

The authors of the eCASH concept point to neurophysiological monitoring as something to be considered for patients who require deeper sedation than those who can be followed through the use of clinical scales (Fig. 6.1) [3].

One of the main purposes of the use of neurophysiological monitoring systems is to avoid the occurrence of brain activity suppression: burst suppression (BS)—alternating high-voltage, low-frequency (<15 Hz), and low-voltage (<5 mV) phases—and flat line. Although the significance of BS phases is not fully understood, these neurophysiological phenomena generally occur under conditions of cerebral hypoxia, septic encephalopathy, hypothermia, conditions of severe brain damage such as hemorrhage and ischemia, and under deep sedation (Fig. 6.2).

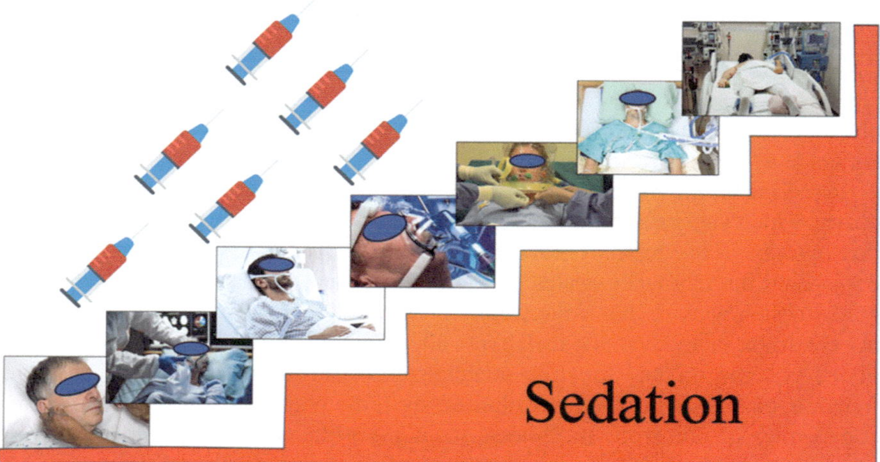

Fig. 6.1 The modulation of sedation in relation to clinical need

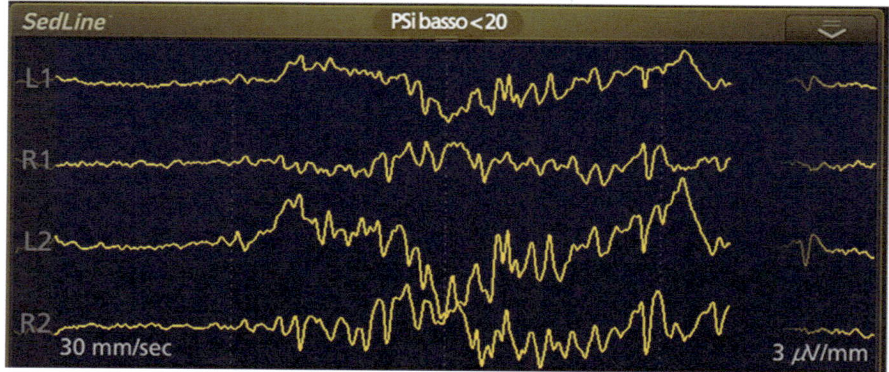

Fig. 6.2 The phenomenon of burst suppression

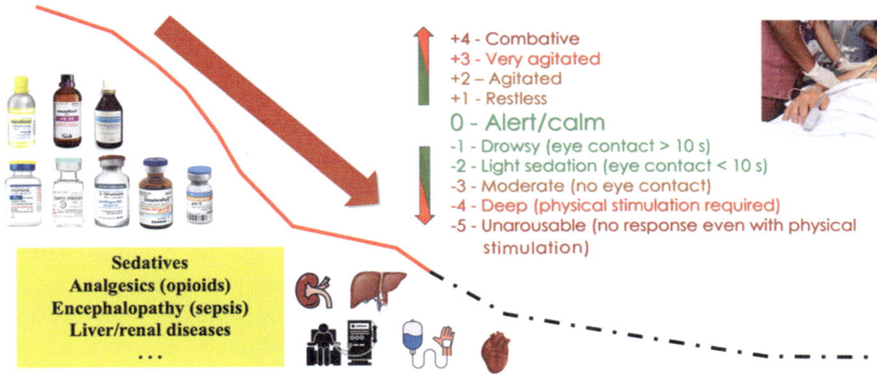

Fig. 6.3 Comparison of clinical scales and neurophysiological monitoring in relation to the depth of sedation

The American guidelines consider brain monitoring systems particularly useful in those patients who require deep sedation associated with neuromuscular blockade but also emphasize the importance in the case of less deep levels of sedation of better adjusting sedation administration when clinical scales cannot be used [1] (Fig. 6.3).

Two studies published in 2008 and 2014 demonstrated increased mortality at 30 days, 6 months, and 1 year, as well as increased incidence and duration of delirium in those patients who had shown greater periods of unintentional suppression of brain electrical activity during ICU admission [8, 9].

In light of what we can understand from the literature, logic, and pathophysiology, we can conclude that avoiding suppression phenomena through the use of pEEG monitors can be an important therapeutic target throughout the period during which deep sedation is actually necessary.

Even under conditions of "clinically explorable" sedation (e.g., RASS −2 and −3), the use of pEEG can help for a number of reasons:

1. Clinical monitoring is discontinuous and generates awakening that is not always useful.
2. Continuous monitoring can reduce the workload of the personnel assigned to monitor sedation.
3. The sedative state fluctuates over 24 h by being able to expose to deeper states than deemed necessary (fluctuations are due to circadian sleep/wake rhythms and changes in serum concentrations of analgo-sedative drugs).

6.4   The pEEG Systems for Monitoring Sedation

EEG is not a routine monitoring practice in the ICU because EEG tracing, as compared with other investigative methods (e.g., electrocardiography) is complex and requires specific preparation. EEG still remains a "black box," and to make it easier for non-specialists to use EEG for optimizing anesthetic-hypnotic-sedation administration, since 1994 (the year the bispectral index was introduced into clinical practice), companies have released a simplified frontal EEG recording system with "auto analysis" of the trace (processed EEG–pEEG) that delivers a dimensionless index that helps the operator to quickly identify the level of depth of anesthesia and sedation.

Very importantly, the subcortical regions of the brain (e.g., the thalamus) generate small potentials that cannot be identified and recorded by electrodes placed on the scalp because an electric field decreases in amplitude with the square of the distance of its origin. Nevertheless, by virtue of the continuous interconnections with the deep layers, the electrical activity detectable at the level of the frontal surface reflects the cortical–sub-cortical interaction. The systems available today offer different information to clinicians [10, 11] (Fig. 6.4):

1. The raw frontal mono- or bilateral EEG trace: It represents the summation of potentials of cortical postsynaptic neurons recorded through sensors placed on the frontal skin surface. Macroscopic currents recorded on the skin represent the summation of microscopic currents generated by individual contributors (electrically active cells).
2. The dimensionless depth of anesthesia/sedation index: Through the application of proprietary algorithms, these monitors analyze and process the raw EEG trace generating a dimensionless number representing the depth of sedation and anesthesia. Following the administration of the hypnotic, with a quantifiable delay of 20–30 s, which is necessary for the machine to analyze a sufficiently long period of EEG, the numerical value indicative of hypnosis-anesthesia decreases according to changes in EEG patterns from a value of 100 (fully awake patient) to a value appropriate for anesthesia (PSI: 25–50; SE, qCON, and BIS: 40–60). In case of absence of brain electrical activity (isoelectric), the number may drop to 0. The complex analytical capability of these systems comes from the cooperation of neuroscientists, biostatisticians, mathematicians, bioengineers, and a large number of databases and libraries, thousands of clinical cases, and traces of healthy volunteers. As previously pointed out, potential sources of electrical disturbances are numerous: electromyography (EMG), electro-oculography (EOG), ECG, neuro-muscular block monitoring systems (e.g., Train of Four), active heating systems (e.g., thermal air blanket), wall "powerline" signals, and roller pumps (e.g., renal replacement therapy machines).
3. Density Spectral Array (DSA): By deriving the signal from the channels and exploring the frontal electrical activity bilaterally, these monitors generate a visualization of hemispheric electrical activity of rapid interpretation. Through the use of a set of colors (from warm colors such as red and orange to cool colors such as blue, light blue, and green) the frequencies that make up the raw EEG

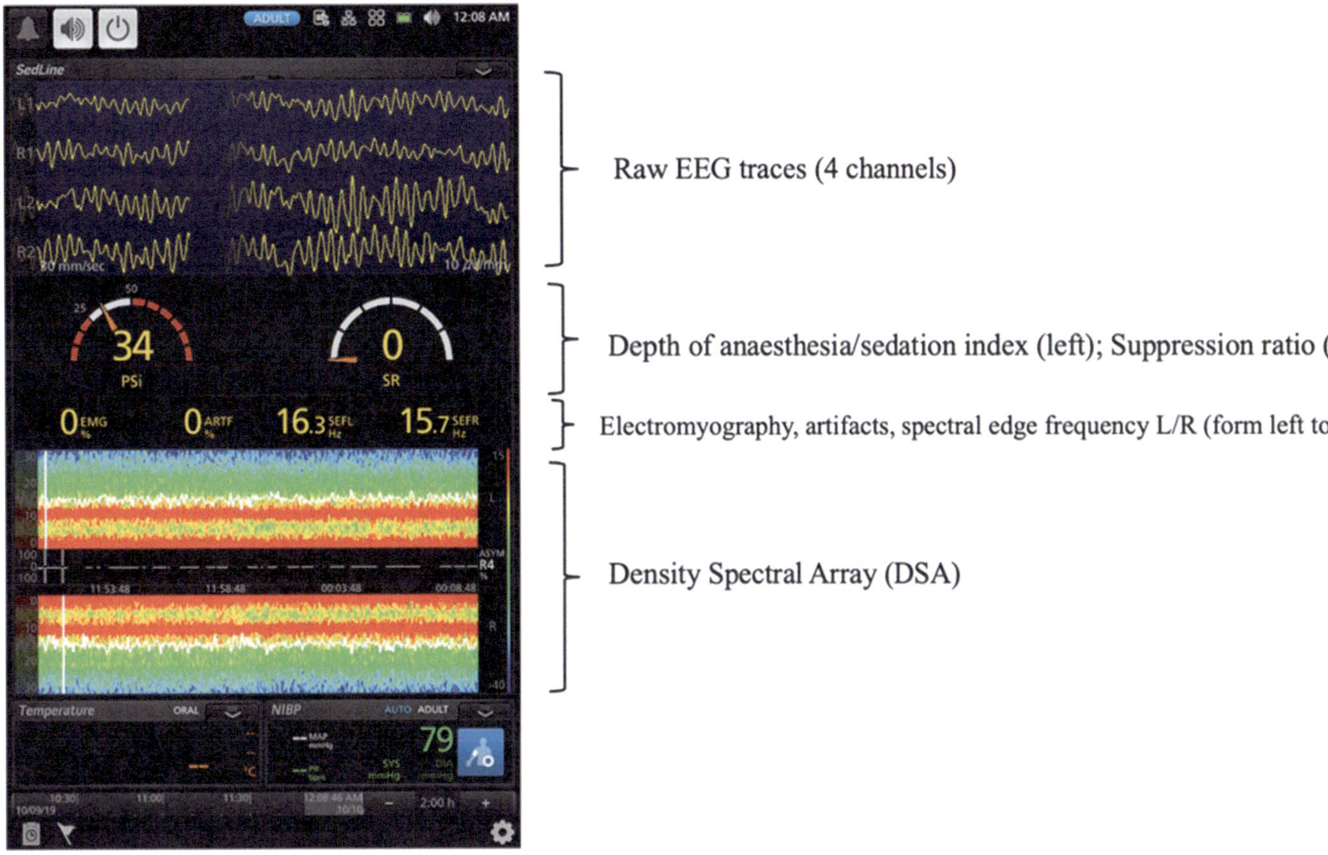

Fig. 6.4 Processed EEG (Masimo SedLine®)

traces are represented. In practice, through the application of the fast Fourier transform, a raw trace is decomposed into its component sinusoids. Once the constituent components of the raw trace have been isolated, they are reported. The DSA, in turn, is the colored representation of the frequency distribution on a graph in which the Y-axis represents the frequencies, while the Z-axis represents the amplitude over time (X-axis; Fig. 6.4).

6.5 Not Only Excessive Sedation: The Phenomenon of Awakenings in Patients with Paralysis in ICUs

Two recent papers published in *Critical Care Medicine*, aimed at investigating the incidence of awakening with recall (awareness with recall) in patients admitted to the emergency department and ICU after intubation and paralysis, showed that awareness/awakening with paralysis (curarization) is a frequent phenomenon in mechanically ventilated patients, eventually leading to long-term psychological sequelae [12, 13]. Hundreds of thousands of patients require mechanical ventilation each year between emergency rooms and ICUs, and, so far, the analysis of awakenings with recall during paralysis has been studied exclusively in the anesthesia and surgery area, demonstrating an incidence of about 0.1%. These recent new studies demonstrate a global incidence of awareness with paralysis outside the operating room of over 3.0%. According to the study, the main risk factors for awakening during curarization include: the under-dosing of sedatives; the lack of monitoring/protocol of the depth of sedation; the use of neuromuscular blocking agents; the use of intravenous anesthetics versus that of inhalation anesthetics; and the use of long-acting drugs for muscle relaxation [12, 13].

In addition, an interesting editorial pointed out that awakening during paralysis in these patients is probably related to the fear of the association between the depth of sedation and hemodynamic instability, prolonged duration of mechanical ventilation, ICU stay, hospital stay, and increased mortality [14]. The editorial reports data from the *National Emergency Airway Registry*, which suggest that more than 20% of intubated patients in emergency departments receive no sedation after the procedure [14].

Before concluding this section on sedation monitoring in the ICU, it is worth mentioning that patients who do not receive muscle relaxants may show electromyographic activity of about 30–45 Hz that could falsely elevate the EEG processing value because of an overlap with the higher electroencephalographic frequencies characterized by beta and gamma waves. This risk is considered by many as one of the major obstacles to monitoring by pEEG in patients admitted to the ICU.

6.6 Summary

We can summarize our efforts toward optimizing sedation monitoring of the ICU inpatient as follows:

1. Light sedation (RASS >−2) is preferable to deep sedation (RASS <−3) in critically ill patients, and clinical scales are the gold standard for monitoring the depth of sedation.
2. EEG tools must be used for monitoring sedation when clinical assessment is difficult or impossible.
3. Avoiding the phenomenon of suppression of brain electrical activity is an important goal to improve the outcome of patients admitted to the ICU.
4. Awakenings with recall during paralysis are unexpectedly frequent phenomena in emergency departments and ICUs; these can be prevented by neuromonitoring.

6.7 Monitoring and the Importance of Sleep

The importance of sleep, in its two components (quantity/duration and quality/structure/architecture) in critically ill patient admitted to the ICU has received much attention in the last few years [15].

Importantly, the latest American guidelines on sedation and analgesia, previously called PAD (pain, agitation, and delirium), have been renamed as PADIS (Clinical Practice Guidelines for the Prevention and Management of Pain, Agitation/Sedation, Delirium, Immobility, and Sleep Disruption in Adult Patients in the ICU) in the 2018 version [1]. As a general principle, what is called "night sedation" should become "sleep promotion" when patients' conditions permit.

Consequences resulting from sleep deprivation include high blood pressure, increased risk of ischemic heart disease, prolonged weaning time from mechanical ventilation, poor blood glucose control, increased thyroid hormones (T3, T4, and TSH), altered thermoregulation mechanisms, fatigue, hallucinations, disorientation, delirium, anxiety, and immunodepression with altered function of natural killer cells and T helper lymphocytes [16–18].

6.8 The Concept of Sleep Disruption and Risk Stratification

Sleep disruption refers to a profound alteration in sleep architecture. It represents a common complication for patients admitted to the ICU and one of the most frequent sources of stress and recollection [15].

Sleep is measured using polysomnography systems (simultaneous recording of multiple physiological parameters during the night using a polysomnography: EEG, EMG, chest and abdominal movements, oronasal flow, and peripheral oxygen saturation). The main data derived by polysomnography are total sleep time (TST), time spent in one of the sleep stages (rapid eye movement [REM], non-REM stage 1, non-REM stage 2, non-REM stage 3), sleep efficiency (TST/polysomnograph recording time), sleep fragmentation, and cortical arousal (stages of cortical awakenings not necessarily corresponding to clinical awakenings—very shallow and disturbed sleep signal; Fig. 6.5).

Sleep Profiler Study Report Table

		NI: Diagnostic 26 Jun 2013	N2: N/A N/A	Normal Range Low / High
Patient Name	Insomnia, Maintenance			
Study Time (Hours)		5.9	N/A	-
Excluded Time (Hours)		0.1	N/A	-
Recording Time (Hours)		5.8	N/A	-
Sleep Time (Hours)		5.6	N/A	5.2 / 7.3
Sleep Efficiency (%)		96.3	N/A	74.2 / 95.5
Sleep Time Supine (%)		58.9	N/A	-
Number of Sleep Cycles		4	N/A	-
Average Sleep Cycle Time (Minutes)		88	N/A	-
Percent (%) Sleep Time				
Stage R (REM)		25.8	N/A	14.1 / 29.9
Stage N1 (NREM 1)		11.0	N/A	1.7 / 9.8
Stage N2 (NREM 2)		44.3	N/A	44.5 / 68.4
Stage N3 (NREM 3 / SWS)		17.8	N/A	1.7 / 29.4
Sleep-NOS		1.2	N/A	-
Total Hours				
Wake		0.2	N/A	-
Stage R (REM)		1.5	N/A	-
Stage N1 (NREM 1)		0.6	N/A	-
Stage N2 (NREM 2)		2.5	N/A	-
Stage N3 (NREM 3 / SWS)		1.0	N/A	-
Sleep-NOS		0.1	N/A	-
Total Minutes				
Sleep Latency		2	N/A	7.0 / 31.0
REM Latency		55	N/A	23.8 / 121.8
Stage N3 Latency		20	N/A	-
Wake after Sleep Onset		11	N/A	-
Average per Hour				
Cortical Arousals		22.0	N/A	7.7 / 23.5
Sympathetic Arousals Overall		53.2	N/A	-
	Non-REM	34.1	N/A	-
	REM	18.8	N/A	-
Movement Arousals		4.6	N/A	-
Awakenings	≥ 30 sec	2.7	N/A	1.8 / 5.9
	≥ 90 sec	0.4	N/A	-
Percent (%) Time Snoring				
> 40 dB Overall		3.7	N/A	-
Supine		6.2	N/A	-
Non Supine		0.0	N/A	-
> 50 dB Overall		0.6	N/A	-
Supine		1.0	N/A	-
Non Supine		0.0	N/A	-
Pulse Rate				
Mean +/–1 S.D.		62+/–8.0	N/A	-
Max/Min		98/48	N/A	-

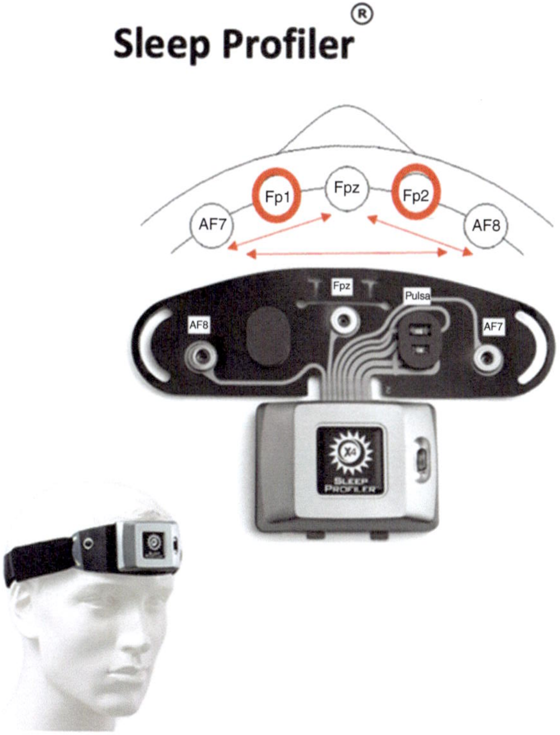

Fig. 6.5 Simplified polysomnography (Sleep Profiler®)

Among the major risk factors associated with sleep disorders in the ICU are some that are not modifiable (e.g., female sex, older age, history of pre-hospitalization sleep disorders, chronic use of hypno-inducing drugs, hypertension, diabetes, cancer, and thyroid disease) and others that are modifiable (pain, environmental stimuli, interruptions of sleep for clinical care, psychological factors, respiratory factors, and treatments that alter sleep quality).

6.9   Preserving the Sleep–Wake Cycle

In full awareness of the alterations in sleep quality, duration, and distribution over the 24-h period (e.g., numerous patients spend most of the daytime hours in superficial stages of sleep), behavioral procedures have been developed to preserve the physiological sleep–wake rhythm as much as possible [19].

Interventions can be divided into non-pharmacological and pharmacological. The literature on these aspects is still highly contradictory, and several trials have brought conflicting results [20]. What predominantly supports the implementation of these strategies is supported by physiology and logic.

Among the main non-pharmacological interventions, we must consider environmental factors:

1. Light is a very strong stimulus to prevent the physiological initiation of sleep. During the day, the lighting level in the ICU is around 30–165 lux, and, during the night, if dedicated night lighting systems are not used, the same level of intensity is frequently applied.
2. Noise, especially that produced by conversations and communications between healthcare professionals, is a significant stimulus. According to the World Health Organization, noise should not exceed 30 dBA, while many studies have shown that in ICUs, noise levels often exceed 53–59 dBA, with peak levels at 67–86 dBA [18].
3. Another environmental, or rather behavioral, factor that strongly alters sleep physiology is the use of physical restraints. For numerous reasons, including the risk of delirium development and maintenance, the use of physical restraints should be excluded from clinical practice.
4. Additional non-pharmacological systems, which are still being studied and evaluated today, are eye masks (further reduction of light penetration), earplugs (reduction of perceived noise), and music therapy [20, 21].

With regard to pharmacological aspects, we must emphasize that from a neurophysiological perspective, drugs commonly used as sedatives in ICUs (GABAergics and opioids) do not generate EEG patterns equivalent to those recorded during physiological sleep [22]. In particular, a very important component of physiological sleep, N3, is missing or extremely rare during sedation with propofol, benzodiazepines, and opioids. Unlike molecules that act on GABA receptors, dexmedetomidine (alpha-2 agonist) has been shown to induce activation of essentially physiological sleep (termed quasi-physiological sleep) [23–25].

Several studies have demonstrated the efficacy of dexmedetomidine in reducing the incidence, or at least the duration, of delirium [25]. Underlying this beneficial effect may, at least in part, be dexmedetomidine's ability to secure that share of N3 sleep that other drugs are unable to generate [25]. In further support of dexmedetomidine's efficacy to ensure quasi-physiological sleep lies the fact that, clinically, patients sedated with the alpha −2 agonist show waking characteristics very similar to those of a sleeping subject.

A study by Romagnoli et al. [18] showed that the use of dexmedetomidine in patients admitted to the ICU ensured better sleep duration and architecture in comparison with patients who showed profound sleep alterations, although they did not appear to need adjuvant sleep medications. Specifically, the study, which used a simplified polysomnography, showed that in the 36 sedated and 36 non-sedated patients, the following sleep characteristics were recorded [18] (Figs. 6.6 and 6.7):

4.5 vs. 1.4 h in N2 ($P < 0.0001$)

68.9 vs. 49.5% in N2 ($P < 0.0001$)

6.5 vs. 3.4 h in TST ($P < 0.0001$)

0.8 vs. 0.1 h in N3 ($P = 0.0035$)

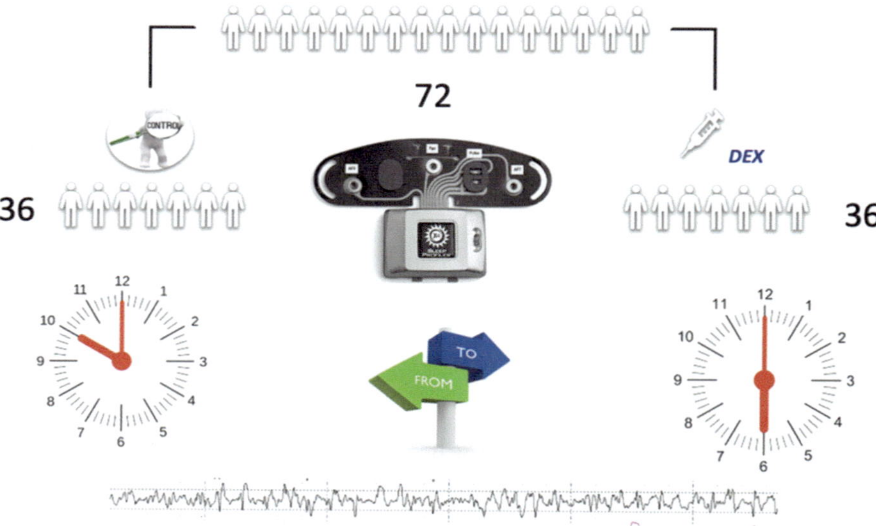

Fig. 6.6 Study design [18]

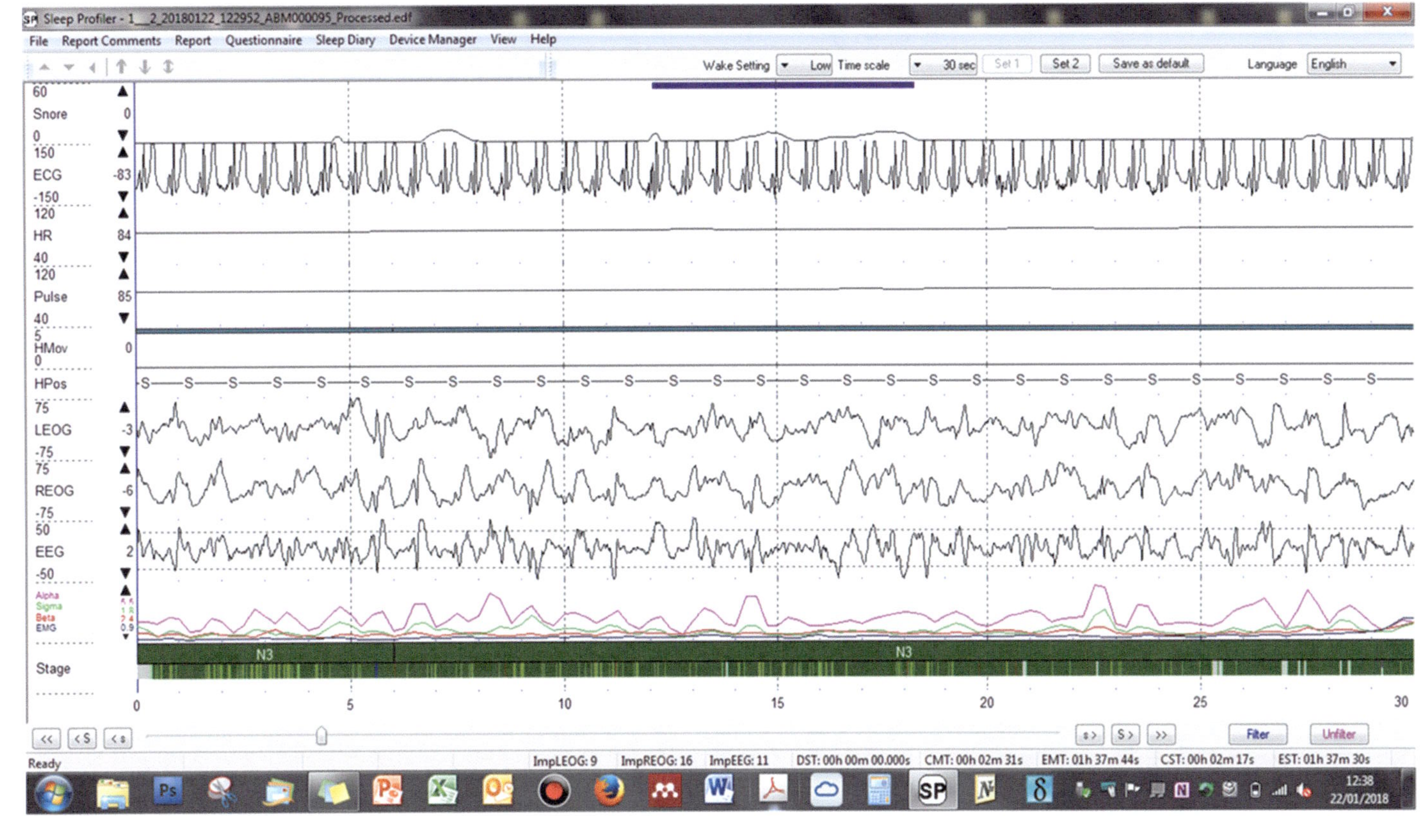

Fig. 6.7 EEG trace from Sleep Profiler®

6.10 Conclusions

In conclusion, we can summarize that

1. Sleep is a key element in preserving the mental balance of patients admitted to the ICU.
2. Changes in sleep quality are among the most frequently reported problems by patients discharged from ICUs.
3. Sleep alterations affect the functionality of many systems.
4. Every effort aimed at preserving the sleep–wake cycle is crucial in clinical practice.
5. Before using medications, many non-pharmacological strategies should be tried. They have shown great potential in improving the quantity and quality of sleep in ICU inpatients.

In conclusion, neuromonitoring for moderate-to-deep sedation in the ICU must become standard practice to avoid oversedation episodes and awareness in paralyzed patients. At the same time, sleep hygiene should be considered an important part of clinical practice. Neuromonitoring of sleep architecture should be implemented in ICU patients.

References

1. Devlin JW, Skrobik Y, Gélinas C, et al. Clinical practice guidelines for the prevention and management of pain, agitation/sedation, delirium, immobility, and sleep disruption in adult patients in the ICU. Crit Care Med. 2018;46:e825–73. https://doi.org/10.1097/CCM.0000000000003299.
2. Baron R, Binder A, Biniek R, et al. Evidence and consensus based guideline for the management of delirium, analgesia, and sedation in intensive care medicine. Revision 2015 (DAS-guideline 2015)—short version. GMS Ger Med Sci. 2015;13:2–42. https://doi.org/10.3205/000223.
3. Vincent JL, Shehabi Y, Walsh TS, et al. Comfort and patient-centred care without excessive sedation: the eCASH concept. Intensive Care Med. 2016;42:962–71. https://doi.org/10.1007/s00134-016-4297-4.
4. Rasulo FA, Hopkins P, Lobo FA, et al. Processed electroencephalogram-based monitoring to guide sedation in critically ill adult patients: recommendations from an international expert panel-based consensus. Neurocrit Care. 2022;38:296. https://doi.org/10.1007/s12028-022-01565-5.
5. Pun BT, Jackson JC, Ely EW, et al. Caring for critically ill patients with the ABCDEF bundle: results of the ICU liberation collaborative in over 15,000 adults. Crit Care Med. 2019;47:3–14. https://doi.org/10.1097/CCM.0000000000003482.Caring.
6. Shehabi Y, Bellomo R, Kadiman S, et al. Sedation intensity in the first 48 hours of mechanical ventilation and 180-day mortality: a multinational prospective longitudinal cohort study. Crit Care Med. 2018;46:850–9. https://doi.org/10.1097/CCM.0000000000003071.
7. Chanques G, Constantin JM, Devlin JW, et al. Analgesia and sedation in patients with ARDS. Intensive Care Med. 2020;46:2342–56. https://doi.org/10.1007/s00134-020-06307-9.
8. Watson PL, Shintani AK, Tyson R, et al. Presence of electroencephalogram burst suppression in sedated, critically ill patients is associated with increased mortality. Crit Care Med. 2008;36:3171–7. https://doi.org/10.1097/CCM.0b013e318186b9ce.

9. Andresen JM, Girard TD, Pandharipande PP, et al. Burst suppression on processed electroencephalography as a predictor of postcoma delirium in mechanically ventilated ICU patients. Crit Care Med. 2014;42:2244–51. https://doi.org/10.1097/CCM.0000000000000522.
10. Romagnoli S, Franchi F, Ricci Z. Processed EEG monitoring for anesthesia and intensive care practice. Minerva Anestesiol. 2019;85:1219. https://doi.org/10.23736/S0375-9393.19.13478-5.
11. Rasulo FA, Togni T, Romagnoli S. Essential noninvasive multimodality neuromonitoring for the critically ill patient. Crit Care. 2020;24:100. https://doi.org/10.1186/s13054-020-2781-2.
12. Pappal RD, Roberts BW, Winkler W, et al. Awareness with paralysis in mechanically ventilated patients in the emergency department and ICU: a systematic review and meta-analysis. Crit Care Med. 2021;49:E304–14. https://doi.org/10.1097/CCM.0000000000004824.
13. Fuller BM, Pappal RD, Mohr NM, et al. Awareness with paralysis among critically ill emergency department patients: a prospective cohort study. Crit Care Med. 2022;50:1449–60. https://doi.org/10.1097/CCM.0000000000005626.
14. Mohr NM, Sharma A. Mr. Sandman, bring me a dream. Crit Care Med. 2021;49:540–4. https://doi.org/10.1097/CCM.0000000000004880.
15. Bluff NEB, Georgia B. Sleep disturbances and critical illness. J Intensive Crit Care. 2017;3:1–5. https://doi.org/10.21767/2471-8505.100098.
16. Rittayamai N, Wilcox E, Drouot X, et al. Positive and negative effects of mechanical ventilation on sleep in the ICU: a review with clinical recommendations. Intensive Care Med. 2016;42:531–41. https://doi.org/10.1007/s00134-015-4179-1.
17. Freedman N, Kotzer N, Schwab R. Patient perception of sleep quality and etiology of sleep disruption in the intensive care unit. Am J Respir Crit Care Med. 1999;159:1155–62.
18. Romagnoli S, Villa G, Fontanarosa L, et al. Sleep duration and architecture in non-intubated intensive care unit patients: an observational study. Sleep Med. 2020;70:79–87. https://doi.org/10.1016/j.sleep.2019.11.1265.
19. Telias I, Wilcox ME. Sleep and circadian rhythm in critical illness. Crit Care. 2019;23:2–5. https://doi.org/10.1186/s13054-019-2366-0.
20. Demoule A, Carreira S, Lavault S, et al. Impact of earplugs and eye mask on sleep in critically ill patients: a prospective randomized study. Crit Care. 2017;21:1–9. https://doi.org/10.1186/s13054-017-1865-0.
21. Engwall M, Fridh I, Johansson L, et al. Lighting, sleep and circadian rhythm: an intervention study in the intensive care unit. Intensive Crit Care Nurs. 2015;31:325–35. https://doi.org/10.1016/j.iccn.2015.07.001.
22. Akeju O, Brown EN. Neural oscillations demonstrate that general anesthesia and sedative states are neurophysiologically distinct from sleep. Curr Opin Neurobiol. 2017;44:178–85.
23. Lu W, Fu Q, Luo X, et al. Effects of dexmedetomidine on sleep quality of patients after surgery without mechanical ventilation in ICU. Medicine (United States). 2017;96:1–5. https://doi.org/10.1097/MD.0000000000007081.
24. Alexopoulou C, Kondili E, Diamantaki E, et al. Effects of dexmedetomidine on sleep quality in critically ill patients: a pilot study. Anesthesiology. 2014;121:801–7. https://doi.org/10.1097/ALN.0000000000000361.
25. Skrobik Y, Duprey M, Hill N, Devlin J. Low-dose nocturnal dexmedetomidine prevents ICU delirium: a randomized, placebo-controlled trial. Am J Respir Crit Care Med. 2018;197:1147–56.

Davide Chiumello and Eleonora Duscio

Laparoscopic robotic surgery can be considered the evolution of traditional laparoscopic surgery. Technological advancement since the introduction of the first prototypes at the end of the 1980s has made it possible to overcome some of the technical limitations of traditional surgery. Nowadays, robotic surgery represents a minimally invasive technique associated with reduced length of stay, better and faster functional recovery, reduced intraoperative blood loss and need for blood transfusions, and finally reduced postoperative pain (George et al., JSLS 22:00039, 2018). The specificities of robotic laparoscopic surgery lead to a series of problems faced by the operating room staff both at the clinical and organizational level. First of all, the anesthesiologist will have to be prepared to face the physiopathological alterations induced by pneumoperitoneum and by "extreme" positions of the operating bed; moreover, the operating room must be equipped to accommodate the instrumentation of robotic surgery. Finally, all personnel must be adequately trained in robotic surgery, so as to be prepared to face the problems of this type of surgery and to act to minimize the associated risks.

D. Chiumello
Department of Anesthesia and Intensive Care, ASST Santi Paolo e Carlo, San Paolo University Hospital, Milan, Italy

Department of Health Sciences, University of Milan, Milan, Italy
e-mail: davide.chiumello@unimi.it

E. Duscio (✉)
Department of Anesthesia and Intensive Care, ASST Santi Paolo e Carlo, San Paolo University Hospital, Milan, Italy
e-mail: eleonora.duscio@gmail.com

D. Chiumello (ed.), *Practical Trends in Anesthesia and Intensive Care 2022*,
https://doi.org/10.1007/978-3-031-43891-2_7

7.1   Surgical Technique

Among the various systems on the market, the da Vinci® robot (Sunnyvale, Cal. USA) is certainly one of the most widespread in the world. It consists of three main elements: a surgical console from which the operator enjoys an immersive three-dimensional view of the operating field and from which, thanks to manual controls and foot pedals, he directs the actions of the robotic arms; a patient trolley consisting of three or more robotic arms; and a vision trolley containing the central processing unit and a full HD video system [1]. Laparoscopic robotic surgery as such relies on the insufflation of carbon dioxide into the abdominal cavity to create the surgical workspace. After the induction of pneumoperitoneum (which can be performed with different methods according to the operator's expertise), and the positioning of the surgical trocars, the so-called docking of the robot to the patient takes place and the robotic arms are connected to the surgical ports. It is of fundamental importance to consider that, once the docking has taken place, it will no longer be possible to mobilize the operating bed and the patient until after *undocking*. In fact, after docking is completed, there is a high risk of tissue damage even in case of small movements.

The da Vinci system, like many other robotic systems on the market, occupies a lot of space in the operating room. Consequently, it is important to emphasize that, for this surgical setting, it will be necessary to have a dedicated operating room in which the robotic and anesthesia equipment (including anesthesia workstation, floor stands, anesthesia trolley) will have to be positioned according to specific procedure diagrams to allow the correct functioning of the equipment and safe access to the patient [2].

From a technical surgical point of view, compared to traditional laparoscopy, the robot gives the operator a three-dimensional view of the operating field and expands the possibilities of movement of surgical instruments up to seven degrees of freedom. Moreover, the instrumentation is able to stabilize the movement, thus eliminating the physiological tremor and allowing the first operator to work far from the operating field, in a comfortable and ergonomic environment where the possibility of concentration is increased [3].

In most cases, the operation is performed by two surgeons: the first operator sits at the console from which he controls the robotic arms, effectively performing the surgical act, while an experienced assistant surgeon sits at the operating table and is responsible for positioning the trocars, performing docking, changing instruments, and moving any additional endoscopic instruments.

The positioning of the patient during the robotic procedure varies according to the type of surgery performed and is aimed at optimizing surgical exposure. In particular, in pelvic surgery (e.g., robotic-assisted prostatectomy and hysterectomy) the patient is positioned in steep Trendelenburg with an inclination of the operating table of up to 18°–25° (in some cases even 45°); in upper abdominal surgery, in contrast, the patient is positioned in anti-Trendelenburg; finally, for some types of surgery (e.g., lung surgery or kidney surgery) the patient is positioned in lateral decubitus.

The field in which the robotic approach has found its greatest application is urological surgery and in particular prostate surgery; to date, in the United States about 85% of radical prostatectomies are performed with this method [4]. Numerous studies have documented how the robotic approach reduces hospital stay, blood loss, and postoperative pain and allows better functional recovery [5]. Today, robotic surgery has many other applications ranging from gynecological surgery, to general surgery, to thoracic surgery, and also head and neck surgery [2, 6–9].

7.2   Pathophysiological Alterations During Robotic Surgery

In laparoscopic surgery, the surgical working chamber is obtained by pressurizing the abdominal cavity thanks to the insufflation of carbon dioxide and the creation of the so-called pneumoperitoneum. The resulting increase in intra-abdominal pressure (IAP) will lead to complex physiological changes at respiratory and cardiovascular levels, the extent of which will vary depending both on the patient's initial conditions and other factors such as the level of IAP, the degree of hypercapnia, and, lastly, the position. The hemodynamic and respiratory impact is generally minimal in the healthy patient, but may be clinically relevant in the patient with reduced cardiopulmonary reserve (Tables 7.1 and 7.2).

Table 7.1 Cardiovascular changes in robotic surgery

Parameter		Causes
SVR and MAP	↑	• Hypercapnia • Neuroendocrine response • Mechanical factors
PVC and PW	↑	• Increased intrathoracic pressures • Increased sympathetic stimulus • Positioning
Cardiac filling volumes	↑/↓	Interaction between • Increased intravascular volume (liver and spleen compression) • Preload and venous return variations • Positioning • Patient's baseline condition
CI	↓=	Interaction between • Increased afterload • Reduction of venous return • Increased intravascular volume • Positioning • Patient's baseline condition
Heart rate	↓	Peritoneal stretch and vagal tone
	↑	• Hypercapnia • Hypoxia • Capnotorax • Embolism

Based on data from Joshi G, Cunningham A. Anesthesia for laparoscopic and robotic surgeries. In: Clinical Anesthesia, 7th ed, Barash PG, Cullen BF, Stoelting RK, et al. (Eds), Lippincott Williams & Wilkins, Philadelphia 2013

SVR, systemic vascular resistance; *MAP*, mean arterial pressure; *PVC*, central venous pressure; *PW*, wedge pressure; *CI*, cardiac index; ↑, increase; ↓ decrease; =, unchanged variable

Table 7.2 Lung changes in robotic surgery

Parameter		Causes
FRC	↓	• Diaphragm elevation • IAP increase • Positioning
Lung compliance	↓	• Atelectasis development
Thoracic cage compliance	↓	• Diaphragm elevation • IAP increase
PaCO$_2$	↑	• CO$_2$ absorption
PaO$_2$	Variable	Interaction between • Atelectasis • Hypoxic vasoconstriction • Basal pulmonary conditions

Based on data from Joshi G, Cunningham A. Anesthesia for laparoscopic and robotic surgeries. In: Clinical Anesthesia, 7th ed, Barash PG, Cullen BF, Stoelting RK, et al. (Eds), Lippincott Williams & Wilkins, Philadelphia 2013

FRC, functional residual capacity; *PaCO$_2$*, arterial partial pressure of carbon dioxide; *PaO$_2$*, arterial partial pressure of oxygen; *IAP*, intra-abdominal pressure; ↑, increase; ↓, decrease

7.3 Hemodynamic Effects

The hemodynamic effects of robotic abdominal surgery are very similar to those observed in laparoscopic surgery. Most of the studies in the literature in this field concern prostate surgery, where the consequences of pneumoperitoneum are associated with those induced by the position in steep Trendelenburg.

The pneumoperitoneum and, in particular, the increase in IAP determine, on the one hand, the activation of neuroendocrine mechanisms (e.g., activation of the renin-angiotensin-aldosterone system and increase in the release of catecholamines) and, on the other hand, a mechanical vascular compression, which have as a consequence an increase in mean arterial pressure (MAP) and an increase in systemic and pulmonary vascular resistance (SVR and PVR) [10–12]. When the pneumoperitoneum is associated with a marked Trendelenburg position (25–45 degrees of inclination), the effect on MAP remains unchanged while the increase in SVR is mitigated, as shown by Lestar et al. in a study conducted on healthy patients undergoing robotic prostatectomy [12]. The same authors demonstrated that cardiac filling pressures, although not influenced by the establishment of the pneumoperitoneum, increased 2–3 times when the patient was placed in Trendelenburg with a 45° inclination. However, an impact of these alterations on the cardiac performance indices, i.e., cardiac output (CO) and cardiac index (CI), was not observed [12]. Moreover, a resolution of the picture and a return to basal hemodynamic values was observed once pneumoperitoneum and Trendelenburg were eliminated.

In contrast, when the position required for the surgical procedure is reverse Trendelenburg (e.g., for operations on the upper abdomen), the most frequent physiopathological alteration, especially if the patient is in a state of hypovolaemia, is a transitory hypotension due to venous pooling in the lower limbs and the consequent reduction in preload [13]. These cardiovascular alterations seem to be transitory with a tendency to return to basal values within a few minutes, as shown by a study conducted on 38 patients undergoing laparoscopic cholecystectomy [14].

Induction of pneumoperitoneum and peritoneal stretch can also trigger significant vagal stimulation and consequently induce severe bradycardia, the risk of which increases especially if the patient is on beta-blocker therapy, if insufflation pressures are high (>15 mmHg), and if target pressures are reached too quickly [11, 15]. Accordingly, a strategy aimed at reducing the risk of hemodynamic complications related to pneumoperitoneum and Trendelenburg relies on slow abdominal insufflation combined with maintenance of an IAP < 15 mmHg [15].

7.4 Regional Perfusion, Central Nervous System, Eye and Splanchnic Organs

Increased intra-abdominal and thoracic pressures, hypercapnia, and Trendelenburg position may increase cerebral blood flow (CBF) and intracranial pressure (ICP) [16, 17]. In the healthy patient, these changes do not result in an alteration of cerebral perfusion and oxygenation, which remains within normal values; however, in the patient who presents with an intracranial mass or significant vascular pathologies (e.g., a cerebral aneurysm), it is advisable to maintain intraoperative normocapnia in order not to increase ICP [18, 19].

Laparoscopy, due to increased intra-abdominal pressure, is inherently associated with the risk of increased intraocular pressure (IOP). In the case of robotic surgery, and in particular when the laparoscopy is associated with the Trendelenburg position, there is an increased risk of high intraocular pressure with potential detrimental consequences for visual function. The mechanisms underlying this risk have been traced back to increased central venous pressure, hypercapnia, and increased airway pressures, which are said to be involved in vasodilation of the choroidal vessels [20, 21]. In robotic prostatic surgery, the observed increase in IOP also seems to be correlated with the duration of surgery. Shirono et al. in a study of 59 patients, 29 of whom had high baseline IOP, observed that the increase in IOP correlated with the duration of surgery. It should be noted that even in patients with high baseline IOP, this remained within a safe range with return to baseline values for console times of less than 4 h [20].

The mechanical and neuroendocrine effects of the pneumoperitoneum already mentioned may reduce the perfusion of the splanchnic organs. However, this reduction is counterbalanced by the vasodilatation induced by hypercapnia, and therefore the final effect will be null [22]. At the renal level, pneumoperitoneum is responsible for a reduction in perfusion and urinary output secondary to parenchymal compression, reduced renal venous flow, and increased vasopressin levels. Deflation of the abdomen, if IAP levels are maintained below 15 mmHg during surgery, will generally result in full recovery of renal function in the absence of parenchymal histological changes [23].

7.5   Respiratory Effects

The pneumoperitoneum, due to the cephalic shift of the diaphragm associated with a cranial shift of the abdominal and mediastinal contents, determines the reduction of the functional residual capacity (FRC) and the reduction of the compliance of the respiratory system. The latter is a consequence of both the increased stiffness of the rib cage and the reduction in lung volumes. On the one hand, this condition predisposes to an increased risk of developing pulmonary atelectasis; on the other hand, an increase in airway pressures may be observed. The need to increase minute volume to ensure proper washout of the absorbed CO_2 into the peritoneal cavity may in turn underlie increased airway pressures [11, 23].

The systemic absorption of CO_2 reaches a plateau in about 10–15 min, and is therefore independent of the duration of the intervention [24]. The increase in arterial CO_2 remains clinically insignificant in patients without respiratory comorbidities, but may be difficult to manage in patients with respiratory disease, particularly those with moderate to severe chronic obstructive pulmonary disease [25].

These alterations may be further exacerbated in the steep Trendelenburg position that is adopted for most pelvic-abdominal robotic surgeries. However, several studies have shown that the impact in terms of increased dead space ventilation and worsened ventilation-perfusion ratio is minimal even in this subtype of surgery [19, 26]. Lestar et al. in a study conducted on patients undergoing robotic radical prostatectomy in the 45° Trendelenburg position, however, showed that the $EtCO_2$ could underestimate the arterial $PaCO_2$ in these cases. Moreover, the same authors showed that, in their study setting, a 40% reduction in pulmonary compliance was observed without, however, a consequent worsening of gas exchange which, on the contrary, was improved probably because of the ventilatory changes adopted during surgery [12].

Finally, the association of pneumoperitoneum and Trendelenburg position determines a cephalic shift of the carina during the intraoperative phase. Consequently, a desaturation or a sudden increase in peak pressures at the ventilator may be a sign of selective intubation of the right main bronchus, which must therefore be ruled out [27].

7.6   Anesthesia Management

7.6.1   Preoperative Evaluation

The surgical indication for robot-assisted surgery is made by the surgeon based on his experience, the existing guidelines for the proposed procedure, and the risk-benefit ratio based on the patient's condition [2]. Regarding exclusion criteria, there are no specific contraindications for robotic surgery. The same considerations applied for laparoscopic surgery should be considered for robotic surgery as well. Therefore, the 2022 European Society of Cardiology (ESC) guidelines for preoperative evaluation are also valid for patients who are candidates for robotic surgery

[28]. Particular attention should be paid to patients with significant heart disease, severe pulmonary disease, and obesity; these categories of patients have a high risk of perioperative complications due to the prolonged duration of surgery and the Trendelenburg position [2, 9, 29].

It is therefore important, during the preoperative anesthesiologic evaluation, to inform the patient about all special aspects of robotic surgery and to identify the presence of any risk conditions.

7.6.2 Intravenous and Volatile Anesthesia

General anesthesia with orotracheal intubation and mechanical ventilation is definitely the anesthesia of choice for robotic surgery. Several studies have attempted to identify the superiority between balanced general anesthesia and total intravenous anesthesia (TIVA) in robotic surgery. The surgical intervention causes an activation of inflammatory response and metabolic/neuroendocrine changes which could promote both an impairment of cell-mediated immunity and an activation of circulating tumor cells, with a possible postoperative recurrence of primary cancer and/or spread of metastasis. In addition to the surgical intervention, general anesthesia itself has been reported to increase the risk of metastasis [24]. Several retrospective studies found that in ovarian, colon, breast, and prostate cancer surgery, regional anesthesia compared to general anesthesia was associated with better oncologic outcomes. However, at the present time data are conflicting [24, 25].

The two most common general anesthesia techniques are total intravenous anesthesia (TIVA), mainly based on propofol and opioid infusion, and balanced general anesthesia (BGA), which is based on the administration of sevoflurane or desflurane in association with opioid.

It has been reported that propofol compared to desflurane is able to decrease the inflammatory response and to induce higher antioxidants effects [26, 27, 30]. Moreover, in a randomized trial comparing TIVA with BGA, the first significantly reduced the incidence of moderate to severe nausea and vomiting during the first postoperative 48 h. This effect was particularly evident during the immediate postoperative period in the recovery room (0% vs. 19%) and in the postoperative 1–6 h (0% vs. 26%) [29]. Roh et al. compared the effects of propofol versus desflurane on inflammation and on postoperative renal function [31]. They found that propofol was associated with a reduced inflammatory response measured as interleukin-6 levels. They also found that intraoperative urine output was significantly higher in the propofol compared to the desflurane group. However, no difference was found regarding postoperative complications and length of hospital stay.

Few studies evaluated the influence of anesthetic agents on the recurrence of prostate cancer. Kim et al. compared the effects of TIVA versus BGA on long-term oncologic outcomes such as biochemical recurrence (BCR) in patients who underwent robot-assisted laparoscopic radical prostatectomy (RALP) [32]. Their study didn't show any significant difference in the incidence of BCR in the two groups (45% in BGA and 39% in TIVA). The only significant predictors for prostate cancer recurrence were the initial PSA levels and the pathologic tumor stage. In contrast, a retrospective cohort study showed that mortality was significantly lower in the TIVA than in the BGA group (1% vs. 7%) during the follow-up [33]. Moreover, lower postoperative recurrence was found in the TIVA group compared with the BGA group (1% vs. 4%). A systematic review searching for randomized controlled trials comparing intravenous anesthesia and volatile anesthesia found only three single-center studies [34]. No clinical difference in postoperative pain between the two types of anesthesia was found at 1–6 h after surgery; it was also suggested that propofol reduced the postoperative nausea and vomiting over a short-term period and the risk for ocular hypertension, although with low quality of evidence [35].

7.6.3 Neuromuscular Blockade

In robotic surgery, continuous quantitative monitoring of neuromuscular blockade is recommended. Regarding the level of curarization required, given the importance of maintaining complete immobility of the patient due to the risk of "displacement" injuries of the robotic arms, maintaining a deep neuromuscular block can be considered. This corresponds to a TOF (train of four) value of zero associated with a post-tetanic count (PTC) of 1–2. A deep neuromuscular blockade allows for a laparoscopic workspace with lower pressures, e.g., 10 mmHg. Many studies have shown that the reduction of pneumoperitoneum pressure can positively affect some of the cardiorespiratory issues related to pneumoperitoneum itself, and can also improve the postoperative outcome, e.g., in terms of pain reduction [36, 37]. This topic is currently the focus of debate, as other studies have not shown any superiority of deep neuromuscular blockade over moderate [2, 38–40].

7.6.4 Positioning

As already mentioned, crucial aspects in robotic surgery are represented by the preparation and positioning of the patient. In fact, the robotic setting means that, due to the spatial encumbrance of the instrumentation, the patient is difficult to access once the robot has been docked. Access to the patient is further complicated by the fact that the position required for many types of surgeries is an "extreme" position (e.g., Trendelenburg vs. anti-Trendelenburg) with both arms stretched across the body. This position will be maintained for the whole surgical time, which on average is longer than in open surgery. In this context, it will be essential to carefully prepare not only the patient, but also the operating room so that quick and safe access to the patient is always guaranteed in case of need [2].

More in detail about the preparation of the patient, the anesthesiologist, according to the characteristics of the subject and the type of procedure, must identify the monitoring and the equipment he needs to perform the operation safely (e.g., vascular accesses, nasogastric tube, electrodes for monitoring, and any equipment to manage pacemakers and defibrillators) and position them before the docking of the robot. In addition, the entire operating room team must pay attention to the protection of the patient from decubitus injuries, slipping and finally eye injuries, whose risk is increased in this type of surgery due to both the position and the prolonged surgical time. Appropriate devices must be chosen for the patient's intraoperative position, such as anti-slip mats that prevent the patient from slipping cranially or caudally, which can be associated with brachial plexus injuries (incidence 0.25–1.8%) [41].

The risk of this type of injury is increased with the use of leg supports and reduced with the use of anti-slip mattresses. Nerve injuries can also affect the lower limb and are correlated with prolonged time, low BMI, and insufficient protection with anti-decubitus pads (0.3–2%) [41]. If the position required is lateral decubitus, this can be achieved by using vacuum mattresses that adapt to the shape and position of the patient's body. Particular attention should be paid to the patient's protruding parts to ensure that they do not come into contact with the robotic arms during their excursions. Contact points, bony prominences, and possible contact with cables and plastic devices should be protected and avoided with anti-decubitus systems and protective draping; the incidence of pressure injuries in this type of surgery is in fact very high (35%) and cases of rhabdomyolysis and compartment syndrome (incidence 0.67–0.95%) have also been described in the literature [41]. Lastly, correct eye protection with suitable devices (e.g., protective mask) is fundamental in this setting to reduce the risk of ocular and corneal injuries (incidence 0.2–3%) [41, 42].

It is important to remember that once the patient has been prepared, the docking of the robot with the connection of the surgical arms to the patient has taken place, and the robotic phase of the operation has started, the position of the operating table and of the patient cannot be changed, otherwise the risk of injury to the wall and internal organs will be high [2].

7.6.5 Ventilation Management

Increased ventilator pressures and reduced compliance induced by pneumoperitoneum and accentuated by the Trendelenburg position very often require adjustment of mechanical ventilation parameters during surgery. The use of protective ventilation, with a tidal volume of 6–8 mL/kg of ideal weight, a positive end-expiratory pressure (PEEP) between 5 and 10 cmH$_2$O, and a respiratory rate aimed at maintaining an EtCO$_2$ between 35 and 45 mmHg may be helpful in reducing the risk of postoperative respiratory complications [43]. The most commonly used mechanical ventilation (MV) mode during RALP is volume-controlled ventilation (VCV), which applies a constant inspiratory flow and guarantees constant tidal volume irrespective of lung conditions [44]. In contrast, pressure-controlled ventilation (PCV) is characterized by decelerating inspiratory flow, and thus tidal volume is dependent on lung conditions. A recent mode of MV is pressure controlled with volume guarantee (PC-VG) which combines the features of both. Three randomized controlled trials compared PC-VG with VCV during RALP [35, 36, 45]. In all these studies oxygenation and hemodynamics were similar between the two groups [46]. Furthermore, the increase in peak and driving pressures during laparoscopy is largely due to a reduction in rib cage compliance and not to a worsening of lung compliance. Consequently, relatively high airway pressures are tolerable during the laparoscopic phase in order to reduce the risk of derecruitment and to maintain adequate oxygenation [37]. The robotic setting, as already mentioned, increases the risk of atelectasis development. Two randomized studies compared a common ventilatory strategy combining low PEEP and tidal volume with a higher PEEP approach ($11-14$ cmH$_2$O) in patients undergoing RALP [38, 39]. The use of high PEEP levels significantly increased oxygenation during the intraoperative and postoperative periods and was associated with reduced rates of patchy or diffuse infiltration at chest X-ray in the following days. Hospital stay was similar between the two groups. In addition to the increase of PEEP, the use of recruitment maneuver (RM) during anesthesia has been suggested to improve both oxygenation and lung function [40]. Choi et al. evaluated the short-term effect of an RM performed before Trendelenburg positioning [40]. Although RM did not improve oxygenation, it significantly decreased the number of patients who developed either postoperative atelectasis or pulmonary complications.

7.6.6 Hemodynamic Monitoring

Regarding hemodynamic monitoring, as for every kind of surgery, this should be proportionate to the perioperative risk identified with the help of numerical scores such as the Lee index [47, 48]. SIAARTI (Società Italiana di Anestesia Analgesia Rianimazione e Terapia Intensiva) consensus for abdominal robotic surgery recommends the use of continuous monitoring of intraoperative stroke volume to maintain adequate oxygen delivery. The same society also recommends that equipment to perform a transesophageal echocardiogram be readily available in the operating room in the event of significant and sustained intra- or postoperative hemodynamic instability [2]. Nevertheless, according to our institution's experience, standard hemodynamic monitoring combined with invasive blood pressure monitoring are more than sufficient for the safe management of any intraoperative hemodynamic and metabolic alterations in the average patient.

Modern management of perioperative fluid therapy follows a goal-directed approach with the goal of zero intraoperative water balance. It is now known that, especially in abdominal surgery, water overload has a major impact on postoperative outcome, while a zero water balance approach is associated with a reduction of complications, including surgical ones [46, 49]. In the patient undergoing robotic surgery in the Trendelenburg position, the prolonged surgical time associated with an excessively positive water balance can lead to facial and conjunctival edema (incidence 43.8%) and also to upper airway edema (incidence 0.7–26%) and in some cases can compromise the patency of the latter [41]. If at the end of the operation significant edema of the facial tissues is evident, a laryngoscopic re-evaluation of the airway or a cuff leak test may be indicated, and in case of negative results, extubation should be delayed [50]. In addition, in urologic robotic surgery, and in particular in prostatic and bladder surgery, excessive water input and the polyuria that may be associated with it may lead to a worsening of the surgical vision at the time of anastomosis sutures [11]. Given these premises, a fluid therapy tailored to the actual needs of the patient is essential, although the reliability of dynamic indicators of fluid responsiveness such as pulse pressure variation (PPV) and stroke volume variation (SVV) in this type of surgery is controversial because of the important cardiovascular changes induced by pneumoperitoneum and Trendelenburg [2, 9, 51].

7.6.7 Postoperative Pain Management

Postoperative pain in laparoscopic robotic surgery is generally lower than in the same surgical procedures performed with the open technique. It has a somatic component from trocar access and a visceral component from surgical manipulation [9, 52]. Moreover, in some cases, shoulder pain of multifactorial origin may occur, also related to diaphragmatic irritation induced by pneumoperitoneum [53]. A multimodal approach that combines systemic medical therapy with locoregional analgesia techniques allows optimal pain management and rapid functional recovery postoperatively. However, pain after RALP is typically from mild to moderate. In an observational study comparing RALP versus retropubic radical prostatectomy, Webster et al. found that the total morphine sulfate equivalent administered in addition to a similar amount of ketorolac was not different between the two groups of patients [54]. Within 24 h after surgery, mean abdominal pain was 3.5 according to the Wong-Baker FACES pain rating scale (where 0 equals "no pain" and 10 "worst pain") [55]. The mean opiate administration was 94 and 41 mg in the following days. Forty-five (73%) patients received immediate postoperative ketorolac.

At the present time there is great heterogeneity concerning perioperative pain management for patients undergoing RALP. A recent UK national survey reported that only 32% of centers provided preoperative analgesia and acetaminophen was the most common drug prescribed [56]. Only 40% of centers routinely provided spinal anesthesia, while the vast majority administered intravenous strong opioids intraoperatively (fentanyl being the most common). A minority of centers performed transversus abdominal plane block (TAPb). In the postoperative period, all centers prescribed acetaminophen and up to 50% administered ibuprofen as an association [56].

As anticipated, acetaminophen, non-steroidal anti-inflammatory drugs (NSAIDs), and opioids are the mainstay of pain management after RALP. Nevertheless, opioid administration may prolong postoperative ileus, may promote nausea and vomiting, and can increase the length of hospital stay.

In contrast, the addition of repeated doses of IV acetaminophen (up to every 6 h), beginning from the induction of anesthesia, significantly reduced length of hospital stay without any significant difference in intraoperative and postoperative administration of opioids as shown in a randomized double-blind placebo-controlled trial [57].

The use of intrathecal morphine has been proposed to improve the quality of recovery and reduce pain after RALP. One randomized clinical trial showed that the use of intrathecal morphine (300 mcg)—with or without bupivacaine—significantly ameliorated the quality of recovery and pain reduction and reduced IV opioids administration in the intra- and postoperative setting [58]. The rate of complications, except for pruritus, did not increase.

TAPb nerve block has been introduced as a component of multimodal pain management in several surgical procedures. TAPb is performed by injecting local anesthetic between the internal oblique and the transversus abdominis muscle along the fascial plane. It is usually performed at the mid-axillary line, halfway between the costal margin and the anterior superior iliac crest. Several randomized trials evaluated intra- and postoperative analgesic efficacy of TAPb during RALP [59–61]. TAPb significantly ameliorated pain score in the immediate postoperative period and 24 h after surgery with a significant reduction in opioid administration [59, 61]. No significant complications related to the use of TAPb have been reported.

The recent Prospect (PROcedure SPEcific Postoperative Pain Management) working group for pain management after prostatectomy recommended systemic analgesia including acetaminophen and COX-2 selective NSAIDs or non-selective NSAIDs drugs. The association of these drugs has the ability to reduce opioid use [52]. It has been suggested that this strategy should begin preoperatively and be continued postoperatively. TAPb is recommended as a first choice for robotic radical prostatectomy [52].

7.7 Intraoperative Complications

Cardiorespiratory changes derived from pneumoperitoneum exacerbated by the pushed Trendelenburg position and positioning complications have been discussed extensively in previous sections. In addition to the usual and site-specific surgical complications, namely vascular and tissue injury, other complications derived from the surgical technique may be observed in robotic surgery.

Subcutaneous emphysema (incidence 0.3–3.9%) may occur if there is inadvertent insufflation of CO_2 into the subcutaneous, preperitoneal, or retroperitoneal tissue, or from extension of extraperitoneal insufflation. Factors favoring the development of subcutaneous emphysema are a surgical time greater than 200 min and the use of more than five surgical accesses [41]. Subcutaneous emphysema is manifested by a characteristic crackling sensation and in most cases remains localized to the subcutaneous tissue and resolves spontaneously. In more extensive cases, with involvement of the neck and facial tissues, it can be the indicator of extremely rare and potentially fatal complications such as capnomediastinum and capnotorax [62]. Venous gas embolism has a low incidence in robotic surgery and rarely causes significant haemodynamic consequences. In particular, in prostate surgery its incidence is lower in procedures performed by robotic than with the open technique. Moreover, the Trendelenburg position, by increasing the pressure in the right atrium, is protective against haemodynamic sequelae from gas embolism [41, 63]. Other possible complications described in the literature are cerebral edema, associated with prolonged operating time, Trendelenburg position and use of an IAP greater than 16 mmHg, and ischemic optic neuropathy related to the Trendelenburg position, high water balance, and pneumoperitoneum [41].

7.8 Conclusion

Robotic surgery is a minimally invasive method that reduces postoperative pain, facilitates postoperative recovery, and allows for a reduction in hospitalization time. The robotic setting requires careful planning of the work of the operating room team in order to ensure patient safety. The anesthesiologist must take into account the changes induced by pneumoperitoneum and Trendelenburg, which are well tolerated and reversible in the healthy patient but can lead to serious consequences in the patient with pre-existing pathologies. The prolonged surgical position and time increases the risk of intra- and postoperative complications.

References

1. Ballantyne GH, Moll F. The da Vinci telerobotic surgical system: the virtual operative field and telepresence surgery. Surg Clin N Am. 2003;83:1293–304.
2. Corcione A, Angelini P, Bencini L, et al. Joint consensus on abdominal robotic surgery and anesthesia from a task force of the SIAARTI and SIC. Minerva Anestesiol. 2018;84:1189–208.
3. Ashrafian H, Clancy O, Grover V, Darzi A. The evolution of robotic surgery: surgical and anaesthetic aspects. Br J Anaesth. 2017;119:i72–84.
4. Carbonara U, Srinath M, Crocerossa F, Ferro M, Cantiello F, Lucarelli G, Porpiglia F, Battaglia M, Ditonno P, Autorino R. Robot-assisted radical prostatectomy versus standard laparoscopic radical prostatectomy: an evidence-based analysis of comparative outcomes. World J Urol. 2021;39:3721–32.
5. D'Alonzo RC, Gan TJ, Moul JW, Albala DM, Polascik TJ, Robertson CN, Sun L, Dahm P, Habib AS. A retrospective comparison of anesthetic management of robot-assisted laparoscopic radical prostatectomy versus radical retropubic prostatectomy. J Clin Anesth. 2009;21:322. https://doi.org/10.1016/j.jclinane.2008.09.005.
6. Finegersh A, Holsinger FC, Gross ND, Orosco RK. Robotic head and neck surgery. Surg Oncol Clin N Am. 2019;28:115. https://doi.org/10.1016/j.soc.2018.07.008.
7. Moon AS, Garofalo J, Koirala P, Vu MLT, Chuang L. Robotic surgery in gynecology. Surg Clin N Am. 2020;100:445. https://doi.org/10.1016/j.suc.2019.12.007.
8. Schwartz G, Sancheti M, Blasberg J. Robotic thoracic surgery. Surg Clin N Am. 2020;100:237. https://doi.org/10.1016/j.suc.2019.12.001.
9. Aceto P, Beretta L, Cariello C, et al. Joint consensus on anesthesia in urologic and gynecologic robotic surgery: specific issues in management from a task force of the SIAARTI, SIGO, and SIU. Minerva Anestesiol. 2019;85:871–85.
10. O'Malley C, Cunningham AJ. Physiologic changes during laparoscopy. Anesthesiol Clin North Am. 2001;19:1. https://doi.org/10.1016/S0889-8537(05)70208-X.
11. Gainsburg DM. Anesthetic concerns for robotic-assisted laparoscopic radical prostatectomy. Minerva Anestesiol. 2012;78:596.
12. Lestar M, Gunnarsson L, Lagerstrand L, Wiklund P, Odeberg-Wernerman S. Hemodynamic perturbations during robot-assisted laparoscopic radical prostatectomy in 45° Trendelenburg position. Anesth Analg. 2011;113:1069. https://doi.org/10.1213/ANE.0b013e3182075d1f.
13. Hirvonen EA, Poikolainen EO, Pääkkönen ME, Nuutinen LS. The adverse hemodynamic effects of anesthesia, head-up tilt, and carbon dioxide pneumoperitoneum during laparoscopic cholecystectomy. Surg Endosc. 2000;14:272. https://doi.org/10.1007/s004640000038.

14. Zuckerman RS, Heneghan S. The duration of hemodynamic depression during laparoscopic cholecystectomy. Surg Endosc Other Interv Tech. 2002;16:1233. https://doi.org/10.1007/s00464-001-9152-0.
15. Atkinson TM, Giraud GD, Togioka BM, Jones DB, Cigarroa JE. Cardiovascular and ventilatory consequences of laparoscopic surgery. Circulation. 2017;135:700. https://doi.org/10.1161/CIRCULATIONAHA.116.023262.
16. Schramm P, Treiber AH, Berres M, Pestel G, Engelhard K, Werner C, Closhen D. Time course of cerebrovascular autoregulation during extreme Trendelenburg position for robotic-assisted prostatic surgery. Anaesthesia. 2014;69:58. https://doi.org/10.1111/anae.12477.
17. Halverson A, Buchanan R, Jacobs L, Shayani V, Hunt T, Riedel C, Sackier J. Evaluation of mechanism of increased intracranial pressure with insufflation. Surg Endosc. 1998;12:266. https://doi.org/10.1007/s004649900648.
18. Closhen D, Treiber A-H, Berres M, Sebastiani A, Werner C, Engelhard K, Schramm P. Robotic assisted prostatic surgery in the Trendelenburg position does not impair cerebral oxygenation measured using two different monitors: a clinical observational study. Eur J Anaesthesiol. 2014;31:104.
19. Kalmar AF, Foubert L, Hendrickx JFA, Mottrie A, Absalom A, Mortier EP, Struys MMRF. Influence of steep Trendelenburg position and CO_2 pneumoperitoneum on cardiovascular, cerebrovascular, and respiratory homeostasis during robotic prostatectomy. Br J Anaesth. 2010;104:433–9.
20. Shirono Y, Takizawa I, Kasahara T, et al. Intraoperative intraocular pressure changes during robot-assisted radical prostatectomy: associations with perioperative and clinicopathological factors. BMC Urol. 2020;20:26. https://doi.org/10.1186/s12894-020-00595-5.
21. Ackerman RS, Cohen JB, Getting REG, Patel SY. Are you seeing this: the impact of steep Trendelenburg position during robot-assisted laparoscopic radical prostatectomy on intraocular pressure: a brief review of the literature. J Robot Surg. 2019;13:35. https://doi.org/10.1007/s11701-018-0857-7.
22. Hatipoglu S, Akbulut S, Hatipoglu F, Abdullayev R. Effect of laparoscopic abdominal surgery on splanchnic circulation: historical developments. World J Gastroenterol. 2014;20:18165. https://doi.org/10.3748/wjg.v20.i48.18165.
23. Baltayian S. A brief review: Anesthesia for robotic prostatectomy. J Robot Surg. 2008;2:59. https://doi.org/10.1007/s11701-008-0088-4.
24. Byrne K, Levins KJ, Buggy DJ. Can anesthetic-analgesic technique during primary cancer surgery affect recurrence or metastasis? Can J Anesth. 2016;63:184. https://doi.org/10.1007/s12630-015-0523-8.
25. Stollings LM, Jia LJ, Tang P, Dou H, Lu B, Xu Y. Immune modulation by volatile anesthetics. Anesthesiology. 2016;125:399. https://doi.org/10.1097/ALN.0000000000001195.
26. Chen RM, Chen TG, Chen TL, Lin LL, Chang CC, Chang HC, Wu CH. Anti-inflammatory and antioxidative effects of propofol on lipopolysaccharide-activated macrophages. Ann N Y Acad Sci. 2005;1042:262. https://doi.org/10.1196/annals.1338.030.
27. Murphy PG, Myers DS, Davies MJ, Webster NR, Jones JG. The antioxidant potential of propofol (2,6-diisopropylphenol)†. Br J Anaesth. 1992;68:613. https://doi.org/10.1093/bja/68.6.613.
28. Halvorsen S, Mehilli J, Cassese S, et al. 2022 ESC Guidelines on cardiovascular assessment and management of patients undergoing non-cardiac surgery: developed by the task force for cardiovascular assessment and management of patients undergoing non-cardiac surgery of the European Society of Cardiology (ESC) endorsed by the European Society of Anaesthesiology and Intensive Care (ESAIC). Eur Heart J. 2022;43:3826–924.
29. Yoo YC, Bai SJ, Lee KY, Shin S, Choi EK, Lee JW. Total intravenous anesthesia with propofol reduces postoperative nausea and vomiting in patients undergoing robot-assisted laparoscopic radical prostatectomy: a prospective randomized trial. Yonsei Med J. 2012;53:1197. https://doi.org/10.3349/ymj.2012.53.6.1197.
30. Runzer TD, Ansley DM, Godin DV, Chambers GK. Tissue antioxidant capacity during anesthesia: propofol enhances in vivo red cell and tissue antioxidant capacity in a rat model. Anesth Analg. 2002;94:89. https://doi.org/10.1213/00000539-200201000-00017.

31. Roh GU, Song Y, Park J, Ki YM, Han DW. Effects of propofol on the inflammatory response during robot-assisted laparoscopic radical prostatectomy: a prospective randomized controlled study. Sci Rep. 2019;9:5242. https://doi.org/10.1038/s41598-019-41708-x.

32. Kim NY, Jang WS, Choi YD, Hong JH, Noh S, Yoo YC. Comparison of biochemical recurrence after robot-assisted laparoscopic radical prostatectomy with volatile and total intravenous anesthesia. Int J Med Sci. 2020;17:449. https://doi.org/10.7150/ijms.40958.

33. Lai HC, Lee MS, Lin KT, Huang YH, Chen JY, Lin YT, Hung KC, Wu ZF. Propofol-based total intravenous anesthesia is associated with better survival than desflurane anesthesia in robot-assisted radical prostatectomy. PLoS One. 2020;15:e0230290. https://doi.org/10.1371/journal.pone.0230290.

34. Herling SF, Dreijer B, Thomsen T, Møller AM. Total intravenous anaesthesia versus inhalational anaesthesia for transabdominal robotic assisted laparoscopic surgery. Cochrane Database Syst Rev. 2014; https://doi.org/10.1002/14651858.CD011387.

35. Park JH, Park IK, Choi SH, Eum D, Kim MS. Volume-controlled versus dual-controlled ventilation during robot-assisted laparoscopic prostatectomy with steep Trendelenburg position: a randomized-controlled trial. J Clin Med. 2019;8:2032. https://doi.org/10.3390/jcm8122032.

36. Choi EM, Na S, Choi SH, An J, Rha KH, Oh YJ. Comparison of volume-controlled and pressure-controlled ventilation in steep Trendelenburg position for robot-assisted laparoscopic radical prostatectomy. J Clin Anesth. 2011;23:183. https://doi.org/10.1016/j.jclinane.2010.08.006.

37. Brandão JC, Lessa MA, Motta-Ribeiro G, et al. Global and regional respiratory mechanics during robotic-assisted laparoscopic surgery: a randomized study. Anesth Analg. 2019;129:1564. https://doi.org/10.1213/ANE.0000000000004289.

38. Girrbach F, Petroff D, Schulz S, et al. Individualised positive end-expiratory pressure guided by electrical impedance tomography for robot-assisted laparoscopic radical prostatectomy: a prospective, randomised controlled clinical trial. Br J Anaesth. 2020;125:373. https://doi.org/10.1016/j.bja.2020.05.041.

39. Zhou J, Wang C, Lv R, Liu N, Huang Y, Wang W, Yu L, Xie J. Protective mechanical ventilation with optimal PEEP during RARP improves oxygenation and pulmonary indexes. Trials. 2021;22:351. https://doi.org/10.1186/s13063-021-05310-9.

40. Choi ES, Oh AY, In CB, Ryu JH, Jeon YT, Kim HG. Effects of recruitment manoeuvre on perioperative pulmonary complications in patients undergoing robotic assisted radical prostatectomy: a randomised single-blinded trial. PLoS One. 2017;12:e0183311. https://doi.org/10.1371/journal.pone.0183311.

41. Maerz DA, Beck LN, Sim AJ, Gainsburg DM. Complications of robotic-assisted laparoscopic surgery distant from the surgical site. Br J Anaesth. 2017;118:492. https://doi.org/10.1093/bja/aex003.

42. Sampat A, Parakati I, Kunnavakkam R, Glick DB, Lee NK, Tenney M, Eggener S, Roth S. Corneal abrasion in hysterectomy and prostatectomy: role of laparoscopic and robotic assistance. Anesthesiology. 2015;122:994. https://doi.org/10.1097/ALN.0000000000000630.

43. Young CC, Harris EM, Vacchiano C, et al. Lung-protective ventilation for the surgical patient: international expert panel-based consensus recommendations. Br J Anaesth. 2019;123:898. https://doi.org/10.1016/j.bja.2019.08.017.

44. Chiumello D, Meli A, Pozzi T, Lucenteforte M, Simili P, Sterchele E, Coppola S. Different inspiratory flow waveform during volume-controlled ventilation in ARDS patients. J Clin Med. 2021;10:4756. https://doi.org/10.3390/jcm10204756.

45. Kim MS, Soh S, Kim SY, Song MS, Park JH. Comparisons of pressure-controlled ventilation with volume guarantee and volume-controlled 1:1 equal ratio ventilation on oxygenation and respiratory mechanics during robot-assisted laparoscopic radical prostatectomy: a randomized-controlled trial. Int J Med Sci. 2018;15:1522. https://doi.org/10.7150/ijms.28442.

46. Joshi GP. Intraoperative fluid restriction improves outcome after major elective gastrointestinal surgery. Anesth Analg. 2005;101:601. https://doi.org/10.1213/01.ANE.0000159171.26521.31.

47. Vincent J-L, Pelosi P, Pearse R, et al. Perioperative cardiovascular monitoring of high-risk patients: a consensus of 12. Crit Care. 2015;19:224.

48. Kristensen SD, Knuuti J, Saraste A, et al. 2014 ESC/ESA Guidelines on non-cardiac surgery: cardiovascular assessment and management: The Joint Task Force on non-cardiac surgery: cardiovascular assessment and management of the European Society of Cardiology (ESC) and the European Society of Anaesthesiology. Eur Heart J. 2014;35:2383–431.
49. Miller TE, Raghunathan K, Gan TJ. State-of-the-art fluid management in the operating room. Best Pract Res Clin Anaesthesiol. 2014;28:261. https://doi.org/10.1016/j.bpa.2014.07.003.
50. McLarney Thomas J, Rose GL. Anesthetic implications of robotic gynecologic surgery. J Gynecol Endosc Surg. 2011;2:75. https://doi.org/10.4103/0974-1216.114077.
51. Scott MJ, Baldini G, Fearon KCH, et al. Enhanced recovery after surgery (ERAS) for gastrointestinal surgery, Part 1: Pathophysiological considerations. Acta Anaesthesiol Scand. 2015;59:1212. https://doi.org/10.1111/aas.12601.
52. Lemoine A, Witdouck A, Beloeil H, et al. PROSPECT guidelines update for evidence-based pain management after prostatectomy for cancer. Anaesth Crit Care Pain Med. 2021;40:100922. https://doi.org/10.1016/j.accpm.2021.100922.
53. Williams WH, Cata JP, Lasala JD, Navai N, Feng L, Gottumukkala V. Effect of reversal of deep neuromuscular block with sugammadex or moderate block by neostigmine on shoulder pain in elderly patients undergoing robotic prostatectomy. Br J Anaesth. 2020;124:164. https://doi.org/10.1016/j.bja.2019.09.043.
54. Webster TM, Herrell SD, Chang SS, Cookson MS, Baumgartner RG, Anderson LW, Smith JA. Robotic assisted laparoscopic radical prostatectomy versus retropubic radical prostatectomy: a prospective assessment of postoperative pain. J Urol. 2005;174:912. https://doi.org/10.1097/01.ju.0000169455.25510.ff.
55. Woldu SL, Weinberg AC, Bergman A, Shapiro EY, Korets R, Motamedinia P, Badani KK. Pain and analgesic use after robot-assisted radical prostatectomy. J Endourol. 2014;28:544–8.
56. Milliken D, Lawrence H, Brown M, Cahill D, Newhall D, Barker D, Ayyash R, Kasivisvanathan R. Anaesthetic management for robotic-assisted laparoscopic prostatectomy: the first UK national survey of current practice. J Robot Surg. 2021;15:335. https://doi.org/10.1007/s11701-020-01105-3.
57. Wang VC, Preston MA, Kibel AS, Xu X, Gosnell J, Yong RJ, Urman RD. A prospective, randomized, double-blind, placebo-controlled trial to evaluate intravenous acetaminophen versus placebo in patients undergoing robotic-assisted laparoscopic prostatectomy. J Pain Palliat Care Pharmacother. 2018;32:82. https://doi.org/10.1080/15360288.2018.1513436.
58. Koning MV, de Vlieger R, Teunissen AJW, Gan M, Ruijgrok EJ, de Graaff JC, Koopman JSHA, Stolker RJ. The effect of intrathecal bupivacaine/morphine on quality of recovery in robot-assisted radical prostatectomy: a randomised controlled trial. Anaesthesia. 2020;75:599. https://doi.org/10.1111/anae.14922.
59. Dal Moro F, Aiello L, Pavarin P, Zattoni F. Ultrasound-guided transversus abdominis plane block (US-TAPb) for robot-assisted radical prostatectomy: a novel "4-point" technique-results of a prospective, randomized study. J Robot Surg. 2019;13:147–51.
60. Cacciamani GE, Menestrina N, Pirozzi M, et al. Impact of combination of local anesthetic wounds infiltration and ultrasound transversus abdominal plane block in patients undergoing robot-assisted radical prostatectomy: perioperative results of a double-blind randomized controlled trial. J Endourol. 2019;33:295. https://doi.org/10.1089/end.2018.0761.
61. Taninishi H, Matsusaki T, Morimatsu H. Transversus abdominis plane block reduced early postoperative pain after robot-assisted prostatectomy: a randomized controlled trial. Sci Rep. 2020;10:3761. https://doi.org/10.1038/s41598-020-60687-y.
62. Joshi GCA. Anesthesia for laparoscopic and robotic surgeries. In: Barash PG, Cullen BF, Stoelting RK, et al., editors. Clin Anesth. 7th ed; 2013. p. 1257–73.
63. Hong JY, Kim JY, Choi YD, Rha KH, Yoon SJ, Kil HK. Incidence of venous gas embolism during robotic-assisted laparoscopic radical prostatectomy is lower than that during radical retropubic prostatectomy. Br J Anaesth. 2010;105:777. https://doi.org/10.1093/bja/aeq247.

Pre-anesthesia Evaluation and Risk Assessment in Adult Patient Candidates for Non-cardiac Surgery

8

Rita Cataldo, Sabrina Migliorelli, and Felice Eugenio Agrò

8.1 Introduction

The pre-anesthesia assessment includes all clinical evaluations that the anesthesiologist will perform to define the patient's physical status, his/her eligibility for the most suitable anesthesia based on the planned surgery, intra- and postoperative management, the related risks, and the strategies to contain them. With a view to optimizing time and resources, the pre-anesthesia evaluation performed on a "prehospitalization" basis, i.e., on an outpatient basis a few days/weeks before admission for elective surgery, should be the gold standard. The assessment should be individualized for each patient, requiring appropriate diagnostic tests and/or specialist consultations and assessment on the basis of age, anesthesiological and surgical risk factors, and planned surgical procedure. Pre-anesthesia evaluation is always required when anesthesiological procedures are planned, including in case of Non-Operating Room Anesthesia (NORA) procedures; it may be omitted/limited only in some uncommon scenarios related to complex emergency situations [1–4].

R. Cataldo (✉) · F. E. Agrò
Fondazione Policlinico Universitario Campus Bio Medico, Rome, Italy

Research Unit of Anesthesia, Intensive Care and Pain Management, Department of Medicine and Surgery, Università Campus Bio-Medico di Roma, Rome, Italy
e-mail: R.Cataldo@policlinicocampus.it

S. Migliorelli
Research Unit of Anesthesia, Intensive Care and Pain Management, Department of Medicine and Surgery, Università Campus Bio-Medico di Roma, Rome, Italy

Graduate School of Anesthesia, Resuscitation, Intensive Care and Pain Management, Fondazione Policlinico Universitario Campus Bio Medico, Rome, Italy

© The Author(s), under exclusive license to Springer Nature Switzerland AG 2024
D. Chiumello (ed.), *Practical Trends in Anesthesia and Intensive Care 2022*,
https://doi.org/10.1007/978-3-031-43891-2_8

The objectives of the preoperative evaluation are:

- Define the patient's physical status according to the American Society of Anesthesiologists (ASA).
- Obtain information that can guide, confirm, reduce, or implement the planned diagnostic-therapeutic procedures.
- Identify situations requiring treatment before surgery.
- Choose the anesthesiological technique and/or share the most appropriate surgical strategy, sometimes in a different form than as initially planned.
- Reduce the risk and/or increase the benefit of the procedure by scheduling and/or modifying, if needed, the patient clinical pathway (e.g., possible ICU stay in the postoperative period) also in order to avoid postponements of the procedure with avoidable social and health costs.
- Inform the patient regarding the risks related to the planned anesthesia, explaining any possible alternatives and any chance to optimize comorbidities and outcome.
- Anticipate possible perioperative complications and act to avoid or contain them.
- Acquire consent effectively informed, from the patient or his or her legal guardian.

The anesthesiological evaluation coordinates and concludes any multidisciplinary approach, helping to identify the most appropriate timing for the planned procedure and its risk-benefit assessment.

8.2 Preoperative Anesthesiology Assessment in Patients Undergoing Non-cardiac Surgery: A General Overview

8.2.1 Physiological Medical History

The approach to the patient should always begin with a thorough physiological medical history, including general information such as age, sex, weight, and height (to calculate the Body Mass Index). The next step is to obtain a comprehensive list of both pharmacological and non-pharmacological allergies (e.g., food, dust, pollen, latex, etc.), describing the clinical manifestations associated with each of them. In case of medication allergies, it should be clarified which active principles of the same pharmacological class can be safely administered to the patient without causing negative effects. Any data suggesting a possible or known latex allergy requires several specific investigations and potential inclusion of the patient in a latex-free protocol [2, 4].

It is important to investigate the patient's home therapy in order to manage it appropriately in the perioperative period. History of transfusions should always be explored.

It is essential to thoroughly investigate the patient's exposure to, use of, and/or abuse of cigarette smoking, alcohol, and/or psychotropic substances. For each substance, it is necessary to highlight the frequency, method of intake, and any addiction. In case of women of childbearing age, it is important to identify any current or previous pregnancies. Finally, it is necessary to know if the patient observes any religious rules that may be of anesthesiological interest (e.g., Jehovah's Witnesses) [4].

8.2.2 Surgical and Anesthesiological Medical History

Information on previous anesthesia and surgeries is important to identify specific problems related to the perioperative management of the patient. It is essential to collect a detailed list of previous surgeries, their indications (functional or oncological pathology), the year they were performed, and the type of anesthesia administered. The interview should be used to highlight any complications that occurred during anesthesia, with particular reference to airway management, individual response to drugs, and the identification of reasons, including family history, suggestive of susceptibility to malignant hyperthermia (MH) or other complications related to anesthesia. In case of suspected MH, the patient should be referred to one of the national MH centers to confirm the diagnosis and then managed by providing "safe anesthesia" at the time of surgery.

The pathological medical history should aim to investigate in particular the presence of cardiovascular, respiratory, neurological, renal, hematological-coagulative, endocrine-metabolic, and gastrointestinal tract diseases, particularly for the presence of gastroesophageal reflux, leading towards a Rapid Sequence Intubation (RSI) or possible precautions in the use of Supra Glottic Airway (SGA) [4].

In this context, it is appropriate to collect data on the previous experience of postoperative nausea and vomiting (PONV) following general or regional anesthesia and to calculate the Apfel Score value (Table 8.1) [5].

8.2.2.1 Airway Assessment

The correct and safe airway management involves preoperative assessment (regardless of the type of anesthesia planned for the patient) of any risk factors for a difficult airway (difficulty of ventilation with face mask and/or with SGA, difficult tracheal intubation, or anticipated difficult emergency Front of Neck Access (eFONA)).

Table 8.1 Characteristics and score of Apfel's Score [5]

Features	Score
Female sex	1
Previous PONV	1
Non-smoking patient	1
Postoperative opioids	1

Prevention of PONV should be carried out in case of score ≥ 2

Only a careful preoperative assessment allows adequate planning of strategies to ensure the oxygenation/ventilation of that specific patient and the timely preparation of useful devices and of the team.

The preoperative assessment consists of an anamnestic interview and a targeted clinical examination. The medical history must pay attention to any difficulties related to previous intubations, as well as traumas, burns, and prior surgical procedures involving the oro-pharyngo-laryngeal structures and the facial bone mass, pathologies potentially related to a difficult airway (e.g., diabetes, obstructive sleep apnea syndrome, pathological obesity, rheumatic diseases, upper airway infections, congenital disorders and chromosomal abnormalities, facial dysmorphisms, and para-physiological conditions such as pregnancy) [6–8]. The clinical examination should be performed with the patient sitting frontally in profile, with open and closed mouth, and aimed at searching for all elements potentially responsible for difficult airways:

- Presence of beard and mustache
- Short and thick neck
- Presence of surgical scars and/or signs of previous radiotherapy
- Reduced neck mobility in extension
- Conformation and dental health, including the presence of fixed implants and/or removable prostheses
- Presence of retrognathia, prognathia, micrognathia
- Poor visibility of pharyngeal structures (Mallampati test)

The following measurements should be taken:

- Inter-incisor distance: If <3 cm, it indicates probable difficulty; if <2 cm, it does not allow the introduction of the laryngoscope blade into the mouth and can also prevent the placement of a SGA.
- Thyromental distance (between the bony chin and the thyroid cartilage in a subject with the neck extended): If <6 cm, it indicates probable difficulty. Alternatively, the sternomental distance (more sensitive and specific) can be measured, which should be >12.5 cm.
- Mobility of the atlanto-occipital joint: The patient is observed from the side as the head moves from the neutral position to the maximum extension position. The maximum extension corresponds on average to an angle of 35°.
- Mallampati test: It should be performed by asking the patient, in a seated position, to open the mouth and protrude the tongue. Based on the visibility of the pharyngeal structures, a class is assigned, and the test is then repeated with phonation, noting any changes in the class. Classes 3 and 4, especially if not modifiable with phonation, are predictive of possible difficult intubation (Table 8.2).
- Upper Lip Bite Test (ULBT): Assesses the ability of a patient to bite their upper lip with the lower dental arch (see Table 8.3). This test has gained increasing specificity and reliability in recent years.

Table 8.2 Classification of Mallampati [9]

Class	Visible structures
I	Soft palate, fauces, ugula, and palatine pillars
II	Soft palate, ugula, and fauces
III	Soft palate and base of the ugula
IV	Only hard palate

Table 8.3 ULBT—Upper Lip Bite Test [7]

Class	
I	Lower incisors bite the upper lip, beyond the vermilion edge
II	The lower incisors bite the upper lip, below the vermilion edge
III	Lower incisor teeth fail to bite the upper lip

- STOP-Bang questionnaire (see Sect. 8.4 and Table 8.12 for further details): If >3, indicates an increased risk of difficult airway.

For obese patients, in addition to the standard indexes, specific indexes to be evaluated include:

- Neck circumference (cut-off >41 cm in women and >43 cm in men)
- Waist-to-hip ratio (cut-off >0.8 in women and 0.9 in men)
- BMI >50 kg/m^2

There are several scores available to predict a difficult airway, and one of the most commonly used is the El-Ganzouri score (see Table 8.4).

8.2.3 Which Preoperative Tests to Request?

Preoperative examinations aim to provide information on the patient's health condition, optimize comorbidities if possible, and tailor surgery and anesthesia to the individual, as part of an individualized preoperative assessment containing the risk for the patient as much as possible.

Commonly preoperative examinations include standard laboratory investigations, electrocardiogram (ECG), and chest X-ray. It is important to remember that preoperative tests represent costs in terms of human and economic resources, a potential source of risk and discomfort for the patient, and the source of possible delays or rescheduling of planned surgeries. Therefore, only tests that are actually able to modify and guide anestesiological planning on the basis of their results should be performed [10–12].

Table 8.4 El-Ganzouri Score [8]

Parameter	Score 0	Score 1	Score 2
Weight (kg)	<90	90–110	>110
Head/neck mobility (°)	>90	90 ± 10	<80
Inter-incisor distance (cm)	≥4	<4	
Prognathism	Possible	Not possible	
Tyromental distance (cm)	>6.5	6–6.5	<6
Mallampati class	I	II	III and IV
Previous difficult intubation	No	Possible	Note

Score ≥ 4: Possible difficult intubation; score < 4: Unlikely difficult intubation

8.2.3.1 Laboratory Tests

Almost all the scientific literature currently agrees that routine use of laboratory tests produces a wide range of altered results, even in essentially healthy patients, and the clinical significance of many of these abnormal findings is uncertain. The ability of routine preoperative tests to predict perioperative complications in asymptomatic patients is poor or absent. Therefore, it should be considered that:

- The number of preoperative tests can be drastically reduced without causing adverse events for the patient.
- Laboratory tests performed before surgery should not serve as screening tests but should be only focused on the surgical/anesthesiological procedure.
- Patients classified as ASA I and II do not require laboratory tests unless based on specific clinical findings and only for high-/very high-complexity surgeries.
- The prescription of additional investigations should be guided by the patient's clinical history.

Based on the evidence in the literature, each local healthcare institution is called upon to formulate internal guidelines for requesting preoperative investigations, tailored to the patient's age, physical condition, and surgical grading, in order to standardize the evaluation of patients undergoing elective surgery within that specific hospital and contain healthcare costs [13].

8.2.3.2 12-Lead Electrocardiogram (ECG)

Baseline preoperative ECG abnormalities are common, and their incidence increases with patient age, but they do not frequently influence the anesthetic management. The detection of myocardial infarction from preoperative ECG is rare (0.25/1000 male patients over 45 years old or female patients over 55 years old). It increases with age and the presence of associated conditions such as diabetes mellitus. More commonly, occasional findings of non-malignant arrhythmias, such as atrial fibrillation, may be encountered [10–12].

Since baseline ECG abnormalities increase with age, as well as the risk of perioperative cardiovascular complications, it is reasonable to establish an age limit for performing preoperative ECG in non-cardiac, asymptomatic patients without risk factors. Current literature suggests differentiated age limits for males (45 years) and females (55 years), considering the different occurrence of ischemic heart disease between the two sexes.

A preoperative resting ECG is indicated in:

- All patients with cardiovascular risk factors (including age $\geq$65 years, as well as diabetes mellitus, high blood pressure, collagen diseases, dyslipidemia, obesity, cigarette smoking, peripheral vascular diseases, and family history of cardiovascular diseases and/or sudden death)
- Presence of a medical history or definite signs and symptoms of cardiovascular diseases, even if undergoing low-risk surgery
- All patients undergoing high-risk or intermediate-risk surgery but with at least one risk factor according to the Revised Cardiac Risk Index (see paragraph 8.7)
- Patients with pacemakers
- Presence of significant electrolyte abnormalities
- Patients receiving therapy with cardiotoxic/nephrotoxic drugs or medications that are commonly associated with electrocardiographic abnormalities (tricyclic antidepressants, phenothiazines, doxorubicin)

8.2.3.3 Chest X-Ray

A chest X-ray result usually does not change perioperative management and does not predict postoperative pulmonary complications. However, performing the X-ray exposes the patient to radiation, which should not be undervalued in terms of radiation protection. Often, the results of the X-ray are expected based on the patient's clinical evaluation and do not modify the anesthetic management. Some suggested indications for preoperative chest radiography include acute respiratory symptoms, clinical signs suggestive of a new lung disease, signs of exacerbation of a previous condition, recent history of chest trauma, neoplastic conditions with a likelihood of lung metastasis, and cardiothoracic surgery [3, 14, 15]. In general, it can be assumed that:

- For patients undergoing low-risk procedures, a chest X-ray is not indicated.
- For patients undergoing high-risk surgery, it is always indicated (mainly intra-thoracic or intra-abdominal surgery).
- For patients undergoing intermediate-risk surgery, if age is <60 years, it is not indicated; if age is >70 years, it is indicated.
- For patients between 60 and 70 years of age, the decision to request a chest X-ray is based on the surgery, whether it is low or high risk.

Table 8.5 and Fig. 8.1 provide recent recommendations for preoperative testing based on surgical complexity and patient.

The time validity of laboratory hematological and biochemical tests is around 3 months. An ECG has a validity of 3 months in cases of high surgical risk and patients with a history of current or previous cardiovascular diseases, and 6 months in cases of

Table 8.5 Preoperative tests [3, 15]

Preoperative examinations and ASA class/type of surgery			
Minor surgery			
Examination	*ASA I*	*ASA II*	*ASA III or ASA IV*
Complete blood count	Non-routine	Non-routine	Non-routine
Coagulation testing	Non-routine	Non-routine	Non-routine
Renal function	Non-routine	Non-routine	Consider whether risk of AKI
ECG	Non-routine	Non-routine	Consider if performed >12 months earlier
Respiratory function/EGA	Non-routine	Non-routine	Non-routine
Intermediate surgery			
Examination	*ASA I*	*ASA II*	*ASA III or ASA IV*
Complete blood count	Non-routine	Non-routine	Consider in case of cardiovascular and renal disease or in case of symptoms not recently evaluated
Coagulation testing	Non-routine	Non-routine	Consider whether hepatopathy. In case of anticoagulant therapy work out individual management. Perform point-of-care testing for coagulation assessment immediately before surgery
Renal function	Non-routine	Consider whether risk of AKI	Yes
ECG	Non-routine	Consider if performed >12 months earlier	Yes
Respiratory function/EGA	Non-routine	Non-routine	Consider urgent anesthesiological evaluation in case of respiratory failure
Major surgery			
Examination	*ASA I*	*ASA II*	*ASA III or ASA IV*
Complete blood count	Yes	Yes	Yes
Coagulation testing	Non-routine	Non-routine	Consider whether hepatopathy. In case of anticoagulant therapy work out individual management. Perform point-of-care testing for coagulation assessment immediately before surgery
Renal function	Consider whether risk of AKI	Yes	Yes
ECG	Consider if performed >12 months earlier	Yes	Yes
Respiratory function/EGA	Non-routine	Non-routine	Consider urgent anesthesiological evaluation in case of respiratory failure

ASA American Society of Anesthesiologists, *ECG* electrocardiogram, *EGA* blood gas analysis, *AKI* acute kidney injury

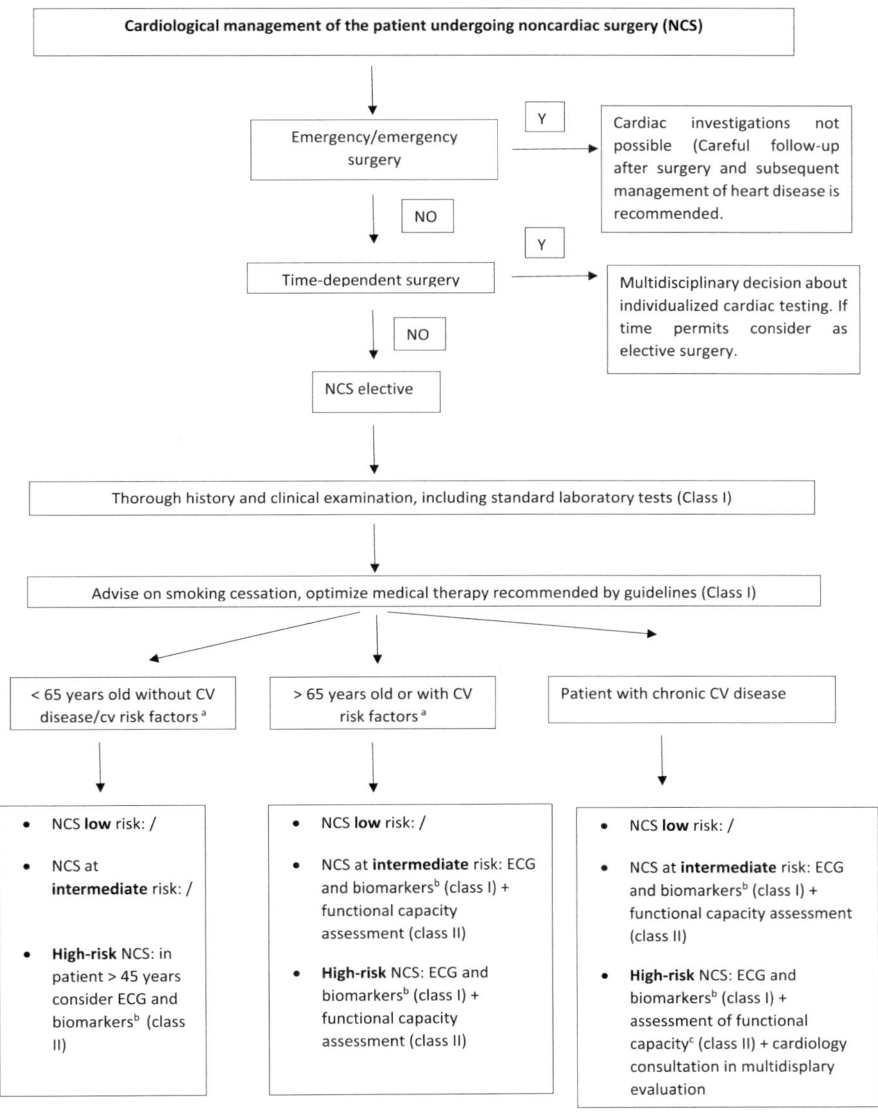

Fig. 8.1 Cardiological management of the patient to undergo non-cardiac surgery (NCS). [a]: Cardiovascular (CV) risk factors: hypertension, smoking, dyslipidemia, diabetes, family history of CVD. [b]: Biomarkers: hs-cTn T/I (class I) and/or or BNP/NT-proBNP (class IIa). If pathological, consult a cardiologist. [c]: Functional ability based on Duke Activity Status Index (DASI) or the ability to climb two flights of stairs. (Excerpted and modified from: S. Halvorsen et al., "2022 ESC Guidelines on cardiovascular assessment and management of patients undergoing non-cardiac surgery: Developed by the task force for cardiovascular assessment and management of patients undergoing non-cardiac surgery of the European Society of Cardiology," Eur. Heart J, 2022, vol. 43, pp. 3826–3924)

low or intermediate surgical risk and patients without a cardiovascular history. Chest X-rays usually have a validity of approximately 1 year. These time limits are valid as long as there have been no active clinical issues since the last examination [14].

8.3 Evaluation of the Cardiovascular System in Patients Undergoing Non-cardiac Surgery

The need for standardization in the preoperative assessment and treatment of cardiac patients undergoing non-cardiac surgery reflects the increase in surgical procedures in progressively older patients. Non-cardiac surgery is associated with a variable rate of complications, including a variable mortality rate; more than 40% of these adverse events are cardiac complications. However, neither human nor instrumental resources are limitless, and there is a need to optimize the use of cardiological assessments to avoid waste, overload, and unnecessary delays in planned procedures.

The ESC/ESAIC guidelines (European Society of Cardiology/European Society of Anaesthesiology and Intensive Care), published in 2022, summarize and evaluate the available evidence, with the aim of assisting healthcare professionals in proposing the best management strategies for individual patients.

8.3.1 Functional Capacity Evaluation

The functional capacity evaluation is a crucial step in preoperative cardiologic assessment and is measured in metabolic equivalents (METs). A MET represents basal metabolic demand (refer to Table 8.6). A MET value below 4 is considered indicative of poor functional capacity and is associated with a higher incidence of postoperative cardiac events. Patients who are unable to perform activities equivalent to at least 4 METs should be evaluated (or reevaluated) by a cardiologist before being referred for surgery. However, patients with MET values above 4 may often avoid a cardiological examination unless they have special acute conditions requiring preparation for high-risk surgery.

Table 8.6 Metabolic equivalents [16]

MET	Physical activity
1	Taking care of one's self (feeding, dressing walking inside the house, walking on level ground at low speed)
4	Light housework (washing dishes, dusting), climbing a floor of stairs
>4	Climbing two flights of stairs, walking on level ground at a fast speed, strenuous household work (moving furniture and mopping floors), moderate sports activity (golf, dancing, tennis)
10	Intense sports activity (swimming, skiing, soccer)

8.3.2 Cardiovascular Risk Factors

Patients can be categorized into three groups based on the presence of cardiovascular risk factors: major, intermediate, and minor (see Table 8.7).

8.3.2.1 Cardiac Risk

In terms of cardiac risk, surgical procedures can be classified as low, intermediate, or high risk (refer to Table 8.8). This classification is based on the estimated incidence of major cardiovascular events (myocardial infarction, stroke, and cardiac death) within 30 days, considering only the specific surgical procedure without considering patient comorbidities. The incidence of adverse cardiac events for each risk category is as follows: low risk <1%, intermediate risk 1–5%, high risk >5%.

In general, it is recommended to optimize the treatment of modifiable cardiovascular risk factors (e.g., blood pressure, dyslipidemia, and blood sugar control) before non-cardiac surgery, if time permits.

Table 8.9 provides an overview of major cardiovascular diseases identified during the preoperative visit and their perioperative management.

Table 8.7 Cardiovascular risk factors [3]

Cardiovascular risk factors	
Major	• Unstable coronary syndromes (unstable or disabling angina) • Acute myocardial infarction (<30 days) with clinical or instrumental evidence of residual ischemia • Decompensated heart failure—NYHA class III or IV • Severe valvulopathies (aortic stenosis, mitral stenosis) • Severe and clinically significant arrhythmias (advanced atrioventricular block, symptomatic ventricular arrhythmias, supraventricular arrhythmias with uncontrolled ventricular response) • PTCA + stent (DES or BMS) in high-risk coronary anatomy or if bioresorbable stents <12 months • PTCA + stent (DES or BMS) performed for acute coronary syndrome (ACS) <6–12 months • Elective PTCA + stent (DES or BMS) in stable coronary artery disease <1–6 months • PTCA without stent in stable coronary artery disease <2 weeks
Intermediate	• Stable or controlled angina • Prior myocardial infarction >30 days • Compensated heart failure—NYHA class I or II or previous heart failure • Pregressed stroke/TIA • Diabetes mellitus • Chronic renal failure (creatinine clearance <60 mL/min/1.73 m^2)
Minor	• Elderly • Abnormal ECG (left ventricular hypertrophy, nonspecific ST tract abnormalities and T wave) • Reduced functional capacity in the absence of history of heart disease • Arterial hypertension not controlled by therapy or untreated

Table 8.8 Degrees of complexity of surgeries in relation to cardiac risk (myocardial infarction, stroke, and cardiac death) [10]

Complexity of surgery		Cardiac risk
Minor surgery	• Superficial surgery (skin lesion exeresis, abscess drainage of superficial structures, superficial lymph node biopsies) • Breast surgery • Dental surgery • Thyroid surgery • Eye surgery • Reconstructive surgery • Minor orthopedic surgery (meniscectomy, arthroscopy) • Gynecologic surgery (hysteroscopy) • Minor urologic surgery (transurethral resection of the prostate or bladder) • Minor lung resection by VATS	<1%
Intermediate surgery	• Intraperitoneal surgery (splenectomy, hiatal hernia surgery, cholecystectomy) • Asymptomatic carotid artery surgery (CAS, CEA) • Symptomatic carotid artery surgery (CEA) • Peripheral arterial angioplasty • Endoscopic vascular surgery • Head and neck surgery (tonsillectomy or adenoidectomy, uvulo-pharyngoplasty) • Neurosurgery and major orthopedic surgery (spine surgery and hip/knee arthroplasty) • Major urologic surgery (radical prostatectomy, nephrectomy) • Major gynecologic surgery (hystero-annessiectomy) • Minor intra-thoracic surgery • Renal transplantation	1–5%
Major surgery	• Aortic and major vascular surgery • Symptomatic carotid artery surgery (CAS) • Open revascularization, amputation, lower extremity thrombectomy • Duodenopancreatic surgery • Liver and biliary tract resection • Esophagectomy • Repair of intestinal perforation Adrenal surgery • Cystectomy • Pneumectomy (VATS or open surgery) • Liver and lung transplantation	>5%

VATS video-assisted thoracoscopic surgery, *CAS* carotid artery stenting, *CEA* carotid endarterectomy

8.3.2.2 Cardiac Arrhythmias

Arrhythmias are a significant cause of morbidity and mortality during the perioperative period. Common arrhythmias such as atrial fibrillation (AF) and ventricular tachycardia (VT) often indicate underlying structural heart disease. Therefore, the detection of such arrhythmias before surgery should prompt specialized cardiologic evaluation.

Table 8.9 Perioperative management of cardiac diseases [10]

Pathology	Preoperative management	Class of recommendation	Level of evidence
Hypertension	• In patients with chronic hypertension undergoing elective NCS, it is recommended to avoid wide fluctuations in blood pressure, especially hypotension, in the perioperative period	I	A
	• In patients to undergo elective major surgery with relief of PAS >180 mmHg or PAD >110 mmHg, deferral of surgery may be considered		
	• Preoperative screening for hypertension-related organ damage and CV risk factors is recommended in newly diagnosed hypertensive patients scheduled for elective high-risk NCS	I	C
	• In the context of isolated hypertension deferring or canceling surgery to perform additional cardiac testing is generally unnecessary or undesirable	III	C
Heart failure (HF)	• In patients with HF suspected or stabilized, assessed by NYHA (New York Heart Association) class, scheduled for intermediate- or high-risk non-cardiac surgery, transthoracic echocardiographic evaluation of left ventricular function and/or NT-proBNP/BNP dosing is recommended	I	B
	• Pharmacological optimization with beta-blockers, ACE-inhibitors/sartanics, anti-aldosteronics, and diuretics is recommended	I	A
	• In patients with HF undergoing NCS, it is recommended that blood volume status and signs of organ perfusion be regularly assessed	I	C
Arrhythmias	• In patients with drug-controlled supraventricular tachycardia, it is recommended to continue using antiarrhythmic drugs during the perioperative period	I	C
	• In patients with atrial fibrillation + acute or worsening hemodynamic instability to undergo NCS, emergency electrical cardioversion is recommended	I	B
	• In patients with symptomatic, monomorphic, sustained VT that recurs despite optimal medical therapy, ablation of the arrhythmia before elective NCS is recommended	I	B

(continued)

Table 8.9 (continued)

Pathology	Preoperative management	Class of recommendation	Level of evidence
Ischemic pathology	• In patients undergoing percutaneous myocardial revascularization (PTCA) with a metal stent (BMS), elective non-cardiac surgery can be performed a minimum of 4 weeks after stent placement and ideally 3 months after implantation	I	B
	• In patients undergoing percutaneous myocardial revascularization (PTCA) with a medicated stent (DES), elective non-cardiac surgery can be performed from 1 year after implantation or 6 months in the case of the latest DES	I	B
	• In patients who have had recent balloon dilatation angioplasty, elective non-cardiac surgery can be performed at least 2 weeks after the procedure	I	B
	• If PTCA before NCS is indicated, next-generation DES is recommended over BMS and balloon angioplasty	I	A
	• Prior myocardial revascularization before high-risk surgery in patients with stable/asymptomatic heart disease may be considered depending on the perfusion deficit induced by surgical stress		
	• Myocardial revascularization before intermediate- and low-risk surgery and in patients with stable heart disease is not recommended	III	B
	• Surgical priority should be discussed by a multidisciplinary *team*, in case of patients who need both urgent revascularization and non-cardiac surgery that cannot be deferred		

Table 8.9 (continued)

Pathology	Preoperative management	Class of recommendation	Level of evidence
Valvular pathology	• Clinical and echocardiographic evaluation (if not recently performed) is recommended in all patients with known or suspected VHD who are scheduled for elective intermediate- or high-risk NCS	I	C
	• Aortic valve repair (surgical or TAVI) is recommended in symptomatic patients with severe aortic stenosis who are scheduled for elective NCS surgery at intermediate or high risk	I	C
	• In patients with symptomatic severe or asymptomatic severe aortic insufficiency and LVESD >50 mm or resting LVEF ≤50%, valve surgery is recommended before elective intermediate- or high-risk NCS	I	C
	• In patients with moderate to severe rheumatic mitral stenosis and symptoms or SPAP >50 mmHg, valve surgery (percutaneous or surgical mitral commissurotomy) is recommended before elective intermediate- or high-risk NCS	I	C
Cerebrovascular pathology	• Preoperative carotid and cerebral imaging is recommended in patients with a history of TIA or stroke in the previous 6 months and who have not undergone ipsilateral revascularization	I	C

NCS non-cardiac surgery, *LVESD* left ventricular end-systolic diameter, *LVEF* left ventricular ejection fraction, *SPAP* systolic pulmonary artery pressure

Patients with implanted pacemaker (PMK) or pacemaker-defibrillator (PMK-I-CD) devices can undergo surgery safely with appropriate precautions. In the preoperative evaluation of these patients, it is important to investigate the reasons behind the device implantation, the frequency of device check-up (annual for PMK or semestral for PMK-I-CD), and the most recent check-up that confirms the proper functioning of the device, battery status, and device settings. In cases where an ICD is present, a preoperative cardiological evaluation is advisable. This ensures that the device can be safely deactivated, reconnected, and/or reevaluated in the postoperative period if considered necessary.

8.3.2.3 Ischemic Disease

The primary goal of prophylactic myocardial revascularization is to prevent potentially fatal perioperative myocardial infarction. Although this procedure is highly effective in treating severe coronary artery stenosis, it does not prevent the rupture of unstable plaques caused by surgical stress, which is responsible for at least half of all fatal perioperative myocardial infarctions. Therefore, the timing of any preoperative revascularization should be discussed in a multidisciplinary meeting involving cardiologists and surgeons. This discussion should also consider the patient's current or planned use of antiplatelet medications and the necessary safety period before elective surgery.

8.3.2.4 Valvular Disease

Patients with valvular disease face an elevated risk of perioperative cardiovascular complications when undergoing non-cardiac surgery. The extent of this risk varies depending on the specific type and severity of the valvular disease, as well as the nature of the non-cardiac surgical procedure. Optimal treatment planning, even with the availability of new minimally invasive procedures, needs the collaboration of a multidisciplinary team including anesthesiologists, cardiologists, heart surgeons, and surgeons.

8.3.2.5 When to Ask for a Cardiological Evaluation?

The decision to request a preoperative cardiological evaluation should be based on criteria that demonstrate effectiveness in reducing the risk of complications. In general, cardiological evaluations for non-cardiac surgery are meaningful only when the cardiologist's opinion is likely to impact the patient's clinical management or the planned anesthesiological and surgical approach. According to recent ESC/ESAIC guidelines, a cardiological evaluation should be considered in the following cases:

1. Presence of predictors of major cardiologic risk, including unstable coronary syndromes (e.g., recent myocardial infarction or unstable angina), congestive heart failure, significant valvular disease (especially aortic stenosis), and hemodynamically significant heart rhythm disorders.
2. High complexity of the planned surgery, which needs proper pharmacological preparation and close postoperative monitoring, particularly within the first 72 h following the procedure.

Table 8.10 provides a summary of the indications for requesting preoperative cardiological evaluation.

Additionally, it is important to consider the necessity of cardiological opinion prior to anesthesia for patients who are on chronic home drug treatment with medications that may have cardiotoxic or cardio-depressant effects. This includes patients receiving tricyclic antidepressants or chemotherapy drugs such as doxorubicin and trastuzumab.

Trans-thoracic Echocardiogram

Routine resting trans-thoracic echocardiography for the evaluation of left ventricular function is not recommended for all patients, especially for asymptomatic ones. Generally, resting echocardiography for assessing left ventricular function is

Table 8.10 The appropriateness of preoperative cardiological evaluation [3]

Predictors	Cardiological risk of surgery		
	High	Intermediate	Low
Higher	Yes	Yes	Postpone surgery
Intermediate	Yes	At discretion (METs <4)[a]	No
Minor	At discretion (METs <4)[a]	Upon specific indication	No
None	No	No	No

[a] If METS >4, cardiology consultation is probably unnecessary [16]

indicated for symptomatic patients who are being considered for high-risk surgery following a cardiological evaluation.

Stress Test

A stress test is not necessary for patients without predictors of cardiac risk who are undergoing low- or intermediate-risk cardiovascular surgery. However, in high-risk patients or high-risk surgery, the decision to perform a preoperative stress test should be made according to the referring cardiologist, following the latest guidelines from ESC/ESAIC.

8.4 Management of Home Drug Therapy

Management of home drug therapy is crucial in the context of preoperative care. The patient's cardiological diseases are often associated with the use of medications, and it is necessary to determine whether certain medications should be discontinued or continued prior to anesthesia for the planned surgery.

Depending on the medication, temporary discontinuation may be required, while it is not recommended to discontinue other medications before surgery. Please refer to Table 8.11 for the recommended discontinuation times for commonly used medications in patients receiving chronic home therapy.

8.4.1 Management of Patients Undergoing Regional Anesthesia While on Anti-thrombotic Medication Treatment

In 2022, joint guidelines were published by the European Society of Anesthesiology and Intensive Care (ESAIC) and the European Society of Regional Anaesthesia (ESRA) regarding the management of anti-thrombotic therapy in patients undergoing loco-regional anesthesia. The primary objective of these guidelines was to minimize the risk of bleeding complications associated with regional neuroaxial anesthesia procedures (e.g., subarachnoid and epidural anesthesia) as well as superficial and deep peripheral nerve blocks. Nerve blocks were categorized as either high risk (neuroaxial and deep peripheral nerve blocks) or low risk (superficial peripheral nerve blocks) in terms of bleeding potential [17].

Table 8.11 Home medication withdrawal times in the case of non-cardiac elective surgery [10]

Timing of discontinuation of home medications in the case of non-cardiac elective surgery		
Home medications	Suspension time	Notes
ACE inhibitors and sartanics	>12 h when used in antihypertensive therapeutic scheme	
	They should not be discontinued when used in the treatment of heart failure	
Beta-blockers	• Continue chronic therapy in the perioperative period, maintaining it until surgery • Abrupt discontinuation of chronic therapy can be harmful • De novo therapy should not be undertaken on the same day as surgery	
Statins	Continue chronic therapy in the perioperative period	
Oral hypoglycemic agents (metformin, peptidase-4 inhibitors, GLP1-agonists, SGLT-2 cotransporter inhibitors)	24–48 h before surgery because of possible side effects, such as the onset of severe lactic acidosis	Goal: To ensure normal glyco-metabolic balance and minimize postoperative complications related to glycemic imbalance, taking into consideration that hyperglycemia represents a normal adaptive response of the patient to the stress that characterizes the perioperative period
Insulin	• Perioperative management can be carried out as per the home treatment until the evening before surgery • In case of overnight or fasting hypoglycemia → reduce the basal insulin dose by 20–30% • For patients with well-controlled type I diabetes mellitus → slight reduction in basal insulin dose by 10–20% • Prandial insulin boluses should be omitted once preoperative fasting has begun	For these patients, multidisciplinary management with the diabetologist following them even in the postoperative period is always advisable. Fast recovery or ERAS protocols that minimize preoperative fasting time and promote early re-feeding are always to be recommended
Corticosteroid medications (>5 days)	Do not discontinue home therapy (regardless of dosage and mode of intake—systemic or topical	Risk of inadequate cortisol production in the perioperative period if suspension

Table 8.11 (continued)

Timing of discontinuation of home medications in the case of non-cardiac elective surgery		
Home medications	Suspension time	Notes
Tricyclic antidepressants (TCAs)	Continuation of home therapy in the perioperative period is recommended in patients with major depression	As with any chronic therapy, however, the risk from decompensation of a severe, adequately treated condition due to discontinuation of therapy versus that of possible drug-related perioperative complications should be carefully evaluated and possibly shared with the referring psychiatrist
Selective serotonin re-uptake inhibitors (SSRIs)	There is insufficient data in the literature to justify their discontinuation	
Monoamine oxidase inhibitors (MAOIs)	It is recommended that irreversible MAOIs be discontinued at least 2 weeks before anesthesia, replacing them with reversible MAOIs to avoid flare-up of the underlying pathology	
Lithium	• Stop at least 72 h before surgery with the possibility of reintroduction of the drug, as per the home treatment, only if hemodynamic stability and normal serum electrolyte levels are present and if diet and oral fluid intake have been restored • Lithium therapy may be continued in patients to undergo minor surgery	
Hydroxychloroquine	≥ 2 weeks	The protocol should always be shared with the referring specialist
Cyclosporine	The day before surgery in case of general anesthesia	
Anti-TNF monoclonal antibodies (infliximab, Etanercept, adalimumab)	>2–3 weeks before surgery because of the risk of postoperative infectious complications	
Methotrexate	2 weeks before surgery and restart 1 week later	

For superficial nerve blocks, it is not generally necessary to discontinue anticoagulant and/or antiplatelet therapy, as bleeding complications are typically limited to bruising and ecchymosis. However, for deep peripheral nerve blocks, the consequences of bleeding can lead to neurovascular damage, while central blocks carry the risk of spinal hematoma, which if not promptly diagnosed (MRI being the gold standard) and treated can result in permanent and even life-threatening complications.

Table 8.12 provides recommendations for the management of chronic antithrombotic drug therapy in these scenarios.

Table 8.12 Management of anti-thrombotic drugs in nerve blocks at high risk of bleeding (deep peripheral blocks and neuroaxial blocks) [17]

Drugs and dose	Time since last intake before surgery	Target value of laboratory tests at the time of surgery	Time elapsed from surgery to next dose of drug	Antidote
Vitamin K anticoagulant inhibitors (VKAs)	Up to normalization of laboratory values: • Acenocoumarol: 3 days • Warfarin: 5 days • Frenprocumone: 7 days	INR (International Normalized Ratio) must be within normal limits		Prothrombin complex concentrate (PCC) based on INR value + Vitamin K (10 mg)
Low-dose oral anticoagulants (NAOs)	• Rivaroxaban, edoxaban: 24 h (30 h if CrCl <30 mL/min) • Apixaban: 36 h	No laboratory test		
High-dose oral anticoagulants (NAOs)	Rivaroxaban, edoxaban, apixaban: 72 h until normalization of laboratory values if CrCl <30 mL/min	Direct factor Xa antagonist (DXA) drug level <30 ng/mL Alternatively: anti-Xa ≤0.1 IU/mL	Low doses: about 6 h. Consider a longer interval in case of a difficult sting	
Low-dose dabigatran	48 h	No laboratory tests		Idarucizumab (monoclonal antibody fragment)
High-dose dabigatran	72 h or until normalization of laboratory values if CrCl <50 mL/min	Direct thrombin inhibitor (DTI) <30 ng/mL Alternatively: thrombin time should be normal	High doses: about 24 h	
Low-molecular weight heparin (LMWH) at low doses (enoxaparin < 4000 UI/day)	12 h (24 h if CrCl <30 mL/min)	No laboratory tests		No

High-dose low-molecular weight heparin (LMWH) (enoxaparin > 4000 UI/die or bidie)	24 h (48 h if CrCl <30 mL/min) or until normalization of laboratory values especially if CrCl <30 mL/min	Anti-Xa ≤0.1 IU/mL	VKA, NAO, high-dose LMWH, and high-dose UFH should not be administered if a deep neuroaxial or peripheral nerve catheter is in situ	No
Unfractionated heparin (UFH) at low doses (≤200 IU/kg/day s.c; ≤100 IU/kg/day e.v)	4 h	No laboratory tests	1 h but validated only for cardiovascular surgery	Protamine (sulfate or chloride)
High-dose unfractionated heparin (UFH)	Until the laboratory value is normal (about 6 h if e.v, 12 h if s.c)	Normal laboratory values for aPTT or anti-Xa (more accurate measure of activity) or ACT (activated clotting time)		
Fondaparinux low dose (≤2.5 mg/day)	36 h (72 h if CrCl <50 mL/min)	No laboratory tests		No
Fondaparinux high dose (>2.5 mg/day)	Until the laboratory value is normal (about 4 days)	Anti-Xa calibrated ≤0.1 IU/mL		No
Low-dose aspirin (≤200 mg/day)	0			
High-dose aspirin	Min 3 days (if normal platelet count), max 7 days (for surgery with high bleeding risk, e.g., intracranial, spinal, or vitreoretinal neurosurgery)	Consider normal platelet count and thromboelastogram	6 h	Platelet transfusion

(continued)

Table 8.12 (continued)

Drugs and dose	Time since last intake before surgery	Target value of laboratory tests at the time of surgery	Time elapsed from surgery to next dose of drug	Antidote
P2Y12 inhibitors	• Tigagrelor: 5 days • Clopidogrel:5–7 days • Prasugrel: 7 days		• Clopidogrel 75 mg: 0 h • Clopidogrel 300 mg: 2 days • Prasugrel and ticagrelor: 24 h	Platelet transfusion
Low-dose aspirin + anticoagulant	Aspirin: 0 + interval time specific to anticoagulant drug used	Specific laboratory tests based on the anticoagulant used	Low-dose aspirin: routinely administered according to therapeutic schedule Anticoagulant: in accordance with therapeutic anticoagulation guidelines (approximately 24 h)	
Low-dose aspirin + antiplatelet (double antiplatelet)	Aspirin: 0 + specific interval time for antiplatelet drug used	Consider specific laboratory tests based on the antiplatelet used		

8.5   Assessment of the Respiratory System

Postoperative pulmonary complications are common adverse events that significantly increase morbidity and mortality rates, especially among patients with pre-existing lung diseases. These complications can be classified as major (acute respiratory failure, need for ventilation and/or intubation for ≥ 48 h, pneumonia, postoperative arrhythmias and/or heart failure, hemodynamic instability in patients with primary vascular disease, clinical worsening of Obstructive Sleep Apnea Syndrome—OSAS) or minor (clinically significant atelectasis, purulent tracheobronchitis, bronchospasm, and/or exacerbation of underlying chronic disease), depending on their potential for mortality [18].

A thorough history and physical examination, followed by targeted diagnostic testing, are essential for assessing the risk of postoperative pulmonary complications during preoperative evaluation. Risk factors for these complications could be patient-related (age, tobacco exposure, COPD, New York Heart Association class II and/or pulmonary hypertension, moderate/severe OSAS, nutritional status) or related to the surgical procedure (surgical site and duration of surgery, surgical regimen—elective, emergency, general anesthesia with neuromuscular blockers).

It is now widely recognized by Enhanced Recovery After Surgery (ERAS) protocols that smoking cessation for at least 4 weeks before surgery reduces postoperative complications and associated mortality. If possible and appropriate for the surgical condition, patients should be given sufficient time to reduce their risk by abstaining from tobacco use starting from the preoperative anesthesia examination.

Routine preoperative chest radiography and spirometry tests are not recommended for patients undergoing extra-thoracic surgery, either in obstructive or restrictive respiratory syndromes, as they rarely impact perioperative management. Instead, preoperative blood gas analysis may be useful to assess baseline functional condition and determine the need for specialist evaluation/optimization.

Screening for Obstructive Sleep Apnea Syndrome (OSAS) should be performed for all candidates undergoing surgery or invasive procedures under sedation, considering the high prevalence of the condition and the number of undiagnosed patients at admission. The STOP-Bang questionnaire is recommended as an easy-to-assess tool for OSAS risk screening (Table 8.13). For patients with a STOP-Bang score greater

Table 8.13 STOP-Bang Questionnaire [19]

Snoring	Does he snore loudly enough to be heard with the door closed?	1
Tiredness	Do you often feel tired/sleepy during daylight hours?	1
Observed apnea	Has enyone observed you stop breathing??	1
Pressure	Do you suffer from hypertension?	1
Body mass index	BMI > 35 kg/m^2	1
Age	Is h/she over 50 years old?	1
Neck circumference	Neck circumference >41 cm for women and >43 cm for men	1
Gender	Male gender	1

Apnea risk: 0–2: Low risk; 3–4: Intermediate risk; ≥ 5: High risk than 5, further diagnostic investigation by overnight pulse oximetry is advisable, with polysomnography reserved for cases where nocturnal desaturations indicate the need for correction with overnight ventilatory therapy. Stratifying postoperative risk related to sleep apnea requires consideration of the severity of OSAS (diagnosed or suspected), type of surgery, type of anesthesia and expected postoperative opioid requirement. Individualized perioperative management based on these factors optimizes time, resources, and, most importantly, patient safety [19–21].

The use of home Continuous Positive Airway Pressure (CPAP), if properly adapted and tolerated, is beneficial for improving preoperative conditions in patients with OSAS. These benefits can also be extended to the postoperative period when CPAP therapy is administered in the recovery room and in the inpatient ward. Severe cases or situations where nocturnal ventilation is not possible may require an ICU stay, which can be anticipated during the pre-anesthesia visit, optimizing the organization of the surgical pathway [22].

8.6 The Preoperative Approach to the Geriatric/ Fragile Patient

Geriatric patients, who are becoming increasingly common in the hospitalized population, are characterized by increased mortality and morbidity, both in elective surgery and, especially, in emergency/urgent surgery [23, 24]. The following factors should be considered for surgical risk assessment:

- Functional status and level of independence: It is necessary to assess the patient's ability to be independent in daily activities.
- Comorbidities: Chronic conditions are found in over 50% of patients aged over 70 years. Advanced age and comorbidities contribute to reduced resistance to surgical stress, making older patients more vulnerable to cardiac and respiratory complications, resulting in increased intra- and postoperative mortality rates.
- Drug therapy: Elderly patients generally take multiple medications, and this, combined with the physiological decline in renal function, increases the risk of accumulation and overdose.
- Cognitive dysfunction: Baseline cognitive assessment should be performed in all patients aged over 65 years.
- Depression: Screening should be conducted during the anesthesiological visit to identify patients at risk of depression.
- Risk of postoperative delirium: It depends on the presence of risk factors, the type of surgery, and the perioperative management. Postoperative delirium is responsible for prolonged hospital stays and increased morbidity and mortality. Preventive strategies should be implemented for high-risk patients.
- Sensory impairment: Age-related sensory deficits (visual, auditory) that accompany the aging process significantly impact the patient's evaluation phase and are risk factors for postoperative delirium and depression.

- Malnutrition: Malnutrition is observed in at least 6% of patients over the age of 70, rising to 40% in hospitalized or nursing home patients. This phenomenon is associated with an increased risk of infectious and non-infectious complications, such as postoperative delirium, prolonged hospitalization, and wound dehiscence.
- Frailty: Frailty is defined as a multisystem disorder that is age-dependent (but not always) and caused by reduced resistance to stressful agents. It is associated with physiological decline, comorbidity, disability, risk of death, and increased perioperative risk. Early recognition of key elements of frailty during the anesthesiological evaluation (e.g., malnutrition, inappropriate therapies, the need for psychological and social support) allows targeted interventions to be implemented.

Validated screening tools and rating scales for different factors, along with collaboration with geriatric specialists, aid in the management of frail patients in a multimodal setting, starting from the preoperative evaluation.

8.7 ASA PS Score and International Risk Scores

Upon completing the patient's comprehensive medical history, clinical examination, laboratory tests, and diagnostic assessments, it is possible to assign the patient to one of the five classes of the American Society of Anesthesiologists—Physical Status (ASA PS Score—2015 version). This classification helps to estimate the patient's anesthesiological risk. Additionally, the risk of perioperative complications within 30 days after surgery can be estimated using clinical risk scores, which are becoming more widely used and available [25].

8.7.1 ASA PS Score

The occurrence of complications during the perioperative period is influenced by both the planned surgical procedure and the presence of pre-existing medical conditions. The ASA PS Score (American Society of Anesthesiologists—Physical Status, 2015 version) is an internationally recognized classification system that defines patients based on their overall health status and comorbidities. It provides valuable information regarding the patient's physical condition and correlates with the anesthesiological risk, although it does not directly measure it (Table 8.14). Additionally, the surgical regimen (elective, urgent, or emergency) in which the procedure is performed represents an additional factor that can further increase the risk of perioperative complications [25, 26].

8.7.2 International Risk Scores

In recent years, various risk scores have been developed based on multivariate analyses of observational data. These scores aim to establish a relationship between the

Table 8.14 ASA-PS classification

Description	Class ASA-PS
No organic, biochemical, or psychiatric impairment—healthy patient (no acute or chronic disease, no tobacco habit, no or minimal alcohol consumption)	I
Mild systemic pathology related or unrelated to the reason for surgery (e.g., smoking habit, moderate alcohol consumption, moderate hypertension, well-controlled non-insulin-dependent diabetes mellitus, mild lung disease, mild renal failure, $30 < BMI < 40$, pregnant woman[a])	II
Severe systemic pathology (with organ damage) but not disabling related or unrelated to the reason for surgery (e.g., alcohol dependence/abuse, history (>3 months) of myocardial infarction, TIA or ischemic heart disease ± coronary stents, implanted pacemaker, moderate reduction in left ventricular ejection fraction, insulin-dependent diabetes mellitus, chronic obstructive pulmonary disease, renal failure on dialysis, BMI ≥40, active hepatitis)	III
Severe systemic pathology impairing survival regardless of surgery (e.g., history (<3 months) of myocardial infarction, TIA, or ischemic heart disease ± coronary stents, heart failure with severe reduction in left ventricular ejection fraction, unstable angina, severe cardiac valvular dysfunction, severe respiratory or renal failure not on dialysis, decompensated diabetes mellitus with severe complications in other organs, myocarditis, sepsis, disseminated intravascular coagulation)	IV
Dying patient with expected exitus within 24 h who undergoes surgery as an *extreme ratio* (abdominal/thoracic aortic aneurysm rupture with hypovolemic shock, head injury with cerebral edema or massive intra-cranial bleeding with "mass effect," severe polytrauma, massive pulmonary embolism, intestinal ischemia)	V
Any surgery that cannot be deferred and that does not allow for a complete preoperative evaluation of the patient and correction of any clinical abnormalities	E[b]

Excerpted and revised from: https://www.asahq.org/standards-and-guidelines/asa-physical-status-classification-system

[a] Although pregnancy is not a disease, the physiological state of the pregnant woman is significantly altered, and hence the assignment of ASA 2 for a woman with an uncomplicated pregnancy

[b] An *emergency* is when a delay in treating the patient would result in a significantly increased threat to life or part of the body

planned surgical procedure, clinical and laboratory characteristics of the patient, and the occurrence of mortality and morbidity in the perioperative period. Table 8.15 provides a summary of the most commonly used risk scores. By considering multiple variables included in these scores, an integrated analysis can provide individualized estimates of potential postoperative complications. These estimates range from the risk of mortality to the likelihood of experiencing major cardiovascular, infectious, pulmonary, or acute kidney injury complications. The scores can also predict the need for re-intervention, the involvement of nursing and rehabilitation staff in patient management, and the days of hospital stay [27].

Table 8.15 Surgical risk calculators [10, 27]

	Portsmouth Physiological and Operative Score for enUmeration of Mortality and Morbidity (P-POSSUM) (1998)	Revised Cardiac Risk Index (RCRI)—Lee's Score (1999)	Surgical Risk Calculator (2011)	The American College of Surgery National Surgical Quality Improvement Program (ACS NSQIP) (2013)	Surgical Outcome Risk Tool (SORT) (2014)	The American University of Beirut (AUB)-HAS2 Cardiovascular Risk Index (2019)
Outcomes	% 30-day mortality and morbidity	Myocardial infarction, cardiac arrest and death at 30 days	Myocardial infarction, intraoperative and 30-day cardiac arrest	Serious complications and any complications at 30 days	30-day mortality	Death, myocardial infarction, or stroke at 30 days
Link	http://www.riskprediction.org.uk/index-pp.php	https://www.mdcalc.com/revised-cardiacrisk-index-preoperative-risk	http://www.surgicalriskcalculator.com/miorcardiacarrest	https://riskcalculator.facs.org	http://www.sortsurgery.com	

8.8 Conclusions

In conclusion, it is evident that preoperative assessment plays a crucial role in ensuring the quality and safety of surgical and anesthesiological care for patients across all age groups. The guidelines emphasize the importance of a comprehensive patient assessment, which combines clinical risk factors and preoperative test outcomes with the anticipated stress of the surgical procedure and associated risks. The ultimate aim is to perform an individualized risk assessment that enables the optimization of the patient's perioperative conditions. Therefore, we can strive to minimize perioperative complications, subsequently reducing the associated social and healthcare costs. Moreover, this approach allows for a more efficient use of available resources.

References

1. Miller RD, et al. Miller's anesthesia. Elsevier Health Sciences Division; 2019.
2. Groves P. Handbook of clinical anaesthesia. 2nd ed. CRC Press Taylor & Francis Group; 2018.
3. Raffaele De Gaudio A, et al. Anesthesia, resuscitation, intensive care, pain (ARTID). Idelson Gnocchi; 2020.
4. Longnecker ED, et al. Anesthesiology. McGraw Hill Education; 2018.
5. Tong JG, et al. Fourth Consensus Guidelines for the management of postoperative nausea and vomiting. Anesth Analg. 2020;131(2):411–48. https://doi.org/10.1213/ANE.00000000004833.
6. Law JA, et al. Canadian Airway Focus Group updated consensus-based recommendations for management of the difficult airway: Part 2. Planning and implementing safe management of the patient with an anticipated difficult airway. Can J Anesth. 2021;68:1405–36. https://doi.org/10.1007/s12630-021-02007-0.
7. Faramarzi E, et al. Upper lip bite test for prediction of difficult airway: a systematic review. Pak J Med Sci. 2018;34(4):1019–23. https://doi.org/10.12669/pjms.344.15364.
8. Corrente A, et al. A new simple score for prediction of difficult laryngoscopy: the EL.GA+ score. Anaesthesiol Intens Ther. 2020;52:206–14. https://doi.org/10.5114/ait.2020.97775.
9. Stutz EW, et al. Mallampati score. StatPearls Publishing; 2022. PMID: 36256766
10. Halvorsen S, et al. 2022 ESC Guidelines on cardiovascular assessment and management of patients undergoing non-cardiac surgery: developed by the task force for cardiovascular assessment and management of patients undergoing non-cardiac surgery of the European Society of Card. Eur Heart J. 2022;43:3826–924. https://doi.org/10.1093/eurheartj/ehac270.
11. De Hert S, et al. Pre-operative evaluation of adults undergoing elective noncardiac surgery. Updated guideline from the European Society of Anaesthesiology. Eur J Anaesthesiol. 2018;35:407–65. https://doi.org/10.1097/EJA.0000000000817.
12. Lee A, et al. 2014 ACC/AHA guideline on perioperative cardiovascular evaluation and management of patients undergoing noncardiac surgery. Circulation. 2014;130:278–333. https://doi.org/10.1161/CIR.0000000000106.
13. Cartabellotta A, et al. Guidelines for the appropriate request of preoperative tests in elective surgery. Evidence. 2017;9:1–4.
14. Excellence C, et al. Routine preoperative testing for elective surgery: NICE (2016). BJU Int. 2018;121(1):12–6. https://doi.org/10.1111/bju.14079.
15. Admass BA, et al. Preoperative investigations for elective surgical patients in a resource limited setting: systematic review. Ann Med Surg. 2022; https://doi.org/10.1016/j.amsu.2022.104777.

16. de Almeida Mendes M, et al. Metabolic equivalent of task (METs) thresholds as an indicator of physical activity intensity. PLoS One. 2018; https://doi.org/10.1371/journal.pone.0200701.
17. Kietaibl S, et al. Regional anasthesia in patiens on antithrombotic drugs: Joit ESAIC/ESRA guidelines. Eur J Anaesthesiol. 2022;39:100–32. https://doi.org/10.1097/EJA.000000001600.
18. Cheng MCF, et al. Pre-operative screening for sleep disordered breathing: obstructive sleep apnoea and beyond. Breathe. 2022; https://doi.org/10.1183/20734735.0072-2022.
19. Chung F, et al. STOP-Bang questionnaire: a practical approach to screen for obstructive sleep apnea. Chest J. 2016;149:631–8. https://doi.org/10.1378/chest.15-0903.
20. Cataldo R, et al. The perioperative management of the patient with obstructive sleep apnea syndrome (OSA). SIAARTI Good Clinical Practices; 2019. www.siaarti.it/standardclinici
21. Ojeda D, et al. STOP-BANG questionnaire as predictor of difficult airway management during anesthesia. Rev Méd Chile. 2022;150:450–7. https://doi.org/10.4067/S0034-98872022000400450.
22. Berezin L, et al. The effectiveness of positive airway pressure therapy in reducing postoperative adverse outcomes in surgical patients with obstructive sleep apnea: a systematic review and meta-analysis. J Clin Anesth. 2023; https://doi.org/10.1016/j.jclinane.2022.110993.
23. Cappe M, et al. Preoperative frailty screening, assessment and management. Curr Opin Anesthesiol. 2023;36:83–8. https://doi.org/10.1097/ACO.00000000001221.
24. De Blasio E, et al. Perioperative strategies: taking care of the elderly with severe comorbidities and advanced stage of disease with acute surgical pathology. SIAARTI Good Clinical Practices- SIAARTI/SIC sharing; 2019. www.siaarti.it/standardclinici
25. Hurwitz EE, et al. Adding examples to the ASA-Physical Status classification improves correct assignments to patients. Anesthesiology. 2017;126:614–22. https://doi.org/10.1097/ALN.000000001541.
26. Mayhew D, et al. A review of ASA physical status-historical perspectives and modern developments. Anaesthesia. 2019;74:373–9. https://doi.org/10.1111/anae.14569.
27. Prytherch, et al. POSSUM and Portsmouth POSSUM for predicting mortality. Br J Surg. 1998;85:1217–20. https://doi.org/10.1046/j.1365-2168.1998.00840.x.

Purification Techniques

9

Luigi Tritapepe, Benedetta Cirulli, Stefania Bove,
Naike Amato, and Aurora Smeriglia

9.1 Introduction

Insufficient organ function inevitably leads to the loss of the depurative/metabolic capacity to which that organ is deputed. In this case, and especially in the critically ill patient in the ICU, it is essential to carry out a purification through the use of dedicated filters that can normalize the parameters altered by the organ dysfunction and, through this depurative bridge phase, allow the restoration of the native function of the organ itself. This can result in the reversibility of the pathology, or if it becomes chronic, chronic purification can be considered.

The most common case involves the kidney, but the lung and liver can also go through situations requiring extracorporeal depurative support.

9.2 Acute Renal Failure

The incidence of acute renal failure is steadily increasing in hospitalized patients, especially in ICU inpatients. This incidence is estimated to be around 5–20% with peaks of up to 60% in ICU patients. The presence of acute renal failure in the critically ill contributes to increased morbidity and mortality. In addition, the use of the

L. Tritapepe (✉)
Sapienza University of Rome, Rome, Italy

AO San Camillo Forlanini, Rome, Italy
e-mail: luigi.tritapepe@uniroma1.it

B. Cirulli · S. Bove · N. Amato
AO San Camillo-Forlanini, Rome, Italy

A. Smeriglia
School of Specialization in Anaesthesia and Intensive Care, Sapienza University of Rome, Rome, Italy

149

D. Chiumello (ed.), *Practical Trends in Anesthesia and Intensive Care 2022*,
https://doi.org/10.1007/978-3-031-43891-2_9

many new biomarkers of renal damage now makes it possible to highlight those situations, still clinically silent, of organic damage with the prospect of acute renal failure (subclinical acute kidney damage).

The definition of acute kidney injury (AKI) is complex and can be identified as the loss of depurative homeostasis of the kidney with increased azotemia and creatininemia (Cr), as well as dysionemia, water retention with oligoanuria. Clearly, such a clinical definition appears somewhat crude to make the definition of AKI homogeneous and allow effective staging of the condition.

Expert groups in numerous international fora have attempted to use identifiable criteria that have resulted in three basic classifications of kidney damage, RIFLE, AKIN, and KDIGO consensus expression.

The RIFLE criteria are based on changes in serum creatinine and urinary output, identifying classes of severity and outcome (risk, injury, failure, loss, end-stage renal disease) based on the duration of renal dysfunction/failure.

To make the intercept of renal injury even more sensitive, AKIN (Acute Kidney Injury Network) used minor changes in serum creatinine alteration, but considered rapid within the 48-h time frame. The use of renal replacement therapy (RRT) regardless of changes in diuresis and creatinine place the patient in an advanced degree of severity.

A review of previous classifications generated the Kidney Disease: Improving Global Outcomes (KDIGO) classification, which defines and identifies the evolution of AKI by considering rapid temporal changes in creatinine (48 h), acute reduction in diuresis, but also reduction in glomerular filtrate (GFR) in the previous week (Table 9.1).

Table 9.1 Classification criteria of AKI

	Serum creatinine			Diuresis
RIFLE	*AKIN*	*KDIGO*		
Risk Cr increase × 1.5 from baseline or reduction of GFR > 25%	*Stage 1* Cr increase × 1.5–2 from baseline or increase Cr ≥0.3 mg/dL	*Stage 1* Cr increase × 1.5–1.9 from baseline or increase Cr ≥0.3 mg/dL		<0.5 mL/kg/h from 6 to 12 h
Injury Cr increase × 2 from baseline or reduction of GFR > 50%	*Stage 2* Cr increase × 2–3 from baseline	*Stage 2* Cr increase × 2–2.9 from baseline		<0.5 mg/kg/h ≥ 12 h
Failure Cr increase × 3 from baseline or Cr >4 mg/dL with increase >0.5 mg/dL from baseline or reduction of GFR > 75%	*Stage 3* Cr increase >3 from baseline or Cr ≥4 mg/dL with increase from baseline of 0.5 mg/dL opp. RRT	*Stage 3* Cr ≥ 3 increase from baseline or Cr ≥4 mg/dL or RRT		<0.3 mg/kg/h ≥ 24 h or anuria ≥12 h
Loss Complete loss of kidney function >4 weeks				
End-stage renal disease Complete loss of renal function >3 months				

A stage of subclinical AKI, unrevealable through changes in many biomarkers, identifies what is now called renal damage that, in particular functional (hypovolemia) or metabolic (iodinated contrast, drugs, inflammatory cytokines in sepsis) situations, results in a temporary reduction of GFR with increased Cr and reduced diuresis that can return to normal if early interventions to prevent renal damage are put in place.

The etiology of AKI should be sought in a multifactorial origin that in the ICU patient gathers around hypoperfusion, inflammation, and renal toxicity, which are frequent simultaneously, rather than in isolation, in many syndromic pictures.

The state of shock represents the pathophysiological paradigm to describe the mechanisms of AKI, and especially septic shock, through immunogenic inflammatory and cytokine damage, which determines the most important renal alterations with distant consequences up to multiorgan dysfunction.

Thus, sepsis-induced AKI, cross-talk syndromes (hepato-, cardio-, and lung-renal), and perioperative AKI represent the most commonly represented pictures in the ICU where conservative treatments such as restoring volemia (with balanced crystalloids), optimizing O_2 availability, and maintaining MAP > 65 mmHg are not always successful in avoiding the use of depurative therapies.

9.3 Renal Replacement Therapies

The purpose of renal replacement therapies (RRTs) is precisely to replace the depurative/emunctory function of the kidney through the use of semi-permeable membranes (filters) that can remove solutes and water, but also adsorb toxic substances.

Today in the ICU it is possible to use very simplified machines for continuous purification in cases of acute renal failure that consist of an extracorporeal circuit equipped with a filter and operated by a blood pump that makes it possible to use the simple venous route.

The key aspect is precisely the filter composed of biocompatible hollow fibers consisting of a porous membrane that interfaces with the patient's blood.

The characteristics of the fibers (length, inner radius, thickness, and porosity) determine their efficiency potential.

Some characteristics of the constituent membranes of filters such as the filtration coefficient, given by the ratio of ultrafiltration flux to applied transmembrane pressure, should be known.

This coefficient distinguishes high-flow (coefficient > 25 mL/h/mmHg), medium-flow (coefficient between 10 and 25 mL/h/mmHg), and low-flow (coefficient < 10 mL/h/mmHg) membranes with regard to water permeability.

Then there is the mass transport coefficient, which represents the resistive limitation to the diffusion of a solute across the entire membrane surface expressed in mL/min, and the more important Sieving coefficient, which is the ratio of the concentration of a solute removed through a convective mechanism to the average of its concentrations at the inlet and outlet of the hemofilter. The Sieving coefficient is specific to each solute and each membrane and can vary with the changes the membrane undergoes during treatment.

It is then important to know the membrane cut-off represented by the molecular weight of the smallest solute not affected by transmembrane removal. It depends essentially on the porosity of the membrane. High cut-off membranes are those with Sieving coefficient for albumin >0 before exposure to blood.

During dialysis therapy, membrane performance is reduced as a result of the progressive loss of permeability due to protein deposition with partial pore obstruction due to coagulative phenomena and formation of a protein layer on the inner membrane surface with increased transmembrane pressure, which should be carefully monitored.

The different methods of CRRT (continuous renal replacement therapy) basically all work by drawing, from a double-lumen central venous catheter, blood that flows through a circuit and a purifying filter and back into the patient by the action of a pump.

In the filter, blood is purified and concentrated depending on the flow rate, which varies from 20 to 400 mL/min depending on venous access. It is necessary to anticoagulate the blood (usually with heparin) to avoid coagulation of the filter, which would make dialysis treatment ineffective, both because of the reduced performance of the filter and the shortened filter life.

Through the filter, purification (transport of water and solutes) occurs by three different mechanisms:

(a) Diffusion (solute transport)
(b) Ultrafiltration (water transport)
(c) Convection (solute transport)

Through diffusion, solutes are removed according to a concentration gradient that also depends on the characteristics of the membrane and the diffusivity coefficient of the solute. This is the working mechanism of hemodialysis.

Diffusive exchange occurs between blood and dialysate flowing counter-currently with the possibility of bidirectional passage of solutes according to a concentration gradient.

The removal rate of a solute depends on its molecular weight, the concentration gradient across the semi-permeable membrane, the surface area of the hemofilter, the rate of blood flow, and the duration of treatment. Small solutes are effectively removed by hemodialysis.

Water passes through membrane pores undergoing hydrostatic and osmotic forces that result in a blood-filter pressure gradient, called transmembrane pressure. Ultrafiltration is thus influenced by membrane properties (ultrafiltration coefficient) and transmembrane pressure. Ultrafiltration results in fluid removal and can be an isolated method to achieve a negative water balance, with solute removal in terms of mass rather than concentration.

Convection, on the other hand, results in the passage of solutes entrained by ultrafiltration fluid movement due to the transmembrane pressure gradient (hydrostatic and osmotic). Clearly, only solutes with a smaller size than the porosity of the membrane will pass through.

The method that allows simultaneous removal of fluids and solutes by convection is hemofiltration.

This method does not use dialysis fluid, but basically removes plasma volume that can also be partly replaced to avoid plasma solute concentration. Reinfusion of solutions can occur before or after the filter (predilution or postdilution) with different efficacy on solute removal and complications (more effective postdilution, but higher filter hemoconcentration).

The combination of hemodialysis with hemofiltration generates the method of hemodiafiltration in which diffusive and convective mechanisms are involved.

It involves the use of highly permeable membranes and the need for reinfusion in both pre- and postdilution.

In addition to convective and diffusive purification mechanisms, solutes can be removed from the blood by either selective adsorption or adhesion to the filter membrane. Certain physicochemical characteristics of membranes allow the adhesion of particular solutes by forming particular cartridges characterized by the amount of specific molecule adsorbed. These particular cartridges allow the removal of specific molecules of large molecular weight by hemoperfusion (on whole blood) or plasmaperfusion (when the method is applied on plasma alone after plasmaseparation).

Hemoperfusion can be combined with other dialysis techniques so as to allow removal of toxins, poisons, cytokines, uremic toxins, hepatotoxic substances, etc. during treatments for AKI.

9.4 How Does an RRT Work?

Based on the frequency and duration of treatments, we have three modes of purification therapy:

(a) Intermittent RRTs
(b) Hybrid RRTs
(c) Continuous RRT (CRRT)

Intermittent therapies include intermittent hemodialysis, intermittent hemofiltration, intermittent hemodiafiltration, and intermittent high-flow hemodialysis.

Interspersed purification sessions (3–4/week) for short periods (3–6 h) are very effective in the rapid removal of water and solutes with minimal need for anticoagulation. Conditio sine qua non is the hemodynamic stability of the patient as rapid filtration of a large amount of plasma exposes the patient to hemodynamic instability.

Hybrid therapies combine the advantages of intermittent and continuous techniques, seeking to minimize, for both, side effects.

In fact, as in CRRT, they use low filtration flows suitable for hemodynamically unstable patients with restrained anticoagulation. This associates the efficacy of CRRTs while having shorter treatment times.

Hybrid methods include prolonged low-efficiency dialysis, slow daily dialysis, intermittent prolonged daily RRT, extended daily dialysis, dialysis with extended daily ultrafiltration, extended dialysis, and accelerated venous-venous hemofiltration. Solute removal occurs by diffusion, although convective mechanisms may be associated.

Prolonged low-efficiency dialysis (SLED) is a widely used method in the ICU because with reduced flows of blood and dialysate, it succeeds in 10–12 h to produce purification benefits, leaving the patient free for the rest of the hours for other therapies (physiotherapy, handling, diagnostics, etc.).

CRRTs provide the greatest hemodynamic stability, fluid removal well tolerated by the ICU patient with a very balanced electrolyte redistribution. CRRT should be continuous over 24 h, in the sense that everything depends on the life of the filters and the efficiency of the venous catheters used.

The undoubted advantages of CRRT can be summarized as hemodynamic stability related to limited changes in plasma osmolarity. In addition, the high efficacy in fluid removal associated with good control of azotemia and acid-base balance make it a highly effective technique in AKI refractory to conventional therapies.

Other positive data include ease of administration of vasoactive drugs and NPT and a limited effect on changes in endocranial pressure.

Depending on the depurative indications required, we may have different therapeutic methods whose increasing complexities, depending on the configurations, result in a broad spectrum of possible therapies.

Continuous slow ultrafiltration (Fig. 9.1) allows fluidic clearance only and is therefore indicated in all cases of fluidic overload associated or not with renal damage. Although a small convective action is possible, solute removal is not achieved with this method.

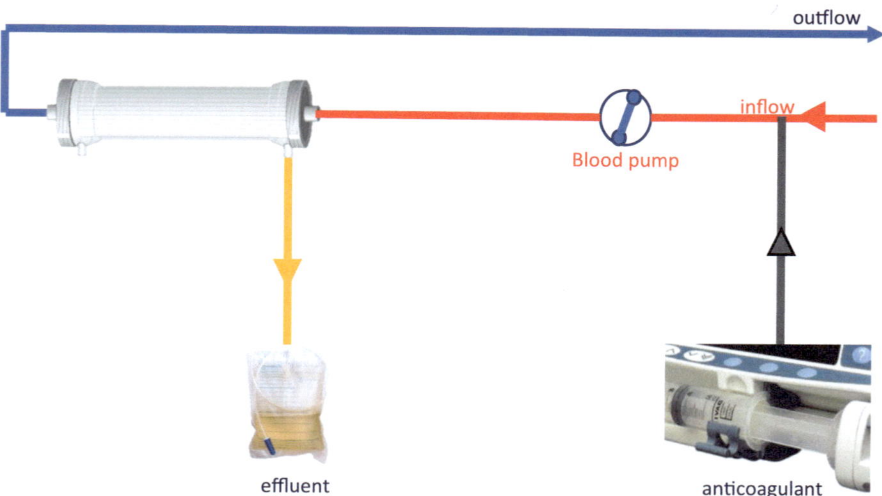

Fig. 9.1 Continuous ultrafiltration

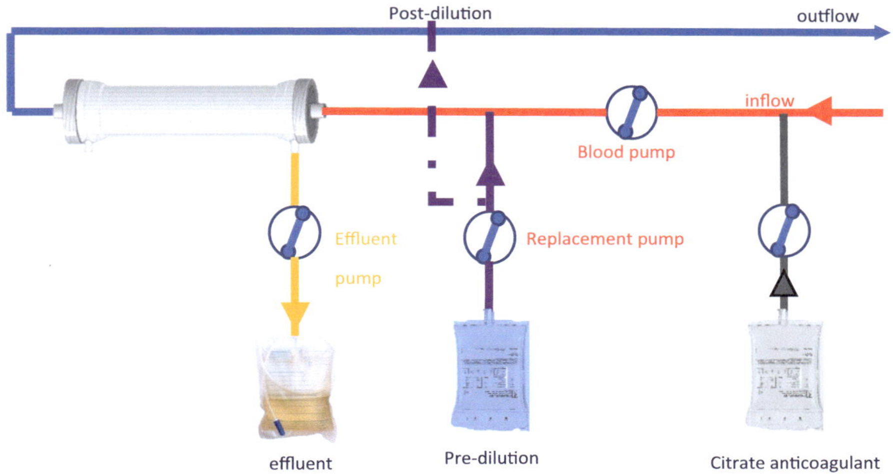

Fig. 9.2 Continuous veno-venous hemofiltration

Continuous veno-venous hemofiltration (CVVH; Fig. 9.2), on the other hand, is a convective clearance method that, through a transmembrane pressure gradient, determines convective clearance of solutes. Sieving's coefficient and transmembrane flow determine the effectiveness of the therapy, which demands the reinfusion of fluid suitable to maintain volemia and the exact concentration of solutes. Such reinfusion can occur pre- or postdilution or both.

Postdilution reinfusion allows increased hemoconcentration with the risk of occlusion of fibers and exchange pores with increased inlet pressures and reduced filter life.

The ultrafiltration flux versus plasma flux, that is, the filtration fraction (FF), should be less than 20–30% so as to avoid the shortened filter and circuit life, thus invalidating the advantage of continuous purification over 24 h.

In this regard, one can think of predilution reinfusion capable of avoiding filter coagulation especially when FF is above 30%. Unfortunately, predilution reinfusion makes solute removal less effective.

Continuous veno-venous hemodialysis (CVVHD; Fig. 9.3) exploits a clearance of solutes in a diffusive manner. The gradient across the membrane depends on dialysate flow, which ranges from 8 to 50 mL/min, and blood pump flow, which can range from 100 to 200 mL/min.

Continuous venous hemodiafiltration (CVVHDF; Fig. 9.4) combines the techniques of hemodialysis and hemofiltration. Pre- or postdilution reinfusion replaces all or part of the ultrafiltrate, while a dialysate flows counter-currently in the hemodiafiltrator.

Diffusive and convective mechanisms result in effective solute clearance even at high blood flows with reinfusion in predilution adequate to reduce filter coagulation.

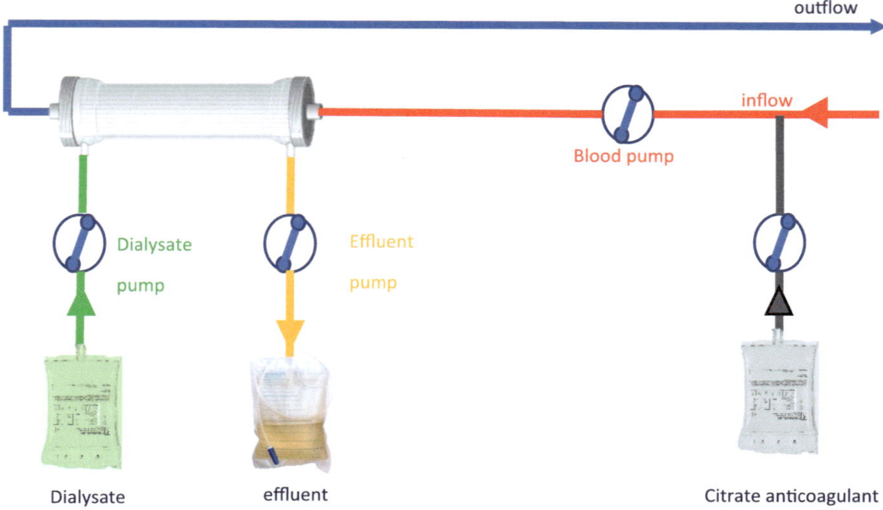

Fig. 9.3 Continuous veno-venous hemodialysis

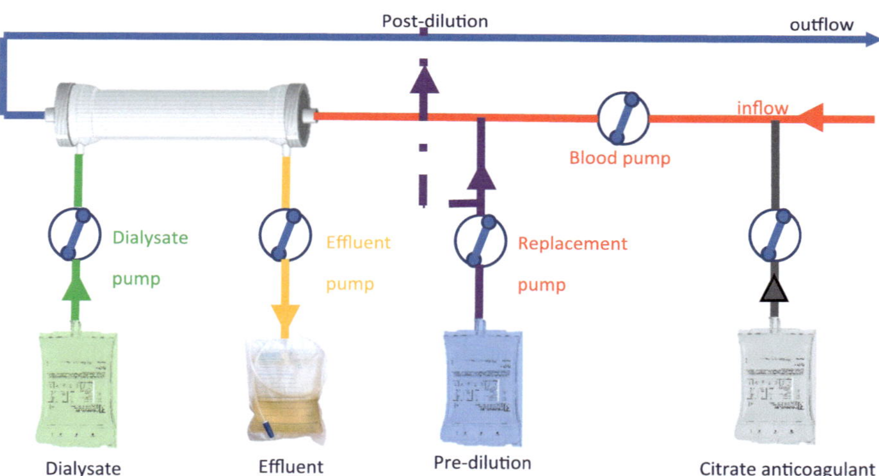

Fig. 9.4 Continuous veno-venous hemodiafiltration

9.5 Anticoagulation in CRRT

As in any extracorporeal circuit, effective anticoagulation must be provided to prevent coagulation of the filter and thus the efficiency of the purification technique.

Two anticoagulation techniques are normally used, a systemic one that uses drugs that coagulate the patient and thus the blood passing through the filter, and a regional one that produces anticoagulation of the filter but does not coagulate the patient.

Systemic anticoagulation is carried out by administering unfractionated or low-molecular-weight heparin.

The use of unfractionated heparin, which is capable of inhibiting thrombin activity by increasing antithrombin activity, is related to the possibility of monitoring its effects and being able to use an antagonist.

Although very effective, especially when infused in prefilter, the area of greatest coagulation activation, systemic heparinization produces side effects such as hemorrhage, heparin-induced thrombocytopenia, and may be ineffective in cases of heparin resistance.

Low-molecular-weight heparins, eliminated renally with increased half-lives in AKI, while effective, suffer from the difficulty of being monitored through anti-Xa activity and thus expose the patient to the risk of overdose.

As simple as systemic anticoagulation with heparin is, it exposes the patient to various risks, for which regional anticoagulation is now widely used.

This involves a method of heparin-protamine administered before and after the filter, so as to return intact blood of clotting capacity to the patient.

The method can be complex in that circuit and patient must be monitored, considering the different half-lives of heparin and protamine, and in addition, adverse effects due to circulating heparin-protamine complexes, such as vasodilation, histamine release, and pulmonary hypertension with following right ventricular dysfunction, are common.

More recently, a regional calcium-citrate anticoagulation method has been introduced. Citrate, by chelating ionized calcium, prevents coagulation, which requires in its cascade the calcium ion. Because chelation reduces circulating calcium levels, coagulation of the filter is prevented, which also removes some of the calcium-citrate complexes as they pass through the filter (up to 50% of the complexes).

The remaining calcium-citrate complexes fed back into the patient are dissociated, and the citrate is metabolized in the liver to bicarbonate. Thus effective anticoagulation in the filter is not achieved in the patient's blood. Citrate should be infused into a proximal prefilter site, and usually a calcium-free predilution reinfusion is associated. The infusion rate of citrate, to make regional anticoagulation effective, must be congruent with the rate of blood flow and must maintain an adequate concentration. Today we have many citrate solutions at different concentrations, but the efficacy of anticoagulation must be governed by the measurement of post-filter calcium concentration, which usually must be within the range of 0.25–0.40 mmol/L, such as to ensure successful anticoagulation in the filter. As the level of ionized calcium, which is essential for systemic coagulation processes, is found to be decreased, calcium should be reinfused, according to well-defined patterns, in the post-filter return line to the patient.

Since the metabolism of citrate to bicarbonate can be altered in some clinical situations, accumulation phenomena may result in metabolic alkalosis, metabolic acidosis, hypernatremia, hypocalcemia, and hypomagnesemia. Therefore, it is essential to monitor calcium and magnesium, control total calcium/ionized calcium ratio (never >2.5), and avoid high citrate administrations (never >25 mmol/L/h).

9.6   When to Start a CRRT?

The increase in CRRT in AKI is related not only to the efficacy of the method in the ICU but especially to the increase in comorbidities that make sepsis, heart failure, liver failure, mechanical ventilation, and cardiac surgery incremental factors of AKI refractory to conventional treatments.

CRRT responds to purely renal reasons, but it is also used for non-strictly renal conditions whose boundaries are not always easily distinguishable.

There are absolute renal indications for the use of CRRT in the ICU, such as water overload refractory to diuretic therapy, hyperazotemia with uremic symptoms, hyperkalemia >6 mmol/L, metabolic acidosis in AKI with pH < 7.20, and intoxication by dialyzable toxicants.

In these conditions, CRRT should be instituted early and possibly within 3 h of indication.

Non-renal indications involve removal of toxicants, poisons, contrast agents, and cytokines that appear dialyzable.

Very controversial, but also much invoked, is the application of CRRT in sepsis. Indeed, because many mediators can be removed during sepsis by continuous hemofiltration or hemodiafiltration methods, these depurative techniques are used as adjunctive therapy to canonical therapies in sepsis. The available data do not support this indication, but it is undeniable that the reduction of water overload associated with the reduction of organ damage may contribute to a more balanced therapeutic management of sepsis.

The timing of CRRT initiation should be individualized and depends on the renal functional reserve, which should not be stressed beyond limits. If the corrective response to initial renal damage produces functional recovery, clearly the strategy of waiting versus instituting CRRT can be considered in AKI. Thus, if metabolic demand is restrained, even more advanced stages of AKI can lead to waiting for CRRT initiation.

The timing of discontinuation of CRRT is equally controversial and should normally be indicated when there is renal functional recovery associated with improvement in the clinical condition that led to dialysis treatment.

It may be indicated to provoke diuresis with furosemide within 24 h of CRRT discontinuation, using this stressor test as a predictive value of renal recovery during hospital stay.

9.7   What Is the Optimal Dosage of CRRT?

The optimal dose of CRRT should predict the effective removal of the solute to be removed. Clearly, a single solute cannot be the marker of dialysis treatment efficiency, considering that multiple solutes accumulate during AKI.

Therefore, the dose of CRRT administered should be indicated with efficiency, intensity, and clinical efficacy in mind.

Efficiency is given by the clearance of a solute in a given time, that is, the clearance of the solute, the value of which should be normalized by the serum concentration.

Thus different methods may have different clearances for that solute, since the clearance represents the instantaneous efficiency of the system.

It is essential to introduce the concept of clearance time, that is, to know the time during which a certain clearance is administered. This describes the intensity of treatment and makes different methods comparable.

The clinical efficacy of RRTs is the result of actual solute removal following a given dosage imposed on a given patient.

Thus, the efficiency of dialysis treatment is represented by the effluent flow per kg of body weight per hour and may vary depending on the method used. In general, according to recent data in the literature, an adequate CRRT treatment is such when it achieves effluent flows equal to or greater than 25 mL/kg/h.

A few points should be considered, however: the prescribed dose, i.e., the theoretical dose of 25 mL/kg/h, should correspond to the current dose, i.e., the instantaneous amount of purification, which, however, due to filtration changes (coagulation and loss of effectiveness of the filter fibers) may result in a necessary adjustment of the set dose to arrive at an administered dose close to the actual dose.

The characteristics then of effective filtration can be assessed by measuring the ratio of effluent azotemia/plasma azotemia, multiplying the value by the effluent volume. It is clear that predilution reduces solute concentration, reducing solute clearance by up to 15%.

For these reasons, also considering the discontinuity of CRRT due to filter/circuit changes, the administered dose should be increased up to 30 mL/kg/h to buffer these losses in filter efficacy by monitoring effluent volumes and the effluent/plasma azotemia ratio (Sieving's coefficient) daily.

9.8 Vascular Access

The choice of vascular dialysis catheter is not of secondary importance because the yield of a CRRT and the filter life depend greatly on the type of catheter and its anatomical position.

The biluminal vascular catheter is presented in various shapes, of which the type with an inflow lumen larger than the outflow lumen is the optimum for initiating CRRT.

Obviously the materials, silicone or polyurethane, determine mechanical issues to be balanced with the advantages. In fact, polyurethane catheters, which are less colonized by bacteria and thermoplastics, have the characteristic of larger internal diameters and softness only after placement, features that recommend their use.

The site of catheter placement also plays an important role in optimizing the function of a CRRT. Preferable, according to the guidelines, to place the dialysis catheter in the right internal jugular vein or femoral vein, while the left internal jugular and subclavian vein are inadvisable (mechanical problems, tortuosity of the vessel, and therefore flow efficiency).

Catheters in right internal jugular should be 12–15 cm in length and femoral 24–25 cm in length.

9.9   Depurative Therapy in Liver Failure

In severe cases of liver failure, reactivation of the excretory, synthetic, and biotrans-forming functions of the liver can be promoted through a special form of purification (MARS: Molecular Adsorbent Recirculating System) that can improve the patient's condition.

The MARS system provides selective removal of albumin-bound and water-soluble toxins produced by liver failure. The result is thus a therapeutic removal of liver toxins such as bilirubin, bile acids, aromatic amino acids, fatty acids (medium and short chains), benzodiazepines, nitric oxide, tryptophan, phenytoin, ammonium, copper, creatinine, urea, iron.

MARS works through recirculation with adsorption of albumin-toxin compounds. Two different dialyzer filters and two adsorbent filters are used in MARS therapy. Water-soluble low-molecular-weight toxins and albumin-bound toxins from the blood circuit are transported to the albumin circuit through the dialyzer in contact with the patient's blood. The second dialyzer is used to remove the low-molecular-weight toxins from the albumin circuit. Toxins bound instead to albumin are removed from the circuit by the two adsorbents in two successive stages of the dialysate pathway. The first stage uses an activated carbon adsorbent capable of binding and eliminating low-molecular-weight and non-polar substances. Other toxins that are still in the albumin are adsorbed in the second stage via an anion exchanger to remove ionic molecules (e.g., bilirubin). Albumin thus treated and detoxified flows back into the dialyzer to capture other toxins from the patient's blood. Indications for MARS are the various forms of acute or chronic decompensated hepatopathy, liver failure after liver transplantation, and all forms of intoxication from potentially albumin-related substances.

9.10   Plasmapheresis

The elementary techniques in apheresis are well represented by three methods of physical separation of blood components: differential centrifugation; membrane filtration; and protein or cell adsorption, from already separated whole blood or plasma. These methods make it quite easy for whole blood to be separated into plasma and corpuscular elements or for the pathogen to be directly separated/adsorbed from the blood or plasma. In the most commonly used therapeutic procedure (plasma exchange), 1–1.5 L of plasma is removed in each individual session, and the volume of plasma removed can be replaced with plasma from donations or other replacement fluids (e.g., albumin). "Plasma exchange" finds particular application in treating hyperviscosity syndrome, caused by the excessive production of para-proteins (abnormal proteins) as occurs in multiple myeloma and Waldenstrom's disease; autoimmune-based diseases, such as myasthenia gravis and Guillain Barré syndrome; and thrombotic microangiopathy syndromes, which are occlusive disorders of small vessels (vascular microcirculation) characterized by anemia and decreased platelet count.

9.11 CPFA

Coupled plasma filtration adsorption (CPFA) is a novel extracorporeal therapy for blood purification during sepsis that nonselectively adsorbs proinflammatory and anti-inflammatory mediators. In vitro studies have demonstrated the efficacy of CPFA in the adsorption of inflammatory mediators such as IL-1β, IL-6, IL-8, IL-10, and tumor necrosis factor α. CPFA has been shown to improve hemodynamic stability, reduce the need for inotropic support, and improve immune response in septic patients. CPFA consists of filtration, adsorption, and hemofiltration. During the filtration step, plasma is separated from blood by a plasma filter. This separated plasma then passes through an absorbent cartridge in which a specific resin allows nonspecific adsorption of pro- and anti-inflammatory mediators and endotoxins. Adsorption is the accumulation of molecules on the surface of an absorbent material depending on membrane material, pH, ionic strength, and pore size. There is no contact of red blood cells, white blood cells, and platelets with the sorbent, thus preventing treatment-induced thrombocytopenia. Plasma filtrate is regenerated and returned to combine with blood, thus preventing unwanted losses. CPFA can be used with a hemofilter for further blood purification and removal of excess fluid in the presence of acute kidney damage. Although studies have shown that CPFA improves hemodynamic stability in septic patients, data are limited because most studies involve very small numbers of patients. CPFA has been shown to be superior to high-volume hemofiltration in septic patients with multiorgan dysfunction syndrome.

9.12 Extracorporeal Removal of CO_2

Mini-invasive extracorporeal carbon dioxide removal devices ($ECCO_2$-R) function similarly to those used for renal replacement therapy.

The main features of these systems are low extracorporeal blood flow (0.4–1 L/min), a filtering membrane that functions like a neonatal lung, the use of a small-caliber (14–18 French) double-lumen catheter, and the need for relatively low doses of heparin (3–19 IU/kg).

The blood, before entering the decapneizer, is diluted (predilution). Inside the decapneizer, a flow of oxygen flows. Then through a gas-only permeable membrane, O_2-CO_2 exchange takes place, exchange driven by the difference in partial pressures of the two gases in the two compartments.

The surface area of the membrane is about $1-3$ m^2 and is able to sustain sufficient exchange, thanks to its connection to a source of O_2 or medical air that causes a pressure gradient within the membrane fibers themselves. Oxygenated blood then passes into the hemofilter, within which excess fluid is removed, while blood leaving the hemofilter is reinfused into the patient.

Double-lumen catheters (13–17 French) similar to those used for dialysis are used.

Arteriovenous systems, on the other hand, are outdated because of major complications.

In contrast to extracorporeal membrane oxygenation (ECMO), ECCO$_2$ R systems remove carbon dioxide (CO_2) without significant effects on blood oxygenation. In fact, ECMO requires very high blood flows (3–5 L/min) and is able to give total respiratory support in terms of both oxygenation and CO_2 removal.

Although carbon dioxide removal has been a known technique since the 1970s, recent improvements regarding the technology of such systems have stimulated a renewed interest that places it as the method of choice in the ultraprotective ventilatory strategy in ARDS.

ECCO$_2$ R has been proposed both in patients with severe hypoxemic acute respiratory failure (ARDS-type) and in patients with hypoxemic-hypercapnic ALI. The rationale in patients with acute respiratory distress syndrome (ARDS) is to allow ventilation with very low tidal volumes ("ultraprotective ventilation") so as to avoid both ventilator-induced lung damage (VILI) and the deleterious effects of hypercapnia that follows reduced minute ventilation (cerebral and systemic vasodilation, cardiovascular depression, arrhythmias, pulmonary vasoconstriction, etc.).

In contrast, in patients with acute hypercapnic respiratory failure secondary to exacerbated COPD, ECCO$_2$ R has been used with fair results both to avoid intubation and to promote early weaning from intubation. Finally, another field of application of ECCO$_2$ R is lung transplant bridge.

9.13 Purification Techniques with Special Filters

9.13.1 Polyethyleneimine Filter and Heparin Coating

The polyethyleneimine and heparin-coated filter set has a three-layer structure with an improved AN-69 membrane with polyethyleneimine surface treatment and heparin coating. This particular structure allows the removal of numerous cytokines and LPS. In vitro and human studies have shown that adsorption of LPS decreases the circulating level of cytokines, systemic inflammation, and vasoplegia, with less detrimental adverse effects on splanchnic perfusion. In addition, polyethyleneimine filter membrane and heparin coating compared with the usual continuous venous hemofiltration membrane could be associated with fewer complications. The ability of polyethyleneimine and heparin-coated filter membrane to clear cytokines and bind LPS suggests that it could be a potential candidate to control the extent of inflammation induced by ischemia-reperfusion processes, so as to prevent or reduce bacterial translocation and progression to multiple organ failure (MOF). The combination of polyethyleneimine filters and heparin coating to renal clearance improves renal function and reduces the inflammatory response during sepsis and AKI. This is not surprising, as the adsorbent membrane of polyethyleneimine and heparin-coated filters is a derivative of the surface-treated AN69 hemofilter with a polyethyleneimine surface coating and an increased amount of preimmobilized heparin. In this way, the polyethyleneimine and heparin-coated filter has antithrombogenic capacity, which is useful for the treatment of acute renal failure during sepsis.

9.13.2 Adsorbent Resin (Styrene-Divinylbenzene)

The disposable adsorbent resin cartridge consisting of small spheres of porous polymer material (styrene-divinylbenzene) coated with polyvinylpyrrolidone, capable of adsorbing hydrophobic molecules of molecular weight between 5 and 55 kDa, is a recently introduced filter. The properties of the polymer result in (a) low flow resistance, (b) high biocompatibility, (c) high hemocompatibility, and (d) absence of hemolysis. It is used for acute treatments for up to 24 h of use per cartridge, although treatments of up to 7 days have been given. The average treatment duration is 48–72 h. It is a sorbent cartridge used as adjuvant therapy in the treatment of SIRS, SEPSIS, septic shock, MOF, liver failure, and rhabdomyolysis. The cartridge enables blood purification in clinical conditions characterized by high concentrations of cytokines and other potentially harmful molecules. Disruption of the cytokine cascade and resumption of homeostasis allow stabilization of the patient's hemodynamics, reduction of inotropic drug use, improvement of fluid balance, normalization of lactate levels, and protection of capillary integrity. The filter is very active in the adsorption of pro- and anti-inflammatory cytokines, mediators of inflammation, bilirubin, and myoglobin. In vitro and in vivo studies have shown that the sorbent is capable of removing additional molecules, including bile acids, ammonium, free hemoglobin, and some drugs.

Adsorption occurs following the concentration-dependent principle, that is, at high concentration of the molecule, there is maximum performance for its removal. The adsorbent resin (styrene-divinylbenzene) operates in isolated hemoperfusion but can adapt to any CRRT, ECMO, or CPB system. In particular, in cases of concomitant renal failure (frequent in this type of patient), the cartridge can be inserted in series on the continuous dialysis circuit.

9.13.3 Adsorbent Cartridge with Polymyxin B

This cartridge is a Polymyxin B hemoperfusion (PMX-HP) filter indicated as a reference therapy for the treatment of endotoxin-mediated septic shock patients unresponsive to conventional therapy. Since its introduction, more than 200,000 patients have been treated with Polymyxin B hemoperfusion (PMX-HP), with a very low incidence of adverse events (<1%) and high tolerability. More than 400 "peer-reviewed" publications are available in the literature, and numerous clinical trials have demonstrated that PMX-HP has a beneficial effect in terms of hemodynamics, organ function, and survival in the septic shock patient. Polymyxin B therapy in hemoperfusion is based on the concept of significantly removing and neutralizing endotoxin by the action of Polymyxin B bound to the polystyrene fibers of the cartridge. The innovative idea of a filter with Polymyxin B (a polycationic antibiotic) through extracorporeal hemoperfusion has made possible the most effective therapy to neutralize endotoxin, a pathogen and real killer when present in the blood stream. Because of its high binding affinity and its ability to remove endotoxin, it enables up to a 90% reduction in circulating endotoxin following two hemoperfusion treatments. Although PMX-HP was designed for endotoxin adsorption, other immunomodulation mechanisms have also been shown in the literature to be involved. Some of these mechanisms are a direct consequence of the elimination of endotoxins, while others involve the direct adsorption of mediators of inflammation, e.g., activated monocytes and neutrophils, and the inactivation of renal pro-apoptotic factors.

9.14 Conclusions

Purification techniques represent therapeutic opportunities not only in acute renal failure in the ICU but also for the nonspecific and specific removal of mediators and toxic substances present in sepsis.

It is important to establish the timing of treatment, the start and end of therapy, and especially the therapeutic method. This makes the method more effective and allows, through tailoring it, to minimize possible side effects.

Further Reading

Bellomo R, Baldwin I, Ronco C, Kellum JA. ICU-based renal replacement therapy. Crit Care Med. 2021;49(3):406–18.

Berlot G, Samola V, Barbaresco I, Tomasini A, di Maso V, Bianco F, Gerini U. Effects of the timing and intensity of treatment on septic shock patients treated with CytoSorb®: clinical experience. Int J Artif Organs. 2022;45(3):249–53.

De Rosa S, Cutuli SL, Ferrer R, Antonelli M, Ronco C. Polymyxin B hemoperfusion in coronavirus disease 2019 patients with endotoxic shock: case series from EUPHAS2 registry. COVID-19 EUPHAS2 Collaborative Group. Artif Organs. 2021;45(6):E187–94.

Garbero E, Livigni S, Ferrari F, et al. High dose coupled plasma filtration and adsorption in septic shock patients. Results of the COMPACT-2: a multicenter, adaptive, randomized clinical trial. Intensive Care Med. 2021;47(11):1303–11.

Gaudry S, Grolleau F, Barbar S, et al. Continuous renal replacement therapy versus intermittent hemodialysis as first modality for renal replacement therapy in severe acute kidney injury: a secondary analysis of AKIKI and IDEAL-ICU studies. Crit Care. 2022;26(1):93. https://doi.org/10.1186/s13054-022-03955-9.

Hellman T, Uusalo P, Järvisalo MJ. Renal replacement techniques in septic shock. Int J Mol Sci. 2021;22(19):10238.

Husain-Syed F, Birk HW, Wilhelm J, et al. Extracorporeal carbon dioxide removal using a renal replacement therapy platform to enhance lung-protective ventilation in hypercapnic patients with coronavirus disease 2019-associated acute respiratory distress syndrome. Front Med (Lausanne). 2020;7:598379.

Kellum JA, Romagnani P, Ashuntantang G, Ronco C, Zarbock A, Anders HJ. Acute kidney injury. Nat Rev Dis Primers. 2021;7(1):52. https://doi.org/10.1038/s41572-021-00284-z.

Kidney Disease Improving Global Outcome KDIGO. Acute kidney injury work group: KDIGO clinical practice guideline for acute kidney injury. Kidney Int Suppl. 2012;2:1–38.

Li R, Gao X, Zhou T, Li Y, Wang J, Zhang P. Regional citrate versus heparin anticoagulation for CRRT in critically ill patients: a meta-analysis of RCTS. Ther Apher Dial. 2022; https://doi.org/10.1111/1744-9987.13850.

Morabito S, Pistolesi V, Tritapepe L. Regional citrate anticoagulation in cardiac surgery patients at high risk of bleeding: a continuous veno-venous hemofiltration protocol with a low concentration citrate solution. Crit Care. 2012;16(3):R111.

Morabito S, Pistolesi V, Tritapepe L, et al. Continuous veno-venous hemofiltration using a phosphate-containing replacement fluid in the setting of regional citrate anticoagulation. Int J Artif Organs. 2013;36(12):845–52.

Morabito S, Pistolesi V, Tritapepe L, Fiaccadori E. Regional citrate anticoagulation for RRTs in critically ill patients with AKI. Clin J Am Soc Nephrol. 2014;9(12):2173–88.

Murugan R, Ostermann M, Peng Z, et al. Net ultrafiltration prescription and practice among critically ill patients receiving renal replacement therapy: a multinational survey of critical care practitioners. Crit Care Med. 2020;48(2):e87–97.

Ostermann M, Bellomo R, Burdmann EA, et al. Controversies in acute kidney injury: conclusions from a Kidney Disease: Improving Global Outcomes (KDIGO) Conference. Kidney Int. 2020;98(2):294–309.

Pistolesi V, Zeppilli L, Fiaccadori E, Regolisti G, Tritapepe L, Morabito S. Hypophosphatemia in critically ill patients with acute kidney injury on renal replacement therapies. J Nephrol. 2019;32(6):895–908.

Ronco C, Reis T. Continuous renal replacement therapy and extended indications. Semin Dial. 2021;34(6):550–60. https://doi.org/10.1111/sdi.12963.

Samoni S, Husain-Syed F, Villa G, Ronco CJ. Continuous renal replacement therapy in the critically ill patient: from garage technology to artificial intelligence. Clin Med. 2021;11(1):172. https://doi.org/10.3390/jcm11010172.

Sanchez-Izquierdo Rieraa JA, Montoiro Allué BR, Tomasa Irriguiblec T, et al. Blood purification in the critically ill patient. Prescription tailored to the indication (including the pediatric patient). Intensive Med. 2016;40(7):434–47.

Shimizu T, Miyake T, Kitamura N, Tani M, Endo Y. Endotoxin adsorption: direct hemoperfusion with the polymyxin B-immobilized fiber column (PMX). Transfus Apher Sci. 2017;56(5):682–8.

Tani T, Shimizu T, Tani M, Shoji H, Endo Y. Anti-endotoxin properties of polymyxin B-immobilized fibers. Adv Exp Med Biol. 2019;1145:321–41.

Zang S, Chen Q, Zhang Y, Xu L, Chen J. Comparison of the clinical effectiveness of AN69-oXiris versus AN69-ST filter in septic patients: a single-center study. Blood Purif. 2021;51:617–29.

Sepsis from SARS-COV2 Infection (COVID-19): Pathophysiology and Clinic of SARS-COV2 Infection and Sepsis

Giorgio Tulli

10.1 The Damage Response Framework (DRF): A New Model to Better Understand the Complexity of Infections

According to this model, sometimes the pathogen might be a mere initiator rather than a current perpetrator, and instead it is the host reactive forces, triggered by the presence of the pathogen, that are the cause of tissue and organ damage. Let us try to better explain what the Damage Response Framework (DRF) represents. The Damage Response Framework (DRF) represents a theory of microbial pathogenesis first proposed by Arturo Casadevall in 1999, which sees host damage as the relevant outcome of host-microorganism interaction and postulates that host damage originates from microbial distinguishing traits or from the immune response and in host tolerance or both [1]. In the DRF, the relationship between damage and immune response is represented by a simple parabola with concavity at the top where host damage is shown on the Y-axis as a function of the complex immune response, ranging from weak immune response on the left to strong immune response on the right of the parabola [2]. The DRF has been and continues to be, even in the pandemic era, very useful in improving the understanding of infectious diseases and providing insight within infectious diseases that occur in situations of either appropriate immune responses or weak or strong responses [3–5]. DRF has also provided and continues to provide information for a better understanding of host susceptibility to infectious diseases and can be a valuable tool in teaching the microbial pathogenesis of infectious diseases [6, 7]. In accordance with the DRF theory, clinical signs and symptoms occur (phenotype) when host damage reaches a threshold beyond which homeostasis is altered . In COVID-19 infection, clinical symptoms range from those

G. Tulli (✉)
Intensive Care and Perioperative Medicine Department of the Florentine Healthcare Trust, Tuscany Region, Italy
e-mail: giotulli@gmail.com

D. Chiumello (ed.), *Practical Trends in Anesthesia and Intensive Care 2022*,
https://doi.org/10.1007/978-3-031-43891-2_10

of mild upper respiratory tract disease to true life-threatening acute respiratory distress syndrome (ARDS) [8]. In the latter pathological situation oxygenation is impaired by lung inflammation, a reflection of host damage. Coronaviruses damage infected cells and trigger the production of pro-inflammatory cytokines that fuel inflammation, which in turn damages host cells and tissues, locally and distantly. Any inflammatory response in the lungs has the potential to knock out the primary function of gas exchange. Lung failure associated with severe cases of COVID-19 is the result of severe lung damage caused by airway inflammation although some neurological mechanisms and immuno-thromboembolism may be contributing factors [9–11]. When the virus is present in large quantities in the lung, SARS-COV2 lung damage is more likely to be due to viral factors than to host factors although the relative contributions to the damage itself are currently unknown. But already in early Chinese observations in Wuhan, advanced age and low lymphocyte counts (lymphopenia), as well as elevated levels of inflammatory markers, were associated with the rapid development of ARDS in patients with COVID-19 [12]. Although the relationship between immunosuppression, inflammatory response, and lung damage in COVID-19 infection remains not fully elucidated, the link between elevated inflammatory markers and respiratory failure has led to the use of immunosuppressive agents ranging from corticosteroids to inhibitors of cytokines, such as IL-6 and other inflammatory mediators [13].

10.1.1 What Are the Clinical and Epidemiological Features of COVID-19 Infection?

The clinical picture of COVID-19, which rapidly evolves over time, has a number of features: the prevalence and severity of the disease increase with age; many, if not most, infections are asymptomatic, pauci-symptomatic, or produce only mild disease; asymptomatic infected individuals may transmit SARS-COV2, thus constituting a major viral spread; individuals with cardiovascular disease, type2 diabetes, obesity, and chronic lung disease have a higher mortality rate; COVID-19 disease is less severe and may be asymptomatic in children, but a minority develop a systemic inflammatory syndrome resembling Kawasaki disease; in young individuals, rapid deterioration with acute progressive lung failure may occur; the incidence and severity of the disease is higher in men than in women; death is usually the result of anoxia due to acute pulmonary failure although there is increasing evidence of dysfunction in other organs, including the heart, kidneys, and tissues affected by dysregulated coagulation and disseminated thrombosis [14, 15].

The DRF highlights that host damage can occur in the condition of either weak or strong immune responses. When considering the strength of immune responses and infectious disease, in the context of the DRF, it emerges that strong immune responses are not necessarily protective; they can damage tissues by inducing exuberant inflammatory responses that are disrespectful of the fact that they eliminate the microorganism. Considering host damage as a function of the immune response ends up being a conceptual approach that provides a roadmap for incorporating viral load and "host inflammation" within the understanding of the clinical manifestations and pathogenesis of COVID-19.

The observation that many SARS-COV2 infections are asymptomatic or result in mild illness implies that the immune response in such individuals controls the virus without causing harm, harm that in turn results in clinical manifestations. Quite differently, the manifestations of COVID-19 that occur in the elderly and/or those with chronic pulmonary, cardiac, endocrine conditions are very likely to reflect a different immune response that may result in a degree of damage that increases the severity of the disease [14–17]. The immune response of patients with comorbidities may be weaker and less effective in eliminating the virus. It is well known that old age is associated with a weaker immune response [7]. Similarly, lung disease, heart disease, and endocrine disease are each associated with organ and tissue damage that can alter local immune responses and increase the likelihood of viral dissemination and disease progression. Men are more vulnerable to many infectious diseases than women; this is due to more effective immune responses in women [18].

In summary, weaker immune responses could explain the observation that COVID-19 is more severe in the elderly, the chronically ill, and the male sex.

The observation that many SARS-COV2 infections are asymptomatic and that asymptomatic individuals can transmit the virus to others has important implications for the pathogenesis of this disease. The problem of asymptomatic transmission of other respiratory microorganisms remains to be studied [19, 20]. The presence of high levels of SARS-COV2 in the upper respiratory tract may explain the efficiency of asymptomatic transmission [21]. Transmission from people without symptoms means that SARS-COV2 replicates at a sufficient level to be acquired by another person without damaging the host tissues and without being able to manifest clinical signs and symptoms. This implies that, for some individuals, repeated rounds of viral replication do not result in damage sufficient to give symptoms. It is important to note that SARS-COV2 antibody levels are lower in hospitalized patients with less severe disease, thus suggesting that there is still much to learn about the relationship between viral load, immune response, and disease manifestations [22].

The main clinical manifestation of severe/critical COVID-19 is lung deterioration. This often occurs in individuals with high levels of pro-inflammatory cytokines, in which a so-called **cytokine storm** may drive the pathogenesis of the disease. Supporting this hypothesis are patients with more severe COVID-19 who have higher serum levels of IL-2r, IL-6, and IL-10, and TNF-alpha than patients with milder disease [23]. However they also have lymphopenia, suggesting that the presence of "cytokine storm" may reflect an insufficiency of cellular immunity to contain the virus. The association of "cytokine storm" with severe disease and subsequent mortality has led to the use of various immunosuppressive agents in patients with elevated inflammatory markers [24]. However, it is still too early to declare that the association of elevated inflammatory markers in severe/critical COVID-19 infection is the cause of clinical deterioration resulting from a strong, exuberant pro-inflammatory response that creates host damage.

COVID-19 is more severe in people who may have crippled or damaged immunity as in the elderly or those with comorbidities [25]. All this reinforces the concept that in such individuals, weak or impaired immune responses may predispose to the development of the disease. Also consistent with this hypothesis are the data associating lymphopenia and low cellular levels of immunity with severe/critical illness and the observation that the prevalence of disease is lower in women, who express stronger immune responses than in men [26]. In contrast, the association of high levels of pro-inflammatory mediators with cytokine storm and disease severity, histologic reports of inflammation and pro-thrombotic inflammatory status, and an absence of viral inclusions in some post-mortem reports suggest that the immune response is itself a major contributor to host damage in COVID-19 [27–30].

With the Damage Response Framework, the responses of asymptomatic or mild disease of young people without comorbidities and children reflect a balanced immune response that eliminates the virus without inducing inflammatory damage. The DRF thus provides an ideal model to further investigate the pathogenesis of COVID-19 by positioning its different clinical manifestations on the axes of the parabola to give due consideration to their occurrence as a function of host susceptibility and immune response.

In the DRF parable adapted to COVID-19 infection, individuals are categorized into three group. *Group 1* consists of individuals with comorbid conditions, or condition of immunodepression or Immonoparalysis, who may have altered their immune response. The response of these individuals is localized on the left side of the parabola, indicating that they may develop higher viral loads and may be at greater risk of progression to severe disease due to the inability to contain the virus in the nasopharynx. In some of these individuals, uncontrolled viral proliferation may trigger an excessive inflammatory response that further damages the lungs and then progresses to true acute respiratory failure. This pathophysiologic event would produce a transition to *Group 3*. In some people, progressive disease is also characterized by hematologic dyscrasia, coagulation abnormality, and multiple organ failure (MOF), which may originate from immune dysregulation. In contrast, those individuals who do not progress to lung failure may be able to manifest an effective response that contains the virus and leads to recovery. *Group 1* also includes immunologically intact individuals who have acquired a large inoculum that overpowers local defences, ultimately resulting in a weak immune response. *Group 2* consists of individuals who are infected with SARS-COV2 but remain asymptomatic or manifest only mild illness. For such individuals, the immune response contains the viral inoculum, and subsequent viral replication occurs without leading to damage that would alter homeostasis. These individuals have mild or no symptoms of COVID-19, although they may transmit virus to others. This group also includes children and teens, many of whom exhibit mild disease or even no manifestation of disease, and possibly some pregnant women who may also be asymptomatic [31]. *Group 3* consists of individuals from *Group 1* whose decompensated disease outcome is the result of an excessive immune response as well as individuals who express an excessive inflammatory response to infection, which results in a cytokine storm, lung failure, and progressive organ damage and possibly death.

It is now generally accepted that the main mode of SARS-COV2 infection is introduction through the respiratory tract. Diagnosis is achieved by detection of the virus by PCR of viral nucleic acids in the upper airway, usually the nasopharynx. To date, definitive assessments about the relationship between nasopharyngeal virus, pneumonia, and disease are difficult to make because PCR testing can be associated with false negative results [32]. With this caveat, we point out that individuals in *Group 1* who are asymptomatic may be positive for nasopharyngeal virus [33, 34]. Individuals in *Groups 2 and 3* show clinical signs and symptoms of illness ranging from dry cough to respiratory failure. To date, the temporal relationship between nasopharyngeal infection and pneumonia is still not well understood, but instead it is clear that in some individuals upper airway infection precedes pneumonia, while in others there is only radiographic or ultrasonographic evidence of pneumonia with nasopharyngeal test results also negative [35]. The relationship between the naso-pharyngeal virus and pneumonia may vary depending on the site of the initial infection. Infection by large droplets (droplets) that end up directly in the upper airway or on fomites and then in the airways could lead to initial nasopharyngeal infection that subsequently spreads to the lungs. Infection by small droplets, which immediately reach the alveoli, would produce initial lung infection that might only later reach the upper airway. The relationship between the site of initial infection in the lung or nasopharyngeal sites and outcomes in *Groups 1 and 3* is unknown, since progression to disease would depend on the rates of virus replication and the nature of the immune response.

Another way of applying DRF to COVID-19 infection is to consider host damage as a function of time. Using this approach, we can organize the outcome of the host-virus interaction into discrete states associated with known outcomes of SARS-COV2 infection. The DRF defines four states to describe the outcome of the host-microorganism interaction: commensalism, colonization, persistence (latency, chronicity), and overt disease [2, 36].

States of colonization and commensalism are identified when the amount of damage produced by host-microorganism interaction is zero. Latency is a recognized state that follows infection with some viruses. Although "colonization" is not a term commonly used to describe viral infections, using the term in this context helps us to define the outcome of host-microorganism interaction and to characterize host damage as a function of time. For SARS-COV2 we can think of the time it takes the virus to replicate in the nasopharynx of an infected individual as representing a state of colonization. During that time, the amount of damage the host experiences is below the threshold for translation into symptoms. Thus, the person is asymptomatic and is still capable of transmitting the virus: he is in a contagious state. This is the reason why it is officially recommended that all people always wear masks in public [37] and maintain a distance to make sure to decrease the possibility that an asymptomatic person can transmit the virus to others. Colonization can initiate an immune response that leads to the elimination of SARS-COV2 and resolution of the infection or a response that leads to progressive host damage and disease. Disease leads to death when host damage is irreparable and severely impairs vital organ function generating multiple organ failure (MOF).

To date, we do not know whether there is a chronic persistent state that may correspond to a state of so-called latency (long Covid).

10.2 Host-Pathogen-Environment Interactions Underlying Knowledge of Infection

We also seek to delve into the interaction between host, pathogen, and environment, an interaction that underlies how to prevent or properly diagnose and treat infectious diseases.

The immediate response of any infectious disease outbreak is to approach it from the perspective of the pathogen, because disease severity is thought to be a direct function of pathogen burden [38]. However, the complexity of SARS-COV2 infection, well expressed by the DRF model, serves as an important "memento" that this perspective is not sufficient to understand infectious disease survival [39]. As in most infections, the virulence of SARS-COV2 manifests itself expressed on a continuum: many individuals who contract the infection experience mild infection, and a subset of individuals progress to the severe or even critical form of the disease: viral sepsis [40]. These severe and critical cases are driven by the host response to infection, resulting in multi-organ dysfunction and severe septic pathology. The pathologies observed in patients with COVID-19 are not necessarily new among infectious diseases. For example, extreme coagulation and multi-organ damage may be the consequence of a different spectrum of infectious conditions progressing gradually to the critical states of sepsis and septic shock. This pandemic has highlighted the need to change our perspective towards infectious diseases so that we can understand what we can do to survive infections. For COVID-19 infection as for all other infectious diseases this perspective will require an understanding of the pathogenesis, pathology, and pathophysiology of the infection: of how pathology and the resulting pathophysiology of pre-existing conditions (beyond changes in immune function) influence susceptibility to disease development once infection has occurred, of the body's intrinsic defence mechanisms that protect against damage and the resulting pathophysiology, and of how to develop treatments that alleviate pathology and pathophysiology and complement antiviral approaches. Since COVID-19 is a multi-systemic condition, understanding the recovery and rehabilitation process in infectious disease survivors is also very important; however, this aspect of infectious disease treatment is currently much neglected. Survivors of severe or critical COVID-19 infection may exhibit a spectrum of morbidity even years after the infections. Efforts should be made to understand how the damage, which results from the infection and any treatment to the patient, affects the development of new conditions in the recovery phase. If we are able to go beyond our focus on the virus, we will learn how to survive the infection and make possible a full recovery of patients, maximizing the duration of health status and quality of life. Metabolism will emerge as a critical regulator of susceptibility to recovery from infection and survival after COVID-19 infection. Infectious diseases and host metabolic processes are intimately linked, and changes in host metabolism occur at all levels: cellular, tissue, organ, physiology, during infection [41–43]. For COVID-19, these changes are clearest at the cellular level, where it is observed that the virus takes over the host cellular machinery to sustain viral replication and promote pathogenesis. However, metabolic responses of the host at the tissue, organ, and physiological levels also occur during viral infection, and it is likely that some of these responses reflect adaptive mechanisms of the host to defend against the infection itself [41, 42].

Although much of the focus has been on understanding how metabolism influences the host resistance response that destroys pathogens, recent scientific evidence from other infectious diseases has shown that metabolic processes are also mediators of host defence mechanisms that protect against the physiological damage that occurs during infections and consequently makes survival possible [44–47]. Furthermore, clinical data on early stage COVID-19 have shown that people with type 2 diabetes and other metabolic conditions that compromise metabolic health have a higher risk of developing a more severe infection pathway than people who are metabolically healthy before acquiring the infection [48]. Although these observations have been widely attributed to the fact that these individuals are more susceptible to viral infection and viral replication, the physiological complications caused by metabolic syndrome and type 2 diabetes probably make individuals more susceptible to developing COVID-19-associated diseases regardless of viral load. Finally, individuals who survive SARS-COV2 infections and other critical illnesses are predisposed to developing metabolic complications during the process of recovery of health status, suggesting that these infections and potentially their treatments could cause long-lasting collateral damage to metabolic health. It is from this perspective that the relationship between the body's metabolism and COVID-19 should be discussed, and why pre-existing metabolic abnormalities that compromise metabolic health, such as type 2 diabetes mellitus and hypertension, may be important risk factors for severe or critical infection cases, highlighting parallels between the pathophysiology of these metabolic abnormalities and the disease course of COVID-19. It should also be studied how metabolism at the cellular, tissue, and organ levels could be exploited to promote a defence against infection, with a focus on mechanisms in addition to resistance to disease tolerance, speculating on the long-term metabolic consequences of COVID-19 survivors.

COVID-19 infection can be classified as either asymptomatic or symptomatic. Asymptomatic individuals account for 25–50% of infected individuals and include those who are healthy carriers for SARS-COV2 and show no symptoms, as well as those who are tested negative for the virus but show seroconversion, indicating previous infection without ever having had symptoms [49]. During infection, these individuals maintain their health, exhibiting a maintenance of the healthy phenotype [50]. Symptomatic individuals include those who exhibit disease after a pre-symptomatic phase without symptoms. Approximately 80% of these people exhibit a mild course of disease, while the other 20% progress to severe or critical stages associated with pneumonia, ARDS and respiratory failure, septic shock, and multi-organ failure [40].

As has already been mentioned, the clinical course for symptomatic individuals can be divided into four stages. *Stage 1* begins when the individual becomes symptomatic. Individuals typically develop a dry cough and fever and may lose their sense of taste and smell, and feel a general malaise. For many people who are careful about their health status, the infection is limited to this stage. *Stage 2* describes the pulmonary phase of the infection. People who enter this stage develop lung inflammation and pneumonia, without hypoxia (stage 2a) or with hypoxia (stage 2b). These people require hospitalization. Patients with prolonged hypoxia tend to require respiratory support by non-invasive and invasive mechanical ventilation. These patients may then progress to *Stage 3*. These patients are in critical condition and may develop ARDS and extrapulmonary systemic hyperinflammatory syndrome. They may also develop shock, vasoplegia, respiratory failure, cardiopulmonary collapse, myocarditis, acute kidney injury, and other extrapulmonary complications. The prognosis of these patients is ominous, and some of them continue to deteriorate to death, while others enter *Stage 4*, the stage of recovery, and survive and exhibit a resilient health phenotype. The metabolic health of an individual is represented by the appropriate functioning of metabolic processes of organs coordinated by multiple physiological systems. Disruption of these systems causes dysfunctional organ metabolic processes and thus a decline in metabolic health. The major risk factor for COVID-19 is poor metabolic health. In past coronavirus epidemics, type 2 diabetes was one of the most common comorbidities in infected individuals [51, 52]. In agreement with these observations, type 2 diabetes, obesity, and hypertension appear to be the major comorbidities in people with COVID-19 and are associated with the most severe, if not critical, COVID-19 disease pathways [53–55]. The reasons behind these observations are likely multifactorial and generally thought to involve immune dysfunction. For example, individuals with metabolic syndrome and type 2 diabetes have impaired immune function [56], and their antiviral response against SARS-COV2 may consequently be impaired. In addition, the physiological complications of type 2 diabetes and metabolic syndrome could also play a synergistic role in the pathogenesis of SARS-COV2 thus making patients more susceptible to the development of severe disease regardless of viral load. Similarly, among people with COVID-19, young obese individuals are much more likely to require hospitalization and develop more severe and critical illnesses [57]. This observation suggests that obesity may complicate COVID-19 infection in more severe and critical cases in young adults. One possible explanation may be that obesity causes physical stress on ventilation by preventing diaphragmatic excursion. In addition, diabetes increases the risk of pulmonary fibrosis, chronic obstructive pulmonary disorder, and reduced respiratory function. When patients with COVID-19 progress to pulmonary stages of infection and develop pneumonia and ARDS, these conditions further complicate patients' respiratory function and hypoxic conditions that then lead to multi-organ damage, sepsis, and septic shock.

10.3 Viral Sepsis: Early Observations of SARS-COV2 Sepsis

In clinical practice, it was noted that many severe or critically ill patients with COVID-19 developed typical clinical manifestations of shock, which included cold extremities and weak peripheral pulses, even in the absence of hypotension. Many of these patients showed severe metabolic acidosis (high lactate values), which was indicative of microcirculatory dysfunction. In addition, some patients had impaired liver and kidney function in addition to severe cardiopulmonary insufficiency. These patients therefore met the diagnostic criteria of sepsis and septic shock according to the new 2016 SEPSIS-3 definition but with the SARS-COV2 infection appearing to be the only infection present. Blood and lower respiratory tract cultures were negative for bacteria and fungi in about 76% of septic patients with COVID-19 infection. To define viral sepsis more accurately, it would be more accurate to describe the clinical manifestations of patients with a severe or critical COVID-19 infection. Understanding the mechanisms of viral sepsis is important because it allows us to better monitor and treat these patients and better apply preventive actions in the time domain.

10.4 Viral Infection and Pathogenesis of COVID-19 Infection in Organs

In biopsies or autopsies, pulmonary pathology in both early and late stages of COVID-19 showed **DAD** (disseminated alveolar damage) with the formation of hyaline membranes, mononuclear cells, and macrophages going to infiltrate the airspaces and widespread thickening of the alveolar wall. Viral particles were observed, by electron microscopy, in type 2 bronchial and alveolar epithelial cells. Also present in some patients were atrophy of the spleen, necrosis of hilar lymph nodes, focal haemorrhages in the kidney, enlarged liver with inflammatory cell infiltration, oedema, and diffuse degeneration of neurons in the brain. SARS-COV2 viral particles have been isolated from respiratory, but also faecal and urine samples, suggesting that multiple organ failure in patients with COVID-19 is partially caused by direct virus attack. However, there are no reports about post-mortem observations of widespread dissemination of viral particles in autopsies. Whether SARS-COV2 can directly target organs other than the lung, especially those organs with high expression of ACE2 and organs with other alternative receptors for SARS-COV2, has yet to be studied. In addition, the question of how SARS-COV2 spreads to extrapulmonary organs remains an enigma. Genomic variants of circulating SARS-COV2 have been observed, and the difference in virulence and behaviour needs further study.

10.4.1 Immune Response to SARS-COV2 and Viral Sepsis

It has been shown that pro-inflammatory cytokines and chemokines including TNF-alpha, IL-1beta, IL-6, and granulocyte colony-stimulating factor (GCSF), interferon gamma-induced protein-10, monocyte chemoattractant protein-1, and macrophage inflammatory protein-1alpha were elevated to significant levels in patients with COVID-19. As in severe influenza infection, cytokine storm could play an important role in the immunopathology of COVID-19. Other studies have revealed that lung epithelial cells, macrophages, and dendritic cells all express cytokines during influenza infection through the activation of PRRs (pattern recognition receptors) that include the Toll-like receptors TLR3, TLR7, and TLR8; the retinoic acid-inducible gene 1; and the NOD like receptor family members. However, still little is known about these mechanisms in COVID-19. It is very important to identify the primary source of the cytokine storm in the SARS-COV2 response and the virological mechanisms underlying the cytokine storm. It would also be important to make clear the kinetics of cytokine activation during SARS-COV2 infection: when the first cytokines would be released, and what these cytokines would be. Also, whether virus-induced tissue damage, systemic cytokine storm, or synergistic effects of both contribute to the multiple organ dysfunction of patients with COVID-19 remains to be elucidated. It has yet to be understood whether blockade of any of these pro-inflammatory mediators can change the clinical outcome. Monoclonal antibody, anti-IL-6, and corticosteroids have been proposed to modulate the inflammatory response. However, IL-6 could play an important role in initiating a preliminary response against viral infection by promoting neutrophil-mediated viral clearance. Indeed, a study in mice revealed that IL-6 or IL-6R deficiency leads to persistence of influenza infection and death. The corticosteroid use is also still controversial.

The dysregulated immune response (contained in the SEPSIS-3 definition) also has a stage of immune suppression that follows the pro-inflammatory phase. This immune suppression is characterized by a sustained and substantial reduction in peripheral lymphocyte counts mainly of CD-4 and CD-8 T-cells in patients with COVID-19 and is associated with a high risk of developing a secondary bacterial infection. This condition, known as lymphopenia, had also been found in severe influenza and other viral respiratory infections. The degree of lymphopenia correlates with the severity of COVID-19. The mechanism underlying lymphopenia still remains unclear. Some studies have shown that SARS-like viral particles and SARS-COV RNA were present in T lymphocytes isolated from samples of peripheral blood, spleen, lymph nodes, and lymphatic tissues of various organs; these findings suggest that SARS-COV2 might be capable of directly infecting T-cells. It can be hypothesized that, in addition to the cell death induced by Pas and Pas ligand interaction as well as TNF-induced apoptosis, SARS-COV2 could directly infect lymphocytes, particularly T-cells, and initiate or promote lymphocyte cell death that would eventually lead to lymphocytopenia and an altered antiviral response. However, this hypothesis needs further study. It is also necessary to identify what types of cell death may occur in lymphocytes after SARS-COV2 infection. In addition, it is noteworthy that lymphocytes lack expression of ACE2, suggesting an alternative mechanism by which SARS-COV2 may compromise T lymphocytes. If alveolar macrophges may or may not phagocytize viral particles and then transfer them to lymphocytes is still an open question.

10.4.2 COVID-19 Infection and Abnormal Coagulation

Some studies found that 71.4% of non-survivors of COVID-19 went on to experience intravascular disseminated coagulation (DIC), so-called overt (>5 points according to ISTH criteria), and showed abnormal coagulation results during the later stages of the disease. Particularly increased was the concentration of D-dimer, and other fibrin degradation products were significantly associated with a poor prognosis. However, the mechanisms simultaneously active in coagulopathy have not yet been fully identified. Still to be explored is whether SARS-COV2 is capable of directly attacking vascular endothelial cells expressing a high level of ACE2 and then leading to abnormal coagulation and sepsis. It should also be mentioned that ACE2 is also an important regulator of blood pressure. High expression of ACE2 in the circulatory system after SARS-COV2 infection could partially contribute to septic hypotension. Many questions have been raised about the use of angiotensin II receptor blocker (ARB) and ACE inhibitor therapy for hypertensive patients affected by COVID-19. Some researchers suggest that ACE inhibitors would promote viral entry through regulation of ACE level 2. However, there is still little clinical evidence on the risk of treating COVID-19 patients with ARBs or ACE inhibitors. Further research is needed to explore whether these drugs inhibit or help viral entry. Based on observations from patients with COVID-19, it is hypothesized that, in mild cases, resident macrophages that initiate lung inflammatory responses are capable of containing the virus after SARS-COV2 infection. Both innate and adaptive responses are effectively operative to limit viral replication so that the patient can recover rapidly. However, in severe and critical cases of COVID-19, the integrity of the epithelial and endothelial barriers of the lung is severely disrupted. In addition to epithelial cells, SARS-COV2 can attack endothelial cells of the lung capillaries, leading to a large influx of plasma components in the form of exudate into the alveolar cavity. In response to SARS-COV2 infection, alveolar macrophages or epithelial cells might produce various pro-inflammatory cytokines and chemokines. Based on this change, monocytes and neutrophils are attracted to the site of infection to clarify and clear these exudates rich in viral particles and infected cells, resulting in uncontrolled inflammation. In this process, due to the substantial reduction and dysfunction of lymphocytes, the adaptive immune response cannot be effectively initiated. Uncontrolled viral infection leads to increased macrophage infiltration and further worsening of the lung injury. At the same time, the direct attack also on other organs by the SARS-COV2 now disseminated everywhere, the immune pathogenesis caused by the systemic cytokine storm, and the microcirculatory dysfunction, all together lead to the occurrence of viral sepsis. Therefore, effective antiviral therapy and measures to modulate the innate immune response and the recovery of the adaptive immune response are essential to breaking the vicious cycle and improving patient outcomes.

10.5 What Has Viral Sepsis from COVID-19 Infection Taught Us About

10.5.1 What Already Did They Know About Bacterial and Fungal Sepsis?

COVID-19 infectious disease itself poses an unprecedented threat to humanity's health, health care systems, and the global economy (syndemic). Since its emergence, clinicians have attempted to extrapolate pathophysiology and treatment strategies from better-known disease processes such as ARDS and other respiratory viral diseases. An important disease paradigm that has been variably applied to COVID-19 disease is precisely sepsis. Although some experts have unequivocally asserted that multiple organ failure that is generated by COVID-19 is sepsis, other case series of severe COVID-19 infection have not been labelled as sepsis despite the fact that patients had established infection and organ dysfunction and therefore entered the 2016 formal definition of sepsis (SEPSIS-3) [8, 58, 59].

Therefore, it deserves to explore this clinical issue more thoroughly and whether it really serves to think of our patients with severe or critical COVID-19 infection as patients with sepsis.

According to the "Third International Consensus Definitions of Sepsis and Septic Shock (Sepsis-3)," sepsis is a dysregulated host response to an infection, causing life-threatening organ dysfunction [60]. Many clinicians only ever associate sepsis with a severe bacterial infection, but this association with bacteria has never been a requirement by any "consensus" on the definition of sepsis. The Sepsis-3 criteria are agnostic about the source of infection but instead emphasize that organ damage in sepsis is due to secondary consequences of complex molecular cascades rather than direct pathogen invasion. Although current knowledge of the mechanisms of organ dysfunction associated with COVID-19 remains incomplete, severe COVID-19 infection appears to include inflammation-mediated organ dysfunction, both internally and externally in the lungs, which is consistent precisely with viral sepsis [61, 62]. Some clinical researchers have documented markedly elevated levels of pro-inflammatory cytokines, observations consistent with a "cytochemical storm" [24, 63]. All anti-inflammatory signals are also present, as occurs in bacterial sepsis. These biochemical cascades are capable of causing organ dysfunction throughout the body, including DAD (diffuse alveolar damage) in the lungs, coagulopathy and microvascular dysfunction, acute cardiac injury, cytopenia, acute kidney injury, and hepatitis. The roles of hypotension and altered tissue oxygenation are less clear in COVID-19 infection than in bacterial sepsis; however, the dysregulated endothelium and microvascular thrombosis typically associated with sepsis are commonly observed in severe cases of COVID-19 infection [64]. Direct viral invasion of the kidneys, heart, and endothelial system has been well reported in studies although not uniformly and so the constellation of data suggests that some part of the organ dysfunction from COVID-19 is immune mediated [65–68].

The observation that nonbacterial organisms can cause sepsis is certainly not new. Fungi are well known as a cause of sepsis and septic shock, and fungal infections have often been included in epidemiological studies of sepsis. Viral sepsis, however, tends not to be well reported in large case histories of sepsis. A recent international point prevalence study attributed only 3.7% of infections in critically ill patients to viruses [69]. This figure is certainly underestimated due to the lack of testing performed, considering that pneumonia is one of the most common causes of sepsis, and one-third or perhaps more of pneumonias in critically ill patients are caused by viruses [70, 71]. A causative organism is not identified in more than one-third of critically ill patients with suspected sepsis, and a fraction of these may be due to undiagnosed viral infections [72, 73].

The potential advantages of "labelling" severe/critical COVID-19 infection associated with organ dysfunction as sepsis are that it emphasizes the severity of the disorder, the imminent threat of death if left without early diagnosis and treatment, the need for intensive observation, care, and intensive care in the time domain.

Mortality in patients with COVID-19 who met Sepsis-3 criteria in a cohort of Chinese patients was 48% [59]. This mortality is much higher than the 15% mortality associated with Sepsis No-COVID [74]. If "labelling" the condition as sepsis helps to estimate the severity of the presentation and the need for aggressive treatment and care, then this is probably of great benefit to the patient. The question of whether severe viral infections can lead to sepsis and septic shock in the absence of secondary bacterial infection echoes a similar discussion during the 2014 Ebola Viral Disease (EVD) outbreak. Members of the Global Sepsis Alliance asserted that the multiple organ dysfunction described with EVD should have been called sepsis and that not doing so could distract from resuscitative efforts and harm international efforts to highlight sepsis as a major unrecognized cause of death [75]. Other experts argued that lumping EVD patients together in the broader category of sepsis could have detrimental implications for the treatment and prognosis of patients with EVD by encouraging early treatment for bacterial sepsis and protocol care and assistance that might not be appropriate for this viral disease [76].

This debate highlights what is considered the strongest argument against "labelling" severe COVID-19 infection as sepsis: that many of the treatments that are reflexively applied to patients with sepsis may be harmful to patients with COVID-19 or better than COVID-19-generated sepsis. It is important to report some of these treatments.

For example, aggressive fluid resuscitation may worsen lung function already borderline in this particular ALI/ARDS. Empirical antimicrobials will expose patients to the risks of antibiotics without a clear promise of benefit since bacterial superinfection in COVD-19 appears to be not uncommon but must absolutely be diagnosed because it is caused in most cases by MDR bacteria. Applying the "label" sepsis may also generate subtle pressure to treat the patient aggressively in all aspects, including early intubation, although this may be harmful to some patients. These concerns about defining severe COVID-19 infection as sepsis highlights a broader issue about sepsis in general. This gives rise to a question concerning all cases of sepsis.

Why has it come to be universally agreed that sepsis is associated with a uniform set of protocolized treatments (blood cultures, serial lactates, aggressive fluid resuscitation, and broad-spectrum antibiotics), the so-called one-hour sepsis bundle?

Even outside of COVID-19 infection, with many bacterial and fungal infections, the essence of sepsis is its heterogeneity. Sepsis contains a broad mosaic of infection sites, causative pathogens, antimicrobial susceptibilities, organ dysfunction, host susceptibility, and treatment responses. The optimal treatment of meningococcal meningitis is radically different from the appropriate treatment for an intestinal perforation with a polymicrobial spillage in the abdomen, which in turn is different from acute *Legionella pneumophila* pneumonia leading to rapid atrial fibrillation and acute exacerbation of congestive heart failure. The best treatment plan for each of these disorders further depends on patients' disease severity; underlying cardiac, pulmonary, and renal function; their history of recent antibiotic exposure; allergies; the presence or absence of invasive devices; and patients' expressed values and preferences. Applying a single common "label" to all these conditions risks leading clinicians to disregard critical analysis on each patient in favour of treating all patients in the same way. A warning sign of this premature short-circuiting in a patient may be when the diagnosis is categorized simply as sepsis and not rather as sepsis due to organism X at body site Y causing organ dysfunction Z. The disadvantages of "labelling" a condition as sepsis can be obviated by making it clear that sepsis is a multifactorial disorder, that its management can be tailored to each patient, and that it is vital to make explicit the name of the suspected pathogen, its characteristics, the site of infection, and the organ dysfunction associated with sepsis. Once these preconditions are accepted, one may well believe that there is substantial value in defining serious infections associated with organ failure, including those due to SARS-COV2, as sepsis, even if they do not all fall under one common pathway of diagnosis and treatment. These preconditions also include drawing clinicians' attention to the vulnerabilities of their patients and the need for careful, patient-centred care and assistance, shedding light on the prognostic implications of a diagnosis of sepsis, and ensuring a more accurate estimate of the epidemiology and burden of sepsis. It can then be well said that, based on these considerations, there should be no argument that SARS-COV2 is an important cause of sepsis and that defining it as such is useful and appropriate. Having outlined these considerations on SARS-COV2 sepsis, let us go into more detail.

Research on the pathogenesis and various treatment options of COVID-19 infection continues to be very active although there are still many unresolved issues. Many patients infected with SARS-COV2 usually show mild or moderate disease, but depending on the viral load, the host's immune system, the host's comorbidities, and underlying or even unknown factors, about 5% of patients develop a critical illness with respiratory failure and organ dysfunction [8]. Pneumonia is the most frequent and severe manifestation of infection, while ARDS is the major complication in critically ill patients. Other complications include coagulopathy, microvascular thrombosis such as myocardial infarction and stroke, arrhythmias, acute cardiac injury, liver injury, acute kidney injury, and shock [8, 77–80].

In a series of 21 critically ill patients admitted to the ICU in the United States, ARDS was observed in most of the patients, and one-third of them also developed cardiomyopathy [79]. Human ACE2 is a functional receptor to which SARS-COV2 attaches for its entry into the cell; quite similar to SARS-COV [81], ACE2 is widely expressed in the nasal mucosa, bronchial mucosa, lungs, heart, oesophagus, kidney, stomach, bladder, and ileum; and these human organs are all vulnerable to SARS-COV2, especially in severe cases with viremia [82].

Viral replication of SARS-COV2 in target organs, as well as the resulting cellular damage, causes a systemic inflammatory response, a cytokine storm, mainly ARDS and multiple organ damage. Some autopsy studies testify to these findings. In an autopsy study of 21 patients with severe COVID-19 infection, the primary cause of death was respiratory failure with diffuse exudative alveolar damage with massive capillary congestion accompanied by microthrombi [83]. In another study performed post-mortem on 12 patients, a high concentration of RNA from SARS-COV2 was found in the lung tissue of all patients, and about half of them had high titres of viral RNA in the liver, kidneys, and heart in addition to viremia [84].

According to the Third International Consensus definitions for sepsis and septic shock (Sepsis-3), as mentioned several times, Sepsis is defined as a life-threatening organ dysfunction caused by dysregulated host response to infection [85]. Considering the multi-systemic clinical and autopsy findings in severe COVID-19 infection patients, viral sepsis would be a much more accurate term to describe the whole clinical picture. If mild-to-moderate COVID-19 infection is considered a "good viral infection," then severe COVID-19 infection is "viral sepsis" or bad viral infection. Viral sepsis can also be caused by a wide variety of viruses, such as herpes simplex virus, influenza virus, enteroviruses, human parechovirus, Ebola virus, and dengue virus [86]. Common features of viral sepsis are intense cytokine release, prolonged inflammation and consequent immunosuppression, T-cell depletion, development of multiple organ damage, and increased susceptibility to secondary bacterial infections. A combination of these concepts has led to a new approach to patients with severe COVID-19 infection as a "subgroup of sepsis," in which particularly profound cellular, immunologic, and metabolic abnormalities are associated with a higher risk of mortality than with infection alone.

10.5.2 What Has COVID-19 Sepsis Taught Us?

Despite research efforts in critical care medicine, these searches for new therapeutic options for sepsis have not yielded great results. However, the COVID-19 infection pandemic showed that effective therapeutic options for the distinct subgroup of viral sepsis from SARS-COV2 infection were found within a few months. What then can be learned from the way COVID-19 is being studied to better understand sepsis in general?

Heterogeneity: In clinical practice, recognition of a broader septic syndrome can improve focus and timely initiation of treatment. However, when new treatment options are sought, this more general approach is less useful. One of the question marks in sepsis research has been, and still is, whether the host response in sepsis represents a final common pathway without respect to the source of infection or the pathogen causing the infection. This would justify looking at a larger population of patients with sepsis, with the added benefit of having larger cohorts of patients to study. However, many believe that the host response is too complex and that a final common pathway just does not exist. The resulting heterogeneity within the septic patient population is therefore considered to be a major limiting factor in finding specific therapies for sepsis. Major efforts have been made to be able to detect homogeneous subgroups of septic patients. Distinct and shared gene expression profiles have been found when, for example, comparing pulmonary sepsis and abdominal sepsis, thus suggesting that some of the heterogeneity in the septic population could be explained by the site of infection or the pathogen invading the host.

Several other studies aiming to find homogeneous subgroups of sepsis through various methods show different distributions of infectious aetiologies across the new subgroups, again implying that infecting organisms are associated with different responses in the host. In contrast to the many different microorganisms and different host responses in sepsis, COVID-19 infection studies show comparable gene expression profiles in the populations studied, as well as upregulation of chemokines and neutrophils. This may be one reason why there have been positive randomized trials with treatment options for COVID-19. For example, dexamethasone treatment lowered 28-day mortality in COVID-19 patients, particularly in patients receiving respiratory support. Perhaps focusing on a single site of infection or infectious agent ends up eliminating much of the heterogeneity present. Those doing sepsis research can learn from this and adapt current research and trial design paradigms in such a way that stratification by infection type is possible and statistically intelligible.

Outcome Measures: In clinical trials on sepsis, outcome measures have been much debated. Trials using new treatment options have not been able to demonstrate a benefit for overall outcomes such as ICU admission rates or mortality. In 2005, the International Sepsis Forum proposed that sepsis researchers broaden the range of outcome measures used in clinical trials: mortality is an attractive outcome measure, but other patient-centred benefits such as quality of life and long-term morbidities should not be neglected. The International Sepsis Forum provided other relevant clinical opportunities to show the benefits of treatment. Nevertheless, the literature on new therapies for sepsis continues to be dominated by the search for benefits on short-term mortality.

For COVID-19, the WHO recognized that a set of outcome measures was needed to study this new infectious disease and be able to compare outcomes globally. The experts who proposed outcome measures for sepsis in 2005 also did so for COVID-19 in 2020.

Another advantage on focusing on a defined disease state such as SARS-COV2 infection, as opposed to all other causes of sepsis, is that site-specific outcome measures can be used. For example, the Murray Score to assess lung injury or diffusing capacity to assess lung function is a valid outcome measure that could potentially be improved by certain specific treatments. Obviously, it does not make sense to assess lung function as an outcome in all septic patients.

Global Collaboration: A few weeks after the start of the COVID-19 outbreak in China, the WHO coordinated a roadmap for global research. Experts from various fields coordinated on key questions and strategies to accelerate research. The WHO launched a Data Platform on COVID-19 in order to collect global data through a predefined "Case Report Form." When patient data were collected with this CRF anywhere in the world, the same variables were documented, and criteria for the diagnosis of COVID-19 (PCR or CT scan) were available. The CRF was widely adopted and created a unique opportunity for global collaborative efforts with minimal data loss or different inclusion criteria. In addition, Global Genomic Alliances are providing insights into how the clinical and immunologic manifestations of infection, and its natural variability, are governed by human genetics. In this case, global collaborations are helping to find specific individuals prone or resistant to the disease, which are especially interesting when trying to shed light on pathophysiological mechanisms. Inevitably, all this research has created many problems. Pressure to publish studies has led to being overly flexible in protocols and trial design with shorter turnaround time (TAT) for peer review in scientific journals and omission of tests in preclinical animal models. Although all these practices have accelerated the research process, one should always beware that they can lead to a lower standard of research, as evident from the withdrawal of several articles even in leading medical journals during the pandemic.

10.5.3 To Understand the Differences Between SARS-COV2 Infection and Other Systemic Disorders

COVID-19 is an infection that is poorly understood to date; so much of our current understanding of organ dysfunction in the SARS-COV2 infection is extrapolated from other disorders that have similar clinical features. Several studies have reported elevated serum concentrations of inflammatory cytokines, including interleukin IL-6, in COVID-19 [63, 87]. These observations have prompted comparisons with other critical illness syndromes that are associated with elevated cytokine concentrations. Examples frequently invoked are ARDS and sepsis [61]. Another comparison of particular interest is made with cytokine release syndrome (CRS) in the setting of CAR-T (chimeric antigen receptor T-cell) therapy because it is an indication approved by many regulatory bodies for the drug tocilizumab [88]. Tocilizumab is a humanized monoclonal antibody against the IL-6 receptor [89]. Based on these comparisons with other diseases, clinical trials with anti-cytokine drugs in patients with COVID-19 are moving forward. The administration of these drugs, including IL-6 antagonists, has become widespread while still awaiting the results of trials [87]. A systematic comparison of the inflammatory milieu in the critical illness associated with COVID-19 and these other disorders could reveal important similarities and differences between these various syndromes and provide greater evidence for the successful application of immune-modulating therapy in COVID-19.

The estimated mean, from a careful study, for IL-6 concentrations in patients with COVID-19 is 36.7 pg/mL (95% CI 21.6–62.3 pg/mL); in contrast, the mean serum IL-6 concentration in patients with CAR-T cell-induced cytokine release syndrome is 3110.5 pg/mL (632.3–15,302.9 pg/mL), almost 100 times higher than in patients with COVID-19 (difference 3074 pg/mL, 95% CI 325–26,735 pg/mL; $p < 0.0001$). Similarly, the mean concentration of IL-6 is 1558.2 pg/mL (525.8–4617.6 pg/mL) in patients with hyperinflammatory ARDS (difference 1521.5 pg/mL, 324.7–26,735.0 pg/mL; $p > 0.0001$) and 983.6 pg/mL (550.1–1758.4 pg/mL) in patients with sepsis (difference 974 pg/mL, 324–2648 pg/mL; $p < 0.0001$). Even in patients with hyperinflammatory ARDS, the mean concentration of IL-6 is 198.6 pg/mL (80.6–489.3 pg/mL), five times higher than the concentration in patients with COVID-19 (difference 162 pg/mL, 16–717 pg/mL; $p = 0.0085$). Patients with ARDS unrelated to COVID-19 have significantly higher concentrations of IL-6 than patients with COVID-19 when analysed as a single disorder (mean 460.1 pg/mL, 216.3–978.7 pg/mL; difference 423.4 pg/mL, 106.9–1438.1 pg/mL; $p < 0.0001$).

IL-6 concentrations in COVID-19 patients showed moderate heterogeneity ($I^2 = 57.7\%$) with a range of 6.5–357.2 pg/mL, and 80% of COVID-19 studies reported a mean IL-6 concentration lower than 100 pg/mL. Heterogeneity was lowest for hyperinflammatory ($I^2 = 0\%$) and hypo-inflammatory ($I^2 = 37.6\%$) ARDS but highest for cytokine release syndrome ($I^2 = 77\%$) and sepsis ($I^2 = 89.3\%$).

10.5.3.1 Other Inflammatory Cytokines

Many other cytokines are low in COVID-19 in comparison with syndromes. For example, the mean concentration of IL-8 (neutrophil chemotactic factor) is 22 pg/mL (95% CI 5–108 pg/mL) in patients with COVID-19 compared with 228 pg/mL in patients with Sepsis (difference 206 pg/mL 95% CI 15–1371 pg/mL; $p = 0.021$) and 196 pg/mL in patients with hyperinflammatory ARDS (difference 174 pg/mL, 5–1436 pg/mL; $p = 0.038$). The mean concentration in patients with cytokine release syndrome is 575 pg/mL; the difference between the mean concentration of IL-8 in patients with cytokine release syndrome versus COVID-19 is not statistically significant in the setting of a large CI (difference 553 pg/mL, −47 to 47,502 pg/mL; $p = 0.11$). However, the estimate for the concentration in patients with hyperinflammatory ARDS is 32 pg/mL, similar to that of COVID-19. TNF-alpha concentrations are available from four studies examining Sepsis ($n = 5320$) and one study examining cytokine release syndrome ($n = 16$) and ten COVID-19 studies ($n = 607$ patients). In comparison with a mean TNF-alpha concentration of 5.0 pg/mL (2.3–10.7 pg/mL) in patients with COVID-19, the mean concentration was 34.6 pg/mL (20.0–59.9 pg/mL) in patients with Sepsis and 52.2 pg/mL (2.0–1390 pg/mL) in patients with cytokine release syndrome. All but one COVID-19 study (92%) had a TNF-alpha concentration lower than 10 pg/mL. IFN gamma concentrations were not high in COVID-19 patients with a mean of 10.8 pg/mL but were very high in patients with cytokine release syndrome, averaging 3722.1 pg/mL (difference 3711 pg/mL, 624–21,838 pg/mL; $p < 0.0001$). The mean concentration of sIL-2R was high in patients with COVID-19, but much less than in patients with cytokine release syndrome (506 pg/mL versus 12,396 pg/mL; difference 11,890 pg/mL, 299–190,957 pg/mL; $p = 0.032$). IL-2 and IL-4 concentrations were not available in every study of the compared disorders, but IL-2 concentration was reported in nine COVID-19 studies and IL-4 concentration in the ten COVID-19 studies. All of these COVID-19 studies reported that these cytokines were within the normal physiological range.

10.5.3.2 Other Inflammatory and Host Response Markers

Acute-phase proteins were substantially elevated in patients with COVID-19. C-reactive protein (CRP) concentrations were comparable in patients with COVID-19 and patients with sepsis and higher in patients with cytokine release syndrome. D-dimer concentrations were available for COVID-19 and sepsis; these studies indicated that patients with COVID-19 had substantially higher D-dimer than patients with sepsis. Mean concentrations of ferritin and lactate dehydrogenase were markedly higher in patients with cytokine release syndrome than in patients with COVID-19, but nevertheless highly elevated in patients with COVID-19. In contrast, procalcitonin concentrations were not elevated in patients with COVID-19 but were elevated in patients with sepsis. Absolute and relative lymphopenia were common in patients with COVID-19, but there were no comparable data in the compared groups.

10.5.3.3 COVID-19 Severe Versus COVID-19 Critical Versus Other Disorders

The mean concentration of IL-6 in patients with critical COVID-19 was 55.3 pg/mL and was not statistically greater than in patients with severe COVID-19 (mean 37.3 pg/mL, $p = 0.94$). This mean IL-6 concentration in patients with critical COVID-19 was again significantly lower than in the other no-COVID disorders compared. Most of the within-COVID-19 heterogeneity in the primary analysis appeared to be driven by the group with critical COVID-19, in which the I^2 was 55.7% compared with 1.1% in the group with severe COVID-19. The mean IL-6 concentration among studies of patients with critical COVID-19 showed a range from 22.3 to 136.8 pg/mL, with six of ten studies reporting a mean concentration lower than 100 pg/mL.

Other cytokine measures in the subgroup of patients with critical COVID-19 were similar to those observed in the primary analysis. In contrast, abnormalities of non-cytokine biomarkers appeared to be exaggerated in the group with critical COVID-19 versus severe COVID-19.

10.5.3.4 The Peak of IL-6 in COVID-19 Versus the Other Disorders

Among COVID-19 studies reporting peak IL-6 concentration (six studies, $n = 245$ patients), the mean IL-6 concentration was 61.3 pg/mL in patients with COVID-19, significantly lower than in patients with sepsis, cytokine release syndrome, and hyperinflammatory ARDS. The results were similar when comparing peak IL-6 concentrations in patients with critical COVID-19 alone (mean 78.1 pg/mL) with those with other disorders. Plasma or serum concentrations of IL-6 are borderline, an order of magnitude lower than those reported in studies of patients with CAR-T cell-induced cytokine release syndrome, sepsis, and ARDS no-COVID-19. Many other cytokine concentrations demonstrated modest elevation in patients with COVID-19 compared to other disorders. Contrasting nonspecific inflammatory biomarkers appeared relatively comparable between COVID-19 versus patients with no-COVID-19-related ARDS [90].

10.5.4 Pathobiology of COVID-19 [61, 68, 87, 91–97]

Cytokinetic storm does not appropriately describe the milieu in COVID-19-induced organ dysfunction. Autopsy reports repeatedly note extensive dissemination of SARS-COV2 through different tissues. Lymphopenia is common and prognostic. T lymphocytes are directly susceptible to SARS-COV2 infection. In this context, it should be considered that the less pronounced elevation of cytokines in COVID-19 might reflect a regulated or even inadequate inflammatory response to an overpowering viral infection. A predominantly hypo-immune state with subsequent virus-mediated tissue damage and dysregulated inflammation may explain both the apparent clinical and pathological abnormalities in COVID-19 and the high concentrations of circulating acute-phase proteins. In contrast to cytokine concentrations, similar or higher concentrations of several acute-phase proteins and other biomarkers were found in patients with COVID-19. Concentrations of D-dimer are five times higher in patients with critical COVID-19 than in patients with sepsis, suggesting that the reported associations between D-dimer and severity in COVID-19 are a consistent signal of distinction. The ability of D-dimer and procalcitonin to discriminate COVID-19 from other infections causing respiratory distress may warrant further exploration. Importantly, although the mortality benefit reported with dexamethasone treatment in patients with COVID-19 goes to inform clinical practice, it is difficult to attribute the benefit in a causal sense to IL-6 suppression. Of the myriad effects of glucocorticoids relevant to critical illness (e.g., inotropism, vasoconstriction in more than 60% of critically ill patients with COVID-19 requiring vasopressor support), perhaps the most relevant is the ability of corticosteroids to suppress late-onset fibrosis leading to irreversible lung damage in ARDS. Of note, the large effect in the RECOVERY trial of dexamethasone was achieved entirely in patients who were randomized more than 7 days after the onset of symptoms.

10.5.5 Pathobiology of COVID-19 ARDS (C-ARDS) [98–100]

Because it originates from many precipitating causes, ARDS is associated with numerous pathobiological processes. Central to its pathogenesis is an acute inflammatory insult that leads to pulmonary epithelial and endothelial injury. To what extent these lesions are observed may depend on the site of the insult. For example, circulating markers of epithelial injury are higher in patients with direct causes (e.g., pneumonia, aspiration) than in those from indirect causes (e.g., pancreatitis, peritonitis) of ARDS. Conversely, indirect causes are associated with higher concentrations of markers of endothelial injury. Distinct hypo-inflammatory and hyper-inflammatory phenotypes of ARDS have been identified that differ on the basis of systemic inflammatory profiles. The hyperinflammatory phenotype is associated with increased concentrations of IL-6 and IL-8 and the soluble TNF receptor, but low concentrations of protein C. In patients with COVID-19, the relative contributions of endothelial and epithelial injuries remain unknown. Since viral pneumonia is a direct cause of lung injury, epithelial injury might be predicted as predominant. Several post-mortem studies in patients with severe COVID-19 have identified diffuse alveolar damage (DAD). These studies also describe severe endothelial damage and coagulopathic features in the pulmonary microvasculature. These studies require cautious interpretation because they are subject to selection bias, and sample sizes are still small. In a prospective study, the pro-inflammatory phenotype of ARDS was observed in 11–20% of patients with COVID-19 versus 35% of patients with no-COVID-19 ARDS. These data substantiate the results of this meta-analysis by suggesting that circulating inflammatory responses are generally lower in patients with COVID-19 ARDS than in patients with hyperinflammatory ARDS.

10.5.6 Pathobiology of Sepsis [101–103]

Sepsis is defined as a life-threatening organ dysfunction caused by a dysregulated host response to infection. The syndrome has several infectious causes and host substrates, which probably underlie the great heterogeneity of its manifestations. The precise biological events that precipitate the transition from regulated to dysregulated host response remain unknown to this day. The "sine qua non" of sepsis is organ dysfunction, often remote from the infectious source. Abnormalities include vasodilatory shock, ARDS, coagulopathy and renal, hepatic, microcirculatory, and endocrine dysfunction. Immune dysfunction is another hallmark of sepsis, but conceptualizing this dysfunction as hyperinflammation is probably too simplistic. While inflammatory cytokine concentrations are often exceptionally high, sepsis is also associated with marked immunosuppression by T-cell depletion, hyporesponsiveness of neutrophils to cytokine stimulation, impaired phagocytosis of cells of innate immunity, and pathogen killing by cells of innate immunity. Elevated cytokines coupled with altered immune effector function is a pattern that explains the peripheral resistance observed in the multiple endocrine axes in sepsis. Therefore, whether inflammatory cytokine elevations in sepsis reflect a driver, a marker, or even an adaptive response to the disease remains unknown to this day. Unanswered questions about the mechanistic role of cytokine elevations are shared between sepsis and COVID-19. However, despite much lower concentrations of systemic cytokines, ex vivo stimulated blood mononuclear cells from patients with COVID-19 produce half as much TNF-alpha and IFN gamma as do cells from patients with sepsis and critical illness without infection (SIRS). Therefore, immunosuppression might be even more pronounced in patients with COVID-19 than the paradoxical suppression frequently observed in sepsis. The innate clearance capacity of microorganisms has not been investigated in patients with severe COVID-19 and is probably a key question for future studies, given the high risk of secondary infection even by MDR bacteria among patients admitted to the ICU.

10.5.7 Pathobiology of CAR-T Cell-Induced Cytokine Release Syndrome [104–111]

Unlike sepsis and ARDS, "CAR-T cell-induced cytokine release syndrome" has a well-defined pathophysiology. After infusion, CAR-T cells encounter antigen, which leads to activation, proliferation, and lysis of target cells with the release of inflammatory cytokines. CAR-T cell infusion is associated with fever, hypotension, coagulopathy, and, in severe cases, multiple organ dysfunction that may also include reversible neurotoxicity. In most patients, cytokine release syndrome develops briefly after infusion and resolves in the following week with supportive therapy alone or in combination with tocilizumab or corticosteroid treatment. However, severe or prolonged cytokine release syndrome is associated with extraordinarily high serum concentrations of inflammatory cytokines that include IFN gamma, IL-6, IL-10, IL-15, the p55TNF receptor, and chemokines such as IL-8. The prompt resolution of fever and often hypotension after tocilizumab suggests that IL-6 contributes to the pathobiology of CAR-T cell-induced cytokine release syndrome, although evidence from randomized trials is still lacking. Laboratory studies suggest that monocytes and macrophages are a major source of IL-6 after CAR-T cell therapy. IL-1 release appears to precede IL-6 release so that targeting IL-1 could mitigate or prevent cytokine release syndrome. Ferritin concentrations rise substantially in patients with severe cytokine release syndrome, which could signify macrophage activation. The elevation in ferritin, CRP, and cytokines such as IL-6 in patients with COVID-19 has led to comparisons to CAR-T cell-associated cytokine release syndrome. However, low concentrations of IL-6 and the absence of substantial elevations of IFN gamma in patients with COVID-19 limit this analogy to cytokine release syndrome. Conversely, low IL-6 concentrations and high ferritin in patients with COVID-19 lead to a similarity with hemophagocytic lymphohistiocytosis or macrophage activation syndrome. However, the similarities are again limited because of the absence of substantial IFN gamma elevations in patients with COVID-19. Some researchers have proposed different immunophenotypes of COVID-19: some patients show Immonoparalysis and others a pattern similar to that of macrophage activation syndrome. However, under this paradigm, the macrophage activation syndrome-like phenotype represents a minority of patients (<15%). Insufficient high-quality data on cytokine patterns in hemophagocytic lymphohistiocytosis or macrophage activation syndrome preclude the inclusion of these diagnoses in analyses to date. There are many doubts about the widespread off-label use of cytokine blockade in the treatment of COVID-19 before there are clear results from randomized trials. Cytokine blockade has not been effective in bacterial sepsis and ARDS, in which inflammatory cytokine concentrations are much higher. Elevation of IL-6 has a role in activating the endothelium and precipitating pulmonary immuno-thrombosis, so that in some trials still in progress it could eventually be shown that anti-cytokine treatment may be beneficial in some patients with COVID-19. However, the use of these agents in the absence of clear evidence may be considered premature. Many guidelines, including that of the Infectious Disease Society of America (IDSA), do not recommend the use of tocilizumab in patients with COVID-19-associated ARDS outside the context of clinical trials, but antagonists against IL-6 and IL-1 have been administered in nearly 20% of patients with COVID-19 admitted to the ICU. The intense focus on cytokine blockade has attracted substantial investment. This focus may have discouraged clinical exploration of other hypotheses such as immunosuppressive therapy. There are in fact 20 trials of various IL-6 antagonists, in contrast to a single trial of recombinant IL-7, which had been effective in several other trials on severe other viral infections. There are four trials with interferons despite the fact that there is evidence that inhibition of IFN-1 signalling is an intrinsic mechanism of immune-evasion by SARS-COV2.

There is a single registered trial of all CTLA-4 and PD-1 or PDL1 blocking agents in which patients are randomized to pembrolizumab (a checkpoint inhibitor) and tocilizumab together versus standard care. Although cytokine concentrations are elevated in patients with severe or critical COVID-19, the degree of cytokinaemia is markedly lower than that seen in other disorders associated with elevated cytokines. With these observations in mind, the described cytokine storm in COVID-19 is very problematic as an activator of organ failure, and alternative mechanisms of organ dysfunction must be considered. The evidence brought by ongoing trials will determine whether cytokine blockade improves outcome in patients with severe and critical COVID-19. In contrast, immune-activating treatments (e.g., interferons, IL-7, or checkpoint inhibition) deserve further study, but there are still too few trials. Thus, the immune characteristics of COVID-19 still remain too poorly elucidated.

Deepening the pathobiological understanding of severe SARS-COV2 infection and host response must be given the highest priority.

10.6 Lessons Learned from Bacterial Sepsis Regarding Immunotherapies for COVID-19 Infection [59, 112–132]

Therapeutic approaches to mitigate the severe lung injury associated with SARS-COV2 infection have rapidly entered clinical trials following anecdotal observations and few clinical trials. In parallel with the clinical symptoms related to viral invasion, the reported molecular response known as the cytokinetic storm has attracted, as noted above, the most attention both in the scientific press and among the public as a cause of organ injury. The hypothesis that it might benefit the patient to temper this storm with anti-inflammatory therapies directed at reducing IL-6, IL-1, or even TNF-alpha has led to many more ongoing trials. Anecdotal evidence from uncontrolled clinical trials has suggested a possible beneficial effect, and anti-IL-6 has been shown to be effective in chimeric antigen receptor T (CAR-T) and cytokine release syndrome (CRS).

However, attempts made in past randomized clinical trials to block the cytokine storm associated with other microbial infections and with sepsis have not been successful, and in some cases have even worsened the outcome.

The redundancy of cytokine action, the delayed intervention, and the essential role of these cytokines in recovery and immune surveillance have all been proposed as possible explanations for these failures.

The first report from China placed emphasis on high plasma concentrations of IL-6 and provided a rationale for the introduction of anti-IL-6 therapies (tocilizumab and sarilumab) in randomized clinical trials. But closer evaluation of plasma IL-6 concentrations had provided contradictory data. Results from earlier studies suggested that plasma concentrations of IL-6, although elevated (hundreds of picograms per microlitre) above values obtained from healthy control patients, were modest, especially when compared with the "cytokine storm" associated with septic shock in which concentrations could be as high as thousands of picograms per microlitre. Although more recent, controlled studies indicate that plasma IL-6 concentrations may be in the range seen even in bacterial infections, the time course of their change is very different; in some cases, concentrations in patients with COVID-19 appear to increase over time with disease severity and worsening lung function.

These dynamics clearly distinguish the host response to SARS-COV2 from that seen in sepsis. Moreover, previous studies on sepsis established that IL-6 concentrations could be an indicator of the magnitude of the inflammatory response rather than the cause of organ injury. Therefore, it is important to ask whether current therapeutic approaches are merely running after symptoms or are modulating the disease itself. Little is known about the concentrations of other pro-inflammatory or anti-inflammatory mediators in patients with COVID-19, the landscape offered by the cytokine storm, and especially the chemokines that regulate the distribution and activity of effector cell populations. Interpreting changes in cytokine concentrations, all of which appear elevated, without additional immune cell parameters does not provide clarity about the molecular basis of COVID-19 or for potential treatment strategies. In truth when measured in patients infected with SARS-COV2, concentrations of IL-10 (the most immunosuppressive cytokine in the body) are elevated, which could lead to a different conclusion for therapeutic approaches and in the very understanding of the pathophysiology of the disease. Similarly it is now known that suppressing the innate and adaptive immune systems to target only high concentrations of cytokines such as elevated IL-6 could make unconditioned viral replication possible, suppress adaptive immunity, and delay the recovery process. Lost in the current enthusiasm of anti-inflammatory approaches to SARS-COV2 infection is the growing recognition that potent immunosuppressive mechanisms are prevalent in such patients. This focus is reminiscent of that seen in early investigations of sepsis-induced inflammation, because it was about a decade ago that, by now, the contribution of immunosuppression to the pathology of sepsis was generally accepted. Profound lymphopenia (low absolute lymphocyte counts) often at levels seen in septic shock is almost a uniform finding in critically ill patients with COVID-19 and correlates with secondary infections and mortality.

This loss of immune effector cells occurs in lymphocyte subgroups, including CD8+ and natural killer cells, which have an important antiviral role, and B cells that are essential for making antibodies that inactivate the virus. Autopsy findings revealed an almost complete dissolution of some lymphoid secondary organs. Without any surprise, nosocomial secondary infections often with pathogens usually associated with immunosuppression are present in more than 50% of hospitalized patients. This early immune picture of SARS-COV2 infection is one that shares many similarities with bacterial sepsis, but some differences should be noted. In particular, the modest inflammatory response and the progressive and profound suppression of adaptive immunity in COVID-19 related to sepsis lead one to consider a different therapeutic approach. Then sustaining the host's protective immunity should be considered as an essential component of any therapeutic intervention of equal or perhaps greater importance than going after the cytokine storm alone.

What is the most rational approach to support protective host immunity? Several immunostimulants are available in the clinical armamentarium for patients infected with SARS-COV2. Focusing on agents that target adaptive immunity in general, and T-cell function in particular, appears to be the most rational approach, based on the observation of progressive T-cell loss. Inhibitors of the "programmed death ligand pathway" (PD-1 example), such as nivolumab and pembrolizumab, have been game changers in cancer and some other viral infections. T-cells from patients with COVID-19 show clear evidence of depletion associated with increased expression of CD 279 (PD-1). In addition to checkpoint inhibitors, the pluripotent cytokine IL-7 has been effective in many other viral infections. Precocious clinical trials of both treatments have already been initiated in sepsis and have been shown to be safe and also have biological activity. IL-7 has been shown to be beneficial in increasing lymphocyte counts in septic patients with low ALC and in recovering protective immunity in JC virus-induced progressive multifocal leucoencephalopathy. Its efficacy and that of other immunostimulants in sepsis has recently begun to be explored and should be considered in SARS-COV2 infection. Although immunostimulants such as IL-7 or nivolumab could theoretically potentiate the cytokine storm, both have been given to patients with sepsis with IL-6 concentrations similar to those of patients with COVID-19 without exacerbation of inflammatory responses.

Randomized clinical trials based on the best observational studies remain of great importance to be able to move forward, and it is proposed to start with IL-7. Because of the complexity of the host response and the fact that monotherapies have never worked in sepsis trials in the past, it is suggested that priority be given to biological response modifiers that are pluripotent (such as IL-7) or combination therapies that target multiple immunologic pathways simultaneously (IL-7 and anti-PD1). What treatment approaches for sepsis teach us about COVID-19? Like sepsis, antimicrobials (antivirals in case of COVD) and supportive therapies remain the cornerstone of therapeutic interventions for SARS-COV2 infection. However, if SARS-COV2 infection is similar to other chronic inflammatory and immunosuppressive diseases, as in sepsis, immunostimulants, not anti-inflammatory agents, should be considered as the first-line option. However, we know that the pathophysiology and mechanisms of SARS-COV2 are yet to be elucidated and that there is great uncertainty in predicting the efficacy of current therapeutic approaches. We are only beginning to explore the interplay of virus-mediated endothelial damage, the effects of signals produced by virus receptors (including ACE2), and alterations in haemostasis and coagulation as a basis of the heterogeneous clinical pathologies observed in patients. Undoubtedly there might be a subgroup of patients with exaggerated release of pro-inflammatory cytokines that might benefit from anti-IL6 and anti-IL-1 therapies. However, until better methods are available to determine (among the heterogeneity in clinical phenotypes) which patients meet these criteria, it will be difficult to establish real benefit. Observations from clinical centres with large volumes of patients with COVID-19 show good evidence that patient mortality is directly related to multi-organ failure, including coagulopathy and probably endothelial damage. These patients also have impaired immune function as evidenced by lymphopenia. It is suspected that a balanced, biologically plausible approach would be to provide anti-inflammatory treatment early in the course of the disease coupled with antiviral therapies such as remdesivir. When the disease transitions to a suppressed state, therapies that make the host recover protective immunity should be considered as a high priority for ICU patients with progressive lung injury. What more needs to be considered? Better methods are needed to assess the functional status of immune cells in patients with COVID-19. Circulating cytokine concentrations might reflect the degree of systemic inflammation but are not indicative of the functional status of individual lymphocyte and myeloid cell populations. Readily applicable tests that inform whether the adaptive immune system is depleted or whether myeloid cells are activated or tolerant would better guide the application of drugs that effectively modulate the immune response. Thus, immune therapies balanced towards cells of innate immunity or those of adaptive immunity are more capable of achieving a result. This approach is now used in cancer immunotherapy and has been tested in the treatment of sepsis.

This balanced therapeutic approach will allow more precise use of inhibitory (anti-IL6 and anti-IL-1) or restorative (IL-7 and checkpoint inhibitors) therapies, probably both as adjuvants to antiviral drugs. We need better measures of viral load with rapid turnaround time (TAT). Our ability to identify and quantify bacterial infections in patients with sepsis is still rudimentary, and quantification of viral loads with qPCR has not provided the required precision that has hampered our ability to evaluate the efficacy of interventions. In designing and conducting trials in patients with COVID-19 we need to remember the lessons learned from the sepsis epidemic that kills 250,000 people each year in, for example, the United States but also in countries around the world. Inflammation is often transient, and the Surviving Sepsis Campaign has shown that early recognition and more immediate implementation of best practices can reduce early mortality and organ injury due to cytokine storm. Conversely, immune suppression is prolonged, progressive, and eventually lethal. Effective treatment of patients in this pandemic needs to be balanced, administered precisely to individual patients, and built on knowledge of past failures so that future successes can be achieved.

10.7 Immunoparalysis in COVID-19 Sepsis

While increasingly effective vaccines and increasingly effective antiviral treatments are awaited, understanding the host immune response to a totally unknown virus is of great importance in terms of immuno-surveillance. At the forefront of the immune changes described in the early COVID-19 cohorts were patients who homogeneously presented with an inflammatory response and severe lymphopenia and who showed similarities to the changes seen in sepsis [54, 59, 125, 133, 134].

By international definition, sepsis is defined as a life-threatening organ dysfunction caused by dysregulated host response to infection. In COVID-19, ARDS, an organ dysfunction, can occur in most critically ill patients, and therefore this severe/critical COVID-19 should be considered a viral sepsis. While it has long been believed that sepsis alters immune homeostasis by provoking a very intense systemic inflammatory response, observations as fundamental as they are little emphasized, most of them based on clinical flow cytometry [135] have shown that sepsis induces the concomitant occurrence of both pro-inflammatory and anti-inflammatory mechanisms. As a result, some septic patients enter a stage of protracted immunosuppression [102, 136], but this aspect, as noted above, has been poorly explored in patients with COVID-19. Among the immunological parameters routinely used to monitor septic patients in ICUs, those obtained by flow cytometry have gradually gained interest because they help stratify septic patients for immune-stimulation in randomized trials [137–139] that will need to confirm their importance. Among these parameters, monocyte HLA-DR (m-HLA-DR) is currently considered as the benchmark.

10.7.1 Monocyte HLA-DR as a Pro-/Anti-inflammatory Marker

Monocytes are by their nature extremely plastic cells. They have the ability to discover damage and trigger inflammation and initiate the resolution of inflammation by triggering anti-inflammation. Throughout the progression of a disease, monocytes can be alternately pro- and anti-inflammatory cells. The resultant pro- and anti-inflammatory forces impacting at a given point in time are globally reflected by the level of m-HLA-DR expression on their surface [139].

In sepsis, reduced expression of m-HLA-DR clinically represents the phenomenon of endotoxin tolerance characterized by altered function (e.g., reduced TNF release to secondary infectious challenge) and reflects decreased antigen presentation capacity since HLA-DR molecules belong to the major histocompatibility complex class II (MHCII) system [140, 141]. To date, there is consensus in considering a low level of m-HLA-DR as a marker of sepsis-induced immunosuppression [142, 143]. In clinical trials, the magnitude and persistence over time of m-HLA-DR loss have been shown to be associated with worsening patient [137, 144], i.e., increased mortality and secondary nosocomial infections (even after multivariate analysis including confounding factors). It should be noted that in addition to sepsis, m-HLA-DR has progressively become a popular immune-monitoring tool in other ICU settings (trauma, burns, major surgery) and other clinical areas (gastroenterology, oncology, haematology, transplantation), where it also identifies patients at risk of worsening: mortality, secondary infections, cancer relapse [140]. In contrast, as marked monocyte activation, extremely increased m-HLA-DR values are reported in hemophagocytic lympho-histiocytosis and cytokine release syndrome [145]. In COVID-19 infection, being a disease that progresses step by step to increased severity until the onset of ARDS, m-HLA-DR can provide useful information on the inflammation/immunosuppression status of patients and disease progression.

10.7.2 Clinical Outcomes in Patients with COVID-19-Immunophenotype In-Depth Studies

Dealing with a totally new disease, many exploratory studies not guided by precise hypotheses have been conducted to decipher the immune processes at play in COVID-19. Taken together, these studies have mixed various approaches of flow methods (spectral flow, multicolour flow, time-of-flight mass spectrometry), transcriptomic strategies (transcriptomic signatures, single-cell RNA sequencing), functional testing, and multiple measurements of soluble mediators. The results were most often analysed by multi data/omics algorithms. In this large number of articles, when specifically considering monocytes and HLA-DR expression as keywords, four relevant studies can be identified [146–149].

Without taking into consideration the protocol used, these studies consistently report decreased HLA-DR in patients with COVID-19. This was the clearest phenotype. These studies consistently observed that the depth of this decrease was associated with severity, i.e., values were lower in patients with more severe disease than those with moderate disease. Severity was also associated with depletion of non-classical monocyte subgroups (e.g., $CD14^{basso}$ CD16+) [149, 150]. In addition, monocytes exhibited altered release of inflammatory cytokines when functionally tested [148, 150], indicating a deactivated rather than pro-inflammatory state, which is in line with that observed by other researchers [150] who measured circulating cytokines and reported the absence of a broad cytochemical storm. In agreement other researchers still [147] hypothesized the pulmonary origin of circulating cytokines rather than an exacerbated systemic production. This agrees with the decreased expression of HLA-DR on circulating monocytes since, in cases of enormous monocyte activation, m-HLA-DR should rise to very high levels. Overall, in patients with COVID-19, these data indicate instead an immunosuppressed phenotype of circulating monocytes.

10.7.3 Measurements of HLA-DR on Arrival at the Hospital and Various Severities of Patients

Four articles specifically report the measurement of HLA-DR at hospital admission [148, 151–153]. Patients presented with various levels of severity, and flow cytofluorimetry was routinely performed, and the results were expressed as averages of fluorescence intensities (for the total CD14+ monocyte population), with the problem that the results cannot then be closely compared between centres. Comparing with healthy controls, all studies observed lower expression of m-HLA-DR in patients with COVID-19. This difference was more pronounced in critically ill patients on arrival at the hospital. In addition, some clinicians observed that among the most severely ill patients, those progressing to a critical state (ICU admission) had the lowest expression [9, 151]. Also, as mentioned above, in COVID-19 patients, the proportion of nonclassical monocytes ($CD14^{low}CD16+$) was lower than in controls. Taken together, these results indicate that, on arrival at the hospital, the m-HLA-DR value is closely associated with the severity of COVID-19 and thus can serve as a marker for triaging patients.

10.7.4 Kinetics of HLA-DR Monitoring in Intensive Care Unit Patients

Seven articles report studies in which m-HLA-DR is monitored in patients admitted to the ICU over 1 week to 1 month. Four were based on values obtained using a standardized protocol, and the results are expressed as the number of antibodies bound per cell (AB/C). These studies performed independently by different groups located in different countries provided extremely homogeneous results [154–157]. The initial m-HLA-DR values for patients admitted to the ICU were around 10,000 AB/C, which was lower than controls (>15,000 AB/C) but not as low as those found in septic shock from bacterial infection (around 5000 AB/C). During the ICU stay, the values remained stable or progressively declined further. In some studies, the lowest levels of m-HLA-DR expression (<4000 AB/C) were observed in patients who died. It is interesting to note that m-HLA-DR expression was used to monitor a critically ill COVID-19 patient receiving rhIL-7 therapy [158]. After more than 3 weeks in the ICU and several episodes of recurrent infections along with consistent PCR positivity for SARS-COV2, m-HLA-DR expression was <4000 AB/C. After drug initiation, m-HLA-DR expression rapidly normalized. In addition, although in these studies the reported data were not in AB/C, two other studies are worth noting: in one study decreased m-HLA-DR expression was reported in patients with COVID-ARDS compared with healthy controls, but this value was not as low as that found with bacterial ARDS. Again, this decreased expression of m-HLA-DR was stable for a period of more than 6 days [159]. Finally, some clinicians followed 157 severe patients for 30 days and reported a drop in m-HLA-DR expression in patients who died, and this alteration was observed at each monitoring point in time [160]. These data are extremely homogeneous because all moderately to severely ill COVID-19 patients have decreased m-HLA-DR expression. The depth of m-HLA-DR drop is associated with severity on hospital admission. However, the loss of m-HLA-DR expression is not as marked as that observed in septic shock. In the ICU, a low level of m-HLA-DR is remarkably stable over time or tends to slowly worsen. Loss of m-HLA-DR is associated with functional deactivation of the monocyte (e.g., altered release of inflammatory cytokines). Loss of m-HLA-DR is also accompanied by the disappearance of nonclassical monocytes (CD14^{basso} CD16+), also known as inflammatory monocytes. In some studies, lower m-HLA-DR expression is associated with mortality in the ICU although the question of the association between low m-HLA-DR and mortality in patients who remain in the ICU for a long time still remains an open question for further evaluation. Based on an extensive literature describing immunosuppression and its associated decreased m-HLA-DR expression in sepsis, it seems that it can be reasonably concluded that COVID-19 patients admitted to the ICU, such as septic patients, exhibit features of immunosuppression. In addition to decreased m-HLA-DR, these COVID-19 patients also exhibit profound lymphopenia, low plasmacytoid dendritic cell counts, and altered IFN alpha production [133, 147, 148, 161, 162]. These additional abnormalities are typical features of the process of age-acquired immunosuppression (also called immune-senescence) observed in elderly people who are, by far, the main victims of COVID-19 infection. It can be hypothesized that the evolution of COVID-19 towards organ failure is primarily a consequence of this altered immunologic status and that in the case of occurrence of ARDS, it secondarily amplifies this immunosuppression in a vicious circle as described in sepsis in the elderly [163].

The concomitant absence of an antiviral drug and a stable memory of immune response against a totally novel virus in immunosuppressed elderly patients probably can explain the long ICU stay and the stability of immune changes in patients admitted to the ICU in comparison with other bacterial ARDS for which appropriate antibiotics are available. Despite a moderate inflammatory process that appears to be of local origin [100, 147, 148, 164] which probably illustrates pulmonary spread of the virus instead of a systemic cytochemical storm, immune-stimulation in COVID-19 could be an important therapeutic approach. Only very few studies have explored this option. Decreased m-HLA-DR expression and profound lymphopenia may help in guiding such therapeutic strategies. Since the emergence of COVID-19 disease, the number of patients admitted to the ICU has never stopped rising. Pending effective antiviral treatment, understanding the host immune response to a totally unknown virus through immune surveillance (immune monitoring) is of paramount importance. At the forefront of the immune alterations previously described in COVID-19, patients homogeneously present with severe lymphopenia [59, 165]. Interestingly, bacterial sepsis also profoundly disrupts immune homeostasis by inducing a complex immune response that varies over time and associates a systemic inflammatory response and lymphopenia [166]. Immune monitoring in the first 15 days in COVID-19 patients admitted to the ICU based on markers previously evaluated in bacterial sepsis becomes critical [166]. In one such immune monitoring, 30 patients were included. After 2 weeks, 4 patients (13%) died, 15 patients (50%) had left the ICU, and mechanical ventilation was still required for 11 (37%). Marked lymphopenia present on admission and stable in the first 15 days could be observed. This affected all lymphocyte subgroups as there was no alteration in lymphocyte subpopulation rates or CD4/CD8 ratio. Expression related to m-HLA-DR moderately decreased upon admission and tended to decrease to about 9000 AB/C. Finally, cytokine levels were modestly elevated compared with the findings observed in bacterial septic shock. It is noteworthy that the most severe alterations were found in ARDS patients. Among the 4 patients who died on day 15, 2 had very high IL-6 values (>7000 pg/mL) and 2 had extremely low m-HLA-DR values (<4000 AB/C). The results of this monitoring begin to shed light on the immune response in patients admitted to the ICU for critical COVID-19. The majority of patients (86%) survived and had immune changes that persisted for at least

2 weeks. Overall, the immune response to SARS-CoV-2 infection has similarities with the delayed immunosuppression phase of bacterial sepsis. These include severe lymphopenia affecting all subgroups of lymphocytes; a decreased m-HLA-DR level but not as low as that observed in bacterial septic shock; and a moderate increase in plasma cytokine levels occurring at the same time, both inflammatory (IL-6) and immunosuppressive (IL-10). Thirty percent of these patients manifested secondary infections. It is therefore of paramount importance to always go for secondary bacterial and/or fungal infection in these patients. However, in COVID-19 patients, the remarkable stability of immune system changes (dominated by profound lymphopenia) is unusual compared with bacterial sepsis. It can be hypothesized that the absence of potent antiviral drugs together with immune defects contributes to preventing the body from eradicating the virus and thus explains the long ICU stays reported by many authors. Supporting this hypothesis, one study showed a negative correlation between lymphocyte count and pulmonary viral load [167, 168]. However, this preliminary study has limitations (small cohort size, single centre, incomplete immune profile, and no follow-up of viral load during ICU stay). However, it provides additional information regarding immune response during COVID-19 infection after ICU admission and underscores the importance of persistent immunosuppression that deserves attention and further study.

References

1. Casadevall A, Pirofski L. Host-pathogen interactions: redefining the basic concepts of virulence and pathogenicity. Infect Immun. 1999;67:3703–13.
2. Casadevall A, Pirofski L. The damage-response framework of microbial pathogenesis. Nat Rev Microbiol. 2003;1:17–24.
3. Jabra-Rizk MA, Kong EF, Tsui C, Nguyen MH, Clancy CJ, Fidel PL Jr, Noverr M. Candida albicans pathogenesis: fitting within the hostmicrobe damage response framework. Infect Immun. 2016;84:2724–39.
4. Panackal AA, Williamson KC, van de Beek D, Boulware DR, Williamson PR. Fighting the monster: applying the host damage framework to human central nervous system infections. mBio. 2016;7:e01906–15.
5. Pirofski LA, Casadevall A. Immune-mediated damage completes the parabola: Cryptococcus neoformans pathogenesis can reflect the outcome of a weak or strong immune response. mBio. 2017;8:e02063–17.
6. Pirofski LA, Casadevall A. The damage-response framework as a tool for the physician-scientist to understand the pathogenesis of infectious diseases. J Infect Dis. 2018;218(Suppl 1):S7–S11.
7. Casadevall A, Pirofski LA. What is a host? Attributes of individual susceptibility. Infect Immun. 2018;86:e00636–17.
8. Guan WJ, Ni ZY, Hu Y, Liang WH, Ou CQ, He JX, Liu L, Shan H, Lei CL, Hui DSC, Du B, Li LJ, Zeng G, Yuen KY, Chen RC, Tang CL, Wang T, Chen PY, Xiang J, Li SY, Wang JL, Liang ZJ, Peng YX, Wei L, Liu Y, Hu YH, Peng P, Wang JM, Liu JY, Chen Z, Chen Z, Li G, Zheng ZJ, Qiu SQ, Luo J, Ye CJ, Zhu SY, Zhong NS, China Medical Treatment Expert Group for Covid-19. Clinical characteristics of coronavirus disease 2019 in China. N Engl J Med. 2020;382:1708–20.

9. Giamarellos-Bourboulis EJ, Netea MG, Ruin N, Akinosoglou K, Antoniadou A, Antonakos N, Damoraki G, Gkavogianni T, Adami ME, Katsaounou P, Ntaganou M, Kyriakopoulou M, Dimopoulos G, Koutsodimitropoulos I, Velissaris D, Koufargyris P, Karageorgos A, Katrini K, Lekakis V, Lupse M, Kotsaki A, Renieris G, Theodoulou D, Panou V, Koukaki E, Koulouris N, Gogos C, Koutsoukou A. Complex immune dysregulation in COVID-19 patients with severe respiratory failure. Cell Host Microbe. 2020;27:992–1000.

10. Li YC, Bai WZ, Hashikawa T. The neuroinvasive potential of SARSCoV2 may play a role in the respiratory failure of COVID-19 patients. J Med Virol. 2020;92:552–5.

11. Cui S, Chen S, Li X, Liu S, Wang F. Prevalence of venous thromboembolism in patients with severe novel coronavirus pneumonia. J Thromb Haemost. 2020;18:1421–4.

12. Wu C, Chen X, Cai Y, Xia J, Zhou X, Xu S, Huang H, Zhang L, Zhou X, Du C, Zhang Y, Song J, Wang S, Chao Y, Yang Z, Xu J, Zhou X, Chen D, Xiong W, Xu L, Zhou F, Jiang J, Bai C, Zheng J, Song Y. Risk factors associated with acute respiratory distress syndrome and death in patients with coronavirus disease 2019 pneumonia in Wuhan, China. JAMA Intern Med. 2020;180:934–43.

13. Zhang W, Zhao Y, Zhang F, Wang Q, Li T, Liu Z, Wang J, Qin Y, Zhang X, Yan X, Zeng X, Zhang S. The use of anti-inflammatory drugs in the treatment of people with severe corona-virus disease 2019 (COVID-19): the perspectives of clinical immunologists from China. Clin Immunol. 2020;214:108393.

14. WHO. Novel coronavirus—China. 2020.

15. Wu Z, McGoogan JM. Characteristics of and important lessons from the coronavirus disease 2019 (COVID-19) outbreak in China: summary of a report of 72314 cases from the Chinese Center for Disease Control and Prevention. JAMA. 2020;323:1239–42.

16. Lu R, Zhao X, Li J, et al. Genomic characterization and epidemiology of 2019 novel corona-virus: implications for virus origins and receptor binding. Lancet. 2020;395:565–74.

17. Mason RJ. Pathogenesis of COVID-19 from a cell biologic perspective. Eur Respir J. 2020;55:2000607.

18. Klein SL, Flanagan KL. Sex differences in immune responses. Nat Rev Immunol. 2016;16:626–38.

19. Ip DK, Lau LL, Leung NH, Fang VJ, Chan KH, Chu DK, Leung GM, Peiris JS, Uyeki TM, Cowling BJ. Viral shedding and transmission potential of asymptomatic and paucisymptom-atic influenza virus infections in the community. Clin Infect Dis. 2017;64:736–42.

20. Althouse BM, Scarpino SV. Asymptomatic transmission and the resurgence of Bordetella pertussis. BMC Med. 2015;13:146.

21. Gandhi M, Yokoe DS, Havlir DV. Asymptomatic transmission, the Achilles' heel of current strategies to control Covid-19. N Engl J Med. 2020;382:2158–60.

22. Long QX, Liu BZ, Deng HJ, Wu GC, Deng K, Chen YK, Liao P, Qiu JF, Lin Y, Cai XF, Wang DQ, Hu Y, Ren JH, Tang N, Xu YY, Yu LH, Mo Z, Gong F, Zhang XL, Tian WG, Hu L, Zhang XX, Xiang JL, Du HX, Liu HW, Lang CH, Luo XH, Wu SB, Cui XP, Zhou Z, Zhu MM, Wang J, Xue CJ, Li XF, Wang L, Li ZJ, Wang K, Niu CC, Yang QJ, Tang XJ, Zhang Y, Liu XM, Li JJ, Zhang DC, Zhang F, Liu P, Yuan J, Li Q, Hu JL, Chen J, Huang AL. Antibody responses to SARS-CoV-2 in patients with COVID-19. Nat Med. 2020;26:845–8.

23. Chen G, Wu D, Guo W, Cao Y, Huang D, Wang H, Wang T, Zhang X, Chen H, Yu H, Zhang X, Zhang M, Wu S, Song J, Chen T, Han M, Li S, Luo X, Zhao J, Ning Q. Clinical and immunologic features in severe and moderate coronavirus disease 2019. J Clin Invest. 2020;130:2620–9.

24. Mehta P, McAuley DF, Brown M, Sanchez E, Tattersall RS, Manson JJ. COVID-19: consider cytokine storm syndromes and immunosuppression. Lancet. 2020;395:1033–4.

25. Onder G, Rezza G, Brusaferro S. Case-fatality rate and characteristics of patients dying in relation to COVID-19 in Italy. JAMA. 2020;323:1775–6.

26. Du RH, Liang LR, Yang CQ, Wang W, Cao TZ, Li M, Guo GY, Du J, Zheng CL, Zhu Q, Hu M, Li XY, Peng P, Shi HZ. Predictors of mortality for patients with COVID-19 pneumonia caused by SARS-CoV-2: a prospective cohort study. Eur Respir J. 2020;55:2000524.

27. Zeng F, Guo Y, Yin M, Chen X, Deng G. Association of inflammatory markers with the severity of COVID-19. Int J Infect Dis. 2020;96:467–74.
28. Xu Z, Shi L, Wang Y, Zhang J, Huang L, Zhang C, Liu S, Zhao P, Liu H, Zhu L, Tai Y, Bai C, Gao T, Song J, Xia P, Dong J, Zhao J, Wang FS. Pathological findings of COVID-19 associated with acute respiratory distress syndrome. Lancet Respir Med. 2020;8:420–2.
29. Barton LM, Duval EJ, Stroberg E, Ghosh S, Mukhopadhyay S. COVID-19 autopsies, Oklahoma, USA. Am J Clin Pathol. 2020;153:725–33.
30. Magro C, Mulvey JJ, Berlin D, Nuovo G, Salvatore S, Harp J, Baxter-Stoltzfus A, Laurence J. Complement associated microvascular injury and thrombosis in the pathogenesis of severe COVID-19 infection: a report of five cases. Trans Res. 2020;220:1–13.
31. Sutton D, Fuchs K, D'Alton M, Goffman D. Universal screening for SARS-CoV-2 in women admitted for delivery. N Engl J Med. 2020;382:2163–4.
32. Xiao AT, Tong YX, Zhang S. False-negative of RT-PCR and prolonged nucleic acid conversion in COVID-19: rather than recurrence. J Med Virol. 2020;92:1755–6.
33. Arons MM, Hatfield KM, Reddy SC, Kimball A, James A, Jacobs JR, Taylor J, Spicer K, Bardossy AC, Oakley LP, Tanwar S, Dyal JW, Harney J, Chisty Z, Bell JM, Methner M, Paul P, Carlson CM, McLaughlin HP, Thornburg N, Tong S, Tamin A, Tao Y, Uehara A, Harcourt J, Clark S, Brostrom-Smith C, Page LC, Kay M, Lewis J, Montgomery P, Stone ND, Clark TA, Honein MA, Duchin JS, Jernigan JA, Public Health-Seattle and King County and CDC COVID-19 Investigation Team. Presymptomatic SARS-CoV-2 infections and transmission in a skilled nursing facility. N Engl J Med. 2020;382:2081–90.
34. Luo Y, Trevathan E, Qian Z, Li Y, Li J, Xiao W, Tu N, Zeng Z, Mo P, Xiong Y, Ye G. Asymptomatic SARS-CoV-2 infection in household contacts of a healthcare provider, Wuhan, China. Emerg Infect Dis. 2020;26:1930–7.
35. Long C, Xu H, Shen Q, Zhang X, Fan B, Wang C, Zeng B, Li Z, Li X, Li H. Diagnosis of the Coronavirus disease (COVID-19): rRT-PCR or CT? Eur J Radiol. 2020;126:108961.
36. Casadevall A, Pirofski L. Host-pathogen interactions: the basic concepts of microbial commensalism, colonization, infection, and disease. Infect Immun. 2000;68:6511–8.
37. Centers for Disease Control and Prevention. Use of cloth face coverings to help slow the spread of COVID-19. 2020.
38. Schneider DS, Ayres JS. Two ways to survive infection: what resistance and tolerance can teach us about treating infectious diseases. Nat Rev Immunol. 2008;8:889–95.
39. Ayres JS. Surviving COVID-19: a disease tolerance perspective. Sci Adv. 2020;2020:eabc1518.
40. Siddiqi HK, Mehra MR. COVID-19 illness in native and immunosuppressed states: a clinical-therapeutic staging proposal. J Heart Lung Transplant. 2020;39:405–7.
41. Ayres JS. Immunometabolism of infections. Nat Rev Immunol. 2020;20:79–80.
42. Troha K, Ayres JS. Metabolic adaptations to infections at the organismal level. Trends Immunol. 2020;41:113–25.
43. Ayres JS. The biology of physiological health. Cell. 2020;81:250–69.
44. Wang A, et al. Opposing effects of fasting metabolism on tissue tolerance in bacterial and viral inflammation. Cell. 2016;166:1512–1525.e1512.
45. Schieber AM, et al. Disease tolerance mediated by microbiome E. coli involves inflammasome and IGF-1 signaling. Science. 2015;350:558–63.
46. Rao S, et al. Pathogen-mediated inhibition of anorexia promotes host survival and transmission. Cell. 2017;168:503–516.e512.
47. Sanchez KK, et al. Cooperative metabolic adaptations in the host can favor asymptomatic infection and select for attenuated virulence in an enteric pathogen. Cell. 2018;175:146–158.e115.
48. Bornstein SR, Dalan R, Hopkins D, Mingrone G, Boehm BO. Endocrine and metabolic links to coronavirus infection. Nat Rev Endocrinol. 2020;16:297–8.
49. Yu X, Yang R. COVID-19 transmission through asymptomatic carriers is a challenge to containment. Influenza Other Respir Viruses. 2020;14:474–5.
50. Ayres JS. The biology of physiological health. Cell. 2020;181:250–69.

51. Booth CM, et al. Clinical features and short-term outcomes of 144 patients with SARS in the greater Toronto area. JAMA. 2003;289:2801–9.

52. Yang JK, et al. Plasma glucose levels and diabetes are independent predictors for mortality and morbidity in patients with SARS. Diabet Med. 2006;23:623–8.

53. Deng SQ, Peng HJ. Characteristics of and public health responses to the coronavirus disease 2019 outbreak in China. J Clin Med. 2020;9:E575.

54. Wang D, et al. Clinical characteristics of 138 hospitalized patients with 2019 novel coronavirus-infected pneumonia in Wuhan, China. JAMA. 2020;323:1061–9.

55. Zhang JJ, et al. Clinical characteristics of 140 patients infected with SARS-CoV-2 in Wuhan, China. Allergy. 2020;75:1730–41.

56. Casqueiro J, Casqueiro J, Alves C. Infections in patients with diabetes mellitus: a review of pathogenesis. Indian J Endocrinol Metab. 2012;16(Suppl 1):S27–36.

57. Kass DA, Duggal P, Cingolani O. Obesity could shift severe COVID-19 disease to younger ages. Lancet. 2020;395:1544–5.

58. Tong A, Elliott JH, Azevedo LC, et al. Core outcomes set for trials in people with COVID-19. Crit Care Med. 2020;48(11):1622–35.

59. Zhou F, Yu T, Du R, et al. Clinical course and risk factors for mortality of adult inpatients with COVID-19 in Wuhan, China: a retrospective cohort study. Lancet. 2020;395:1054–62.

60. Singer M, Deutschman CS, Seymour CW, et al. The third international consensus definitions for sepsis and septic shock (Sepsis-3). JAMA. 2016;315:801–10.

61. Li H, Liu L, Zhang D, et al. SARS-CoV-2 and viral sepsis: observations and hypotheses. Lancet. 2020;395:1517–20.

62. Odabasi Z, Cinel I. Consideration of severe coronavirus disease 2019 as viral sepsis and potential use of immune checkpoint inhibitors. Crit Care Explor. 2020;2:e0141.

63. Huang C, Wang Y, Li X, et al. Clinical features of patients infected with 2019 novel coronavirus in Wuhan, China. Lancet. 2020;395:497–506.

64. Connors JM, Levy JH. COVID-19 and its implications for thrombosis and anticoagulation. Blood. 2020;135:2033–40.

65. Su H, Yang M, Wan C, et al. Renal histopathological analysis of 26 postmortem findings of patients with COVID-19 in China. Kidney Int. 2020;98:219–27.

66. Tavazzi G, Pellegrini C, Maurelli M, et al. Myocardial localization of coronavirus in COVID-19 cardiogenic shock. Eur J Heart Fail. 2020;22:911–5.

67. Varga Z, Flammer AJ, Steiger P, et al. Endothelial cell infection and endotheliitis in COVID-19. Lancet. 2020;395:1417–8.

68. Puelles VG, Lutgehetmann M, Lindenmeyer MT, et al. Multiorgan and renal tropism of SARS-CoV-2. N Engl J Med. 2020;383:590–2.

69. Vincent JL, Sakr Y, Singer M, et al. Prevalence and outcomes of infection among patients in intensive care units in 2017. JAMA. 2020;323:1478–87.

70. Choi SH, Hong SB, Ko GB, et al. Viral infection in patients with severe pneumonia requiring intensive care unit admission. Am J Respir Crit Care Med. 2012;186:325–32.

71. Ljungström LR, Jacobsson G, Claesson BEB, et al. Respiratory viral infections are underdiagnosed in patients with suspected sepsis. Eur J Clin Microbiol Infect Dis. 2017;36:1767–76.

72. Shorr AF, Fisher K, Micek ST, et al. The burden of viruses in pneumonia associated with acute respiratory failure: an underappreciated issue. Chest. 2018;154:84–90.

73. van Someren Gréve F, Juffermans NP, Bos LDJ, et al. Respiratory viruses in invasively ventilated critically ill patients—a prospective multicenter observational study. Crit Care Med. 2018;46:29–36.

74. Rhee C, Dantes R, Epstein L, et al. Incidence and trends of sepsis in US hospitals using clinical vs claims data, 2009–2014. JAMA. 2017;318:1241–9.

75. Kissoon N, Daniels R, van der Poll T, et al. Sepsis-the final common pathway to death from multiple organ failure in infection. Crit Care Med. 2016;44:e446.

76. Sueblinvong V, Johnson DW, Weinstein GL, et al. The authors reply. Crit Care Med. 2016;44:e447–8.

77. Zheng S, Fan J, Yu F, et al. Viral load dynamics and disease severity in patients infected with SARS-CoV-2 in Zhejiang province, China, January–March 2020: retrospective cohort study. BMJ. 2020;369:m1443.
78. Bhatraju PK, Ghassemieh BJ, Nichols M, et al. Covid-19 in critically ill patients in the Seattle region—case series. N Engl J Med. 2020;382:2012–22.
79. Arentz M, Yim E, Klaff L, et al. Characteristics and outcomes of 21 critically ill patients with COVID-19 in Washington State. JAMA. 2020;323:1612–4.
80. Guo T, Fan Y, Chen M, et al. Cardiovascular implications of fatal outcomes of patients with coronavirus disease 2019 (COVID-19). JAMA Cardiol. 2020;5:e201017.
81. Jin Y, Yang H, Ji W, et al. Virology, epidemiology, pathogenesis, and control of COVID-19. Viruses. 2020;12:372.
82. Zou X, Chen K, Zou J, et al. Single-cell RNA-seq data analysis on the receptor ACE2 expression reveals the potential risk of different human organs vulnerable to 2019-nCoV infection. Front Med. 2020;14:185–92.
83. Menter T, Haslbauer JD, Nienhold R, et al. Post-mortem examination of COVID19 patients reveals diffuse alveolar damage with severe capillary congestion and variegated findings of lungs and other organs suggesting vascular dysfunction. Histopathology. 2020;77:198–209.
84. Wichmann D, Sperhake JP, Lütgehetmann M, et al. Autopsy findings and venous thromboembolism in patients with COVID-19: a prospective cohort study. Ann Intern Med. 2020;173:268–77.
85. Singer M. The new sepsis consensus definitions (Sepsis-3): the good, the not-so-bad, and the actually-quite-pretty. Intensive Care Med. 2016;42:2027–9.
86. Lin GL, McGinley JP, Drysdale SB, et al. Epidemiology and immune pathogenesis of viral sepsis. Front Immunol. 2018;9:2147.
87. Cummings MJ, Baldwin MR, Abrams D, et al. Epidemiology, clinical course, and outcomes of critically ill adults with COVID-19 in New York City: a prospective cohort study. Lancet. 2020;395:1763–70.
88. England JT, Abdulla A, Biggs CM, et al. Weathering the COVID-19 storm: lessons from hematologic cytokine syndromes. Blood Rev. 2021;45:100707.
89. Moore JB, June CH. Cytokine release syndrome in severe COVID-19. Science. 2020;368:473–4.
90. Sinha P, Matthay MA, Calfee CS. Is a "cytokine storm" relevant to COVID-19? JAMA Intern Med. 2020;180:1152–4.
91. Tan L, Wang Q, Zhang D, et al. Lymphopenia predicts disease severity of COVID-19: a descriptive and predictive study. Signal Transduct Target Ther. 2020;5:33.
92. Wang X, Xu W, Hu G, et al. SARS-CoV-2 infects T lymphocytes through its spike protein-mediated membrane fusion. Cell Mol Immunol. 2020;17:894.
93. Qin C, Zhou L, Hu Z, et al. Dysregulation of immune response in patients with COVID-19 in Wuhan, China. Clin Infect Dis. 2020;71:762–86.
94. Diao B, Wang C, Tan Y, et al. Reduction and functional exhaustion of T cells in patients with coronavirus disease 2019 (COVID-19). Front Immunol. 2020;11:82.
95. Leisman DE, Deutschman CS, Legrand M. Facing COVID-19 in the ICU: vascular dysfunction, thrombosis, and dysregulated inflammation. Intensive Care Med. 2020;46:1105–8.
96. Horby P, Lim WS, Emberson JR, et al. Dexamethasone in hospitalized patients with Covid-19. N Engl J Med. 2021;384:693–704.
97. Matthay MA, Zemans RL, Zimmerman GA, et al. Acute respiratory distress syndrome. Nat Rev Dis Primers. 2019;5:18.
98. Ackermann M, Verleden SE, Kuehnel M, et al. Pulmonary vascular endothelialitis, thrombosis, and angiogenesis in Covid-19. N Engl J Med. 2020;383:120–8.
99. Schaller T, Hirschbuhl K, Burkhardt K, et al. Postmortem examination of patients with COVID-19. JAMA. 2020;323:2518.
100. Sinha P, Calfee CS, Cherian S, et al. Prevalence of phenotypes of acute respiratory distress syndrome in critically ill patients with, COVID-19: a prospective observational study. Lancet Respir Med. 2020;8:1209–18.

101. Singer M, Deutschman CS, Seymour CW, et al. The Third International Consensus Definitions for Sepsis and Septic Shock (Sepsis-3). JAMA. 2016;315:801–10.
102. Hotchkiss RS, Monneret G, Payen D. Sepsis-induced immunosuppression: from cellular dysfunctions to immunotherapy. Nat Rev Immunol. 2013;13:862–74.
103. Remy KE, Mazer M, Striker DA, et al. Severe immunosuppression and not a cytokine storm characterizes COVID-19 infections. JCI Insight. 2020;5:140329.
104. Hay KA, Hanafi LA, Li D, et al. Kinetics and biomarkers of severe cytokine release syndrome after CD19 chimeric antigen receptor-modified T-cell therapy. Blood. 2017;130:2295–306.
105. Brudno JN, Kochenderfer JN. Toxicities of chimeric antigen receptor T cells: recognition and management. Blood. 2016;127:3321–30.
106. Lee DW, Gardner R, Porter DL, et al. Current concepts in the diagnosis and management of cytokine release syndrome. Blood. 2014;124:188–95.
107. Teachey DT, Lacey SF, Shaw PA, et al. Identification of predictive biomarkers for cytokine release syndrome after chimeric antigen receptor t-cell therapy for acute lymphoblastic leukemia. Cancer Discov. 2016;6:664–79.
108. Park JH, Riviere I, Gonen M, et al. Long-term follow-up of CD19 CAR therapy in acute lymphoblastic leukemia. N Engl J Med. 2018;378:449–59.
109. Giavridis T, van der Stegen SJC, Eyquem J, Hamieh M, Piersigilli A, Sadelain M. CAR T cell-induced cytokine release syndrome is mediated by macrophages and abated by IL-1 blockade. Nat Med. 2018;24:731–8.
110. Norelli M, Camisa B, Barbiera G, et al. Monocyte-derived IL-1 and IL-6 are differentially required for cytokine-release syndrome and neurotoxicity due to CAR T cells. Nat Med. 2018;24:739–48.
111. Ramos-Casals M, Brito-Zeron P, Lopez-Guillermo A, Khamashta MA, Bosch X. Adult haemophagocytic syndrome. Lancet. 2014;383:1503–16.
112. Blanco-Melo D, Nilsson-Payant BE, Liu WC, et al. Imbalanced host response to SARS-CoV-2 drives development of COVID-19. Cell. 2020;181:1036–45.e9.
113. Kotch C, Barrett D, Teachey DT. Tocilizumab for the treatment of chimeric antigen receptor T cell-induced cytokine release syndrome. Expert Rev Clin Immunol. 2019;15:813–22.
114. Le RQ, Li L, Yuan W, et al. FDA Approval Summary: tocilizumab for treatment of chimeric antigen receptor T cell-induced severe or lifethreatening cytokine release syndrome. Oncologist. 2018;23:943–7.
115. Chousterman BG, Swirski FK, Weber GF. Cytokine storm and sepsis disease pathogenesis. Semin Immunopathol. 2017;39:517–28.
116. Giamarellos-Bourboulis EJ. Failure of treatments based on the cytokine storm theory of sepsis: time for a novel approach. Immunotherapy. 2013;5:207–9.
117. Luo P, Liu Y, Qiu L, Liu X, Liu D, Li J. Tocilizumab treatment in COVID-19: a single center experience. J Med Virol. 2020;92:814–8.
118. Zhang C, Wu Z, Li JW, Zhao H, Wang GQ. The cytokine release syndrome (CRS) of severe COVID-19 and interleukin-6 receptor (IL-6R) antagonist tocilizumab may be the key to reduce mortality. Int J Antimicrob Agents. 2020;55:105954.
119. Tanaka T, Narazaki M, Kishimoto T. IL-6 in inflammation, immunity, and disease. Cold Spring Harb Perspect Biol. 2014;6:a016295.
120. Wang D, Hu B, Hu C, et al. Clinical characteristics of 138 hospitalized patients with 2019 novel coronavirus-infected pneumonia in Wuhan, China. JAMA. 2020;323:1061–9.
121. Zheng HY, Zhang M, Yang CX, et al. Elevated exhaustion levels and reduced functional diversity of T cells in peripheral blood may predict severe progression in COVID-19 patients. Cell Mol Immunol. 2020;17:541–3.
122. Zheng M, Gao Y, Wang G, et al. Functional exhaustion of antiviral lymphocytes in COVID-19 patients. Cell Mol Immunol. 2020;17:533–5.
123. Zhang W, Zhao Y, Zhang F, et al. The use of anti-inflammatory drugs in the treatment of people with severe coronavirus disease 2019 (COVID-19): the perspectives of clinical immunologists from China. Clin Immunol. 2020;214:108393.

124. Ritchie AI, Singanayagam A. Immunosuppression for hyperinflammation in COVID-19: a double-edged sword? Lancet. 2020;395:1111.
125. Gardiner D, Lalezari J, Lawitz E, et al. A randomized, double-blind, placebo-controlled assessment of BMS-936558, a fully human monoclonal antibody to programmed death-1 (PD-1), in patients with chronic hepatitis C virus infection. PLoS One. 2013;8:e63818.
126. Hotchkiss RS, Moldawer LL. Parallels between cancer and infectious disease. N Engl J Med. 2014;371:380–3.
127. Alstadhaug KB, Croughs T, Henriksen S, et al. Treatment of progressive multifocal leukoencephalopathy with interleukin 7. JAMA Neurol. 2014;71:1030–5.
128. Levy Y, Lacabaratz C, Weiss L, et al. Enhanced T cell recovery in HIV-1-infected adults through IL-7 treatment. J Clin Invest. 2009;119:997–1007.
129. Lu H, Zhao Z, Kalina T, et al. Interleukin-7 improves reconstitution of antiviral CD4 T cells. Clin Immunol. 2005;114:30–41.
130. Francois B, Jeannet R, Daix T, et al. Interleukin-7 restores lymphocytes in septic shock: the IRIS-7 randomized clinical trial. JCI Insight. 2018;3:98960.
131. Fuller MJ, Callendret B, Zhu B, et al. Immunotherapy of chronic hepatitis C virus infection with antibodies against programmed cell death-1 (PD-1). Proc Natl Acad Sci U S A. 2013;110:15001–6.
132. Minter S, Willner I, Shirai K. Ipilimumab-induced hepatitis C viral suppression. J Clin Oncol. 2013;31:e307–8.
133. Huang W, Berube J, McNamara M, Saksena S, Hartman M, Arshad T, Bornheimer SJ, O'Gorman M. Lymphocyte subset counts in COVID-19 patients: a meta-analysis. Cytom Part A. 2020;97A:772–6.
134. Del Valle DM, Kim-Schulze S, Huang HH, Beckmann ND, Nirenberg S, Wang B, Lavin Y, Swartz TH, Madduri D, Stock A, et al. An inflammatory cytokine signature predicts COVID-19 severity and survival. Nat Med. 2020;26:1636–43.
135. Aziz M, Fatima R, Assaly R. Elevated interleukin-6 and severe COVID-19: a metaanalysis. J Med Virol. 2020;92:2283–5.
136. Monneret G, Gossez M, Aghaeepour N, Gaudilliere B, Venet F. How clinical flow cytometry rebooted sepsis immunology. Cytom Part A. 2019;95A:431–41.
137. Venet F, Monneret G. Advances in the understanding and treatment of sepsis-induced immunosuppression. Nat Rev Nephrol. 2018;14:121–37.
138. Meisel C, Schefold JC, Pschowski R, Baumann T, Hetzger K, Gregor J, Weber-Carstens S, Hasper D, Keh D, Zuckermann H, et al. Granulocyte-macrophage colony-stimulating factor to reverse sepsis-associated immunosuppression: a double-blind, randomized, placebo-controlled multicenter trial. Am J Respir Crit Care Med. 2009;180:640–8.
139. Francois B, Jeannet R, Daix T, Walton AH, Shotwell MS, Unsinger J, Monneret G, Rimmele T, Blood T, Morre M, et al. Interleukin-7 restores lymphocytes in septic shock: the IRIS-7 randomized clinical trial. JCI Insight. 2018;3:e98960.
140. Venet F, Demaret J, Gossez M, Monneret G. Myeloid cells in sepsis-acquired immunodeficiency. Ann N Y Acad Sci. 2020;1499:3. https://doi.org/10.1111/nyas.14333.
141. Biswas SK, Lopez-Collazo E. Endotoxin tolerance: new mechanisms, molecules and clinical significance. Trends Immunol. 2009;30:475–87.
142. Wolk K, Docke WD, von Baehr V, Volk HD, Sabat R. Impaired antigen presentation by human monocytes during endotoxin tolerance. Blood. 2000;96:218–23.
143. Pickkers P, Kox M. Towards precision medicine for sepsis patients. Crit Care. 2017;21:11.
144. Galbraith N, Walker S, Carter J, Polk HC Jr. Past, present, and future of augmentation of monocyte function in the surgical patient. Surg Infect. 2016;17:563–9.
145. Mengos AE, Gastineau DA, Gustafson MP. The CD14(+)HLA-DR(lo/neg) monocyte: an immunosuppressive phenotype that restrains responses to cancer immunotherapy. Front Immunol. 2019;10:1147.
146. Remy S, Gossez M, Belot A, Hayman J, Portefaix A, Venet F, Javouhey E, Monneret G. Massive increase in monocyte HLA-DR expression can be used to discriminate between septic shock and hemophagocytic lymphohistiocytosis-induced shock. Crit Care. 2018;22:213.

147. Laing AG, Lorenc A, del Molino Del Barrio I, Das A, Fish M, Monin L, Munoz-Ruiz M, McKenzie DR, Hayday TS, Francos-Quijorna I, et al. A dynamic COVID-19 immune signature includes associations with poor prognosis. Nat Med. 2020;26(10):1623–35.
148. Arunachalam PS, Wimmers F, Mok CKP, Perera R, Scott M, Hagan T, Sigal N, Feng Y, Bristow L, Tak-Yin Tsang O, et al. Systems biological assessment of immunity to mild versus severe COVID-19 infection in humans. Science. 2020;369:1210–20.
149. Silvin A, Chapuis N, Dunsmore G, Goubet AG, Dubuisson A, Derosa L, Almire C, Henon C, Kosmider O, Droin N, et al. Elevated calprotectin and abnormal myeloid cell subsets discriminate severe from mild COVID-19. Cell. 2020;182:1401–1418.e18.
150. Schulte-Schrepping J, Reusch N, Paclik D, Bassler K, Schlickeiser S, Zhang B, Kramer B, Krammer T, Brumhard S, Bonaguro L, et al. Severe COVID-19 is marked by a dysregulated myeloid cell compartment. Cell. 2020;182:1419–1440.e23.
151. Moratto D, Chiarini M, Giustini V, Serana F, Magro P, Roccaro AM, Imberti L, Castelli F, Notarangelo LD, Quiros-Roldan E. Flow cytometry identifies risk factors and dynamic changes in patients with COVID-19. J Clin Immunol. 2020;40:970–3.
152. Gatti A, Radrizzani D, Vigano P, Mazzone A, Brando B. Decrease of non-classical and intermediate monocyte subsets in severe acute SARS-CoV-2 infection. Cytom Part A. 2020;97A:887–90.
153. Peruzzi B, Bencini S, Capone M, Mazzoni A, Maggi L, Salvati L, Vanni A, Orazzini C, Nozzoli C, Morettini A, et al. Quantitative and qualitative alterations of circulating myeloid cells and plasmacytoid DC in SARS-CoV-2 infection. Immunology. 2020;161:345–53.
154. Peruzzi B, Bencini S, Capone M, Mazzoni A, Maggi L, Salvati L, Vanni A, Orazzini C, Nozzoli C, Morettini A, et al. Quantitative and qualitative alterations of circulating myeloid cells and plasmacytoid DC in SARS-CoV-2 infection. Immunology. 2020;16:345–53.
155. Monneret G, Cour M, Viel S, Venet F, Argaud L. Coronavirus disease 2019 as a particular sepsis: a 2-week follow-up of standard immunological parameters in critically ill patients. Intensive Care Med. 2020;46(9):1764–5.
156. Kox M, Frenzel T, Schouten J, van de Veerdonk FL, Koenen H, Pickkers P, on behalf of the RCI-COVID-19 study group. COVID-19 patients exhibit less pronounced immune suppression compared with bacterial septic shock patients. Crit Care. 2020;24:263.
157. Jeannet R, Daix T, Formento R, Feuillard J, Francois B. Severe COVID-19 is associated with deep and sustained multifaceted cellular immunosuppression. Intensive Care Med. 2020;46:1769–71.
158. Spinetti T, Hirzel C, Fux M, Walti LN, Schober P, Stueber F, Luedi MM, Schefold JC. Reduced monocytic HLA-DR expression indicates immunosuppression in critically ill COVID-19 patients. Anesth Analg. 2020;131:993–9.
159. Monneret G, de Marignan D, Coudereau R, Bernet C, Ader F, Frobert E, Gossez M, Viel S, Venet F, Wallet F. Immune monitoring of interleukin-7 compassionate use in a critically ill COVID-19 patient. Cell Mol Immunol. 2020;17:1001–3.
160. Hue S, Beldi-Ferchiou A, Bendib I, Surenaud M, Fourati S, Frapard T, Rivoal S, Razazi K, Carteaux G, Delfau-Larue MH, et al. Uncontrolled innate and impaired adaptive immune responses in patients with COVID-19 ARDS. Am J Respir Crit Care Med. 2020;202:1509–19.
161. Wang F, Hou H, Yao Y, Wu S, Huang M, Ran X, Zhou H, Liu Z, Sun Z. Systemically comparing host immunity between survived and deceased COVID-19 patients. Cell Mol Immunol. 2020;17:875–7.
162. Zhou R, To KK, Wong YC, Liu L, Zhou B, Li X, Huang H, Mo Y, Luk TY, Lau TT, et al. Acute SARS-CoV-2 infection impairs dendritic cell and T cell responses. Immunity. 2020;53:864–77.
163. Acharya D, Liu G, Gack MU. Dysregulation of type I interferon responses in COVID-19. Nat Rev Immunol. 2020;20:397–8.
164. Monneret G, Gossez M, Venet F. Sepsis and immunosenescence: closely associated in a vicious circle. Aging Clin Exp Res. 2019;33:729–32.

165. Zhou Z, Ren L, Zhang L, Zhong J, Xiao Y, Jia Z, Guo L, Yang J, Wang C, Jiang S, et al. Heightened innate immune responses in the respiratory tract of COVID-19 patients. Cell Host Microbe. 2020;27:883–90.
166. Wang D, Hu B, Hu C, et al. Clinical characteristics of 138 hospitalized patients with 2019 Novel Coronavirus-infected pneumonia in Wuhan, China. JAMA. 2020;321:1061–9.
167. Venet F, Lukaszewicz AC, Payen D, Hotchkiss R, Monneret G. Monitoring the immune response in sepsis: a rational approach to administration of immunoadjuvant therapies. Curr Opin Immunol. 2013;25:477–87.
168. Liu Y, Yang Y, Zhang C, et al. Clinical and biochemical indexes from 2019-nCoV infected patients linked to viral loads and lung injury. China Life Sci. 2020;63:364–74.

Nutrition Therapy in Critically Ill Patients

Yaroslava Longhitano, Christian Zanza, Giulia Racca, and Fabrizio Racca

11.1 Introduction

Malnutrition, defined as loss of lean mass and depletion of essential micronutrients, occurs frequently in critically ill patients (20–40% of cases) [1] and is more frequent in patients requiring prolonged hospitalization [2–5]. Therefore, taking into account that caloric-protein deficit is a crucial critical factor in the outcome of patients with prolonged intensive care unit (ICU) hospitalization [6], all patients requiring a length of stay beyond 48 h in the ICU should be considered at risk of malnutrition and should be nutritionally supported [6]. In fact, protein-energy malnutrition is associated with the occurrence of muscle weakness, increased nosocomial infections, delayed wound repair, greater length of stay, and increased morbidity and mortality rates [1, 4, 6, 7].

Nutrition therapy refers to enteral or parenteral provision of calories, protein, electrolytes, vitamins, minerals, trace elements, and fluids. Traditionally, nutrition support in the critically ill population was regarded as adjunctive care designed to provide exogenous fuels to preserve lean body mass and support the patient throughout the stress response. Recently, this strategy has evolved to represent nutrition therapy, in which the feeding is thought to help attenuate the metabolic response to stress, prevent oxidative cellular injury, favorably modulate immune responses, and

Y. Longhitano · C. Zanza · G. Racca
Department of Anesthesiology and Intensive Care, Azienda Ospedaliera SS. Antonio e Biagio e Cesare Arrigo, Alessandria, Italy

F. Racca (✉)
Department of Anesthesiology and Intensive Care, Azienda Ospedaliera SS. Antonio e Biagio e Cesare Arrigo, Alessandria, Italy

Department of Anesthesiology and Critical Care Medicine, Azienda Ospedaliera SS. Antonio e Biagio e Cesare, Alessandria, Italy
e-mail: fracca@ospedale.al.it; fracca7766@gmail.com

support the capacity of skeletal and respiratory muscles leading to improvement in the clinical course of critical illness [6, 8].

Nutrition therapy includes the provision of either enteral nutrition (EN) by enteral access and/or parenteral nutrition (PN) by central or peripheral venous access. Delivering early nutrition support therapy, primarily by the enteral route, is seen as a proactive therapeutic strategy that may reduce disease severity, diminish complications, decrease length of stay (LOS) in the ICU, and favorably impact patient outcomes [6, 9–11].

Most critically ill patients who require nutrition (85–90%) can be fed enterally through gastric or intestinal tubes and then transitioned to an oral diet. However, in approximately 10–15% of such patients, EN is contraindicated [1].

Like any other management strategy in the ICU, nutrition therapy has potential harm, in particular from early and aggressive feeding [12], and should be tailored to the individual patient [9].

This review is intended to provide an update on clinical nutrition in adult critically ill patients expected to require an LOS greater than 2 days in a medical or surgical ICU.

Box 11.1 summarizes the most important concepts to keep in mind.

Box 11.1 Nutrition Therapy: Most Important Concepts to Keep in Mind
1. Initiation of EN should always be considered within 48 h of admission to the ICU in the absence of contraindications, using the gastric route and infusing the preparation by continuous infusion.
2. In all intubated ICU patients receiving EN, the head of the bed should be elevated 30°–45° and the use of chlorhexidine mouthwash twice a day should be considered.
3. Use standard EN formulas (except for diabetic patient and patients with renal insufficiency).
4. During EN monitor gastric residual volume and consider gastric residual volume increased when it exceeds 200 mL/6 h; temporarily suspend EN if gastric residual is >500 mL/6 h.
5. In case of gastric paresis and/or intestinal paralysis use prokinetics and/or laxatives.
6. If severe diarrhea appears during EN reduce infusion rate, search for the cause (rule out infection), discontinue laxatives and prokinetics, and consider enteral formulas containing fiber.
7. In case of contraindication to EN, PN should be started within 3–7 days. Exceptions are severely malnourished patients with contraindication to EN. In these cases, PN should be started as soon as possible starting with 50% of estimated energy requirements and with a gradual increase in caloric intake.

8. The estimated caloric target should be reached in 3–7 days for both PN and EN.
9. In case of supplementary PN to EN, PN should be discontinued when EN covers more than 60% of energy and protein requirements.
10. To avoid refeeding syndrome, the estimated caloric load should never be reached before 3 days after the start of feeding, starting with no more than 20 kcal/kg/day. The initial protein intake should be 0.8–1.2 g/kg/day and then should be gradually increased.

11.2 Pathophysiology of Malnutrition in ICU Patients

The pathophysiology of malnutrition in ICU patients is multifactorial. Malnutrition and muscle wasting generally occur during ICU stay due to the effect of catabolic hormones, an imbalance between intake and requirements, but also as a result of physical immobilization [6]. Despite efforts by intensivists to mitigate lean mass loss, this effect is still an expected occurrence, albeit in varying proportions.

After injury, the acute phase is characterized by catabolism and is composed of an early (1–2 days) and a late period (3–7 days). The early period (the ancient EBB phase) is defined by metabolic instability and severe increase in catabolism. The late period (ancient FLOW phase) is defined by a significant muscle wasting. Then, there is the post-acute phase, which is characterized by anabolism and rehabilitation and which begins as critical illness resolves; this phase is characterized by anabolism exceeding catabolism [6]. However, the post-acute phase may be characterized by a persistent inflammatory catabolic state, leading to prolonged inflammatory and catabolic syndrome [6].

The acute phase of critical illness is associated with catabolic hormonal and cytokine responses. These include increased blood levels of counterregulatory hormones (e.g., cortisol, catecholamines, and glucagon), increased blood and tissue levels of pro-inflammatory cytokines, and peripheral-tissue resistance to endogenous anabolic hormones (e.g., insulin and insulin-like growth factor 1) [1]. This hormonal milieu increases glycogenolysis and gluconeogenesis, causes a net breakdown of skeletal muscle, and enhances lipolysis, which together provide endogenous glucose, amino acids, and free fatty acids (FAs) that are required for cellular and organ function and wound healing. The above-described process can be compared to what occurs during fasting. During the first 24 h, the mechanism of hepatic and muscle glycogenolysis prevails; thereafter, when glycogen stores are depleted, gluconeogenesis (the production of glucose from plasma amino acids) is the main process by which the body's energy demands are met. When both compensatory mechanisms are exhausted or insufficient to meet the increased demands (due to depletion of glycogen stores and the inability to maintain protracted gluconeogenesis) and fasting is prolonged further, the body uses fatty acid reserves (leading to the phenomenon of ketogenesis) in an attempt to preserve the protein quota. Finally, when the fat reserves are also consumed, the body erodes the structural protein reserves present at the muscle level, resulting in loss of muscle mass. Unfortunately, during catabolic response, although plasma substrate levels may be increased, their availability for use by peripheral tissues is blunted because of factors such as insulin resistance [1].

In addition, critically ill patients often have a history of decreased spontaneous food intake before ICU admission and have episodes of abnormal nutrient loss from diarrhea, vomiting, polyuria, wounds, drainage tubes, renal replacement therapy. Bed rest, decreased physical activity, and neuromuscular blockade during mechanical ventilation cause further skeletal-muscle wasting and inhibit protein anabolic responses. Moreover, drugs that are frequently administered to patients in the ICU may themselves increase skeletal-muscle breakdown (e.g., corticosteroids), decrease splanchnic blood flow (e.g., pressor agents), or increase urinary loss of electrolytes, minerals, and water-soluble vitamins (e.g., diuretics). Finally, infection and surgical trauma may increase energy expenditure and protein needs [1]. Therefore, the nutritional status prior to the onset of the critical event and the duration of the fasting phase (deprivation of nutrition) crucially affect the prognosis.

11.3 Comparisons of Enteral to Parenteral Nutrition in Critically Ill Patients

As compared with PN, EN is less expensive, may better maintain intestinal mucosal structure and gut absorptive and barrier functions, and is associated with fewer infectious and mechanical and metabolic complications [1, 6, 13]. In addition, the evidence supports a clinically important reduction in infections and specifically pneumonia when EN is administered early to critically ill patients. The terms "early" and "late" were differently defined in clinical trials, but, essentially, EN was considered early when initiated within 48 h of ICU access and late when introduced in the following days.

The evidence for this approach is higher quality for patients with surgical problems than for patients with medical problems: surgical patients (e.g., trauma, peritonitis, pancreatitis, and burns) were the main focus of the randomized trials and meta-analyses [14, 15], whereas medical patients have primarily been studied in observational studies [2, 16].

The mechanisms by which EN decreases infectious complications are not completely known, but it has been hypothesized that this benefit is mainly attributable to the maintenance of intestinal immune function [17–22].

Pulmonary inhalation and diarrhea are the most frequent complications associated with EN, while central venous catheter-related infections and metabolic changes frequently arise in patients treated with PN.

11.4 When to Start Nutrition Therapy

A protracted low-calorie nutritional intake for 10–15 days is sufficient to induce malnutrition. No specific ICU nutritional score has been validated to assess patients at risk of malnutrition [6]. Anthropometric measures are not reliable in the assessment of nutrition status or the adequacy of nutrition therapy [9]. In addition, in the ICU setting, the traditional serum protein markers (albumin, prealbumin, transferrin, retinol-binding protein) are a reflection of the acute-phase response (increases in vascular permeability and reprioritization of hepatic protein synthesis) and do not accurately represent nutrition status [9]. Ultrasound is emerging as a tool to measure muscle mass and determine changes in muscle tissue at bedside in the ICU, given its ease of use and availability. However, validation and reliability studies in ICU patients are still pending [9]. While waiting for a validated screening tool, every critically ill patient staying for more than 48 h in the ICU should be considered at risk for malnutrition [6]. As a consequence, nutrition therapy in critically ill subjects is recommended when the patient is unable to spontaneously feed adequately within 48 h. Early EN (within 48 h) in critically ill adult patients should be performed whenever possible. In the case of contraindications to EN, PN should be implemented within 3–7 days. However, in the case of severely malnourished patients with contraindications to EN, early (within 1 week) and progressive PN should be provided [2, 6, 9, 23]. According to ESPEN definition [6], patients suffering from malnutrition include those with a BMI < 18.5 kg/m^2 or suffering from an unintentional weight loss >10% irrespective of time, or >5% over the last 3 months combined with either a BMI < 20 if <70 years of age, or a BMI < 22 if <70 years of age.

Contraindications to EN are displayed in Table 11.1. In particular, guidelines discourage early EN in critically ill patients with uncontrolled shock (i.e., if hemodynamic and tissue perfusion goals are not met despite fluids and vasopressors), since such patients may be predisposed to bowel ischemia [6, 9, 10]. Hemodynamic instability by itself is not a contraindication for enteral nutrition, if there is evidence for adequate tissue perfusion. Some conditions previously considered contraindications to EN are no longer considered as such. Examples include hyperemesis gravidarum and the absence of bowel sounds or flatus following routine colorectal

Table 11.1 Contraindications to enteral nutrition [6, 9, 10]

1. Uncontrolled shock (hemodynamic and tissue perfusion goals not achieved)
2. Uncontrolled life-threatening hypoxemia, hypercapnia, or acidosis
3. Uncontrolled high gastro-enteric bleeding
4. Discontinuity of the gastro-enteric tract
5. Overt bowel ischemia
6. Bowel obstruction (mechanical ileus)
7. Abdominal compartment syndrome
8. In patients with high-output intestinal fistula if reliable feeding access distal to the fistula is not achievable
9. If gastric aspirate volume is above 500 mL/6 h despite appropriate use of prokinetic drugs
10. Untreatable vomiting or diarrhea

surgery or surgery for bowel perforation [24–27]. While such patients remain at increased risk for vomiting, EN may confer an overall benefit since it may decrease the risk of infection [27]. In addition, a new gastrointestinal anastomosis distal to the infusion site that the surgeon feels is at risk of dehiscence was once considered a contraindication until more recent data indicated that early feeding strengthens anastomoses [28]. Whether this applies to all anastomoses is unknown, and when the anastomosis is felt to be tenuous, it is better to defer to the surgeon's judgment on whether EN should be early started.

Contraindications to PN include hyperosmolality, severe hyperglycemia, severe electrolyte abnormalities, volume overload, inadequate IV access, and inadequate attempts to feed enterally.

According to the most recent guidelines early EN (within 24–48 h) should be performed in critically ill adult patients [6, 9]. Indeed, the potential benefits of early enteral feeding (e.g., fewer infections, and possibly lower mortality) outweigh its risks [13, 14, 29, 30].

For adequately nourished patients who have contraindications to EN, guidelines recommend not initiating early PN [6, 9]. While the optimal time for starting PN in these patients is unknown, parenteral feeding typically does not start before 1 week has elapsed, and it should be avoided when conditions that temporarily preclude enteral feeding are expected to reverse quickly. This reflects the evidence that early PN may increase the risk of infection and prolong mechanical ventilation, ICU stay, and hospital stay [10, 20]. As a consequence, guidelines recommend that in the case of contraindications to EN, PN should be implemented within 7 days [6, 9]. On the other hand, for patients with malnutrition who have contraindications to EN, PN is suggested as soon as possible [9]. The rationale is that failure to treat starvation in patients with little reserve will result in a worsening of their state of malnutrition, which is associated with increased morbidity. As a consequence, guidelines recommend that in the case of severely malnourished patients with contraindications to EN, early and progressive PN should be provided [6, 9].

The optimal time to initiate supplemental PN in a patient who continues to receive hypocaloric EN is not clear. At some point after the first week of hospitalization, if the provision of EN is insufficient to meet energy requirements, the addition of supplemental PN should be considered, with the decision made on a case-by-case basis. ASPEN guidelines recommend that the use of supplemental PN should be considered after 7–10 days if unable to meet >60% of energy and protein requirements by the enteral route alone [9]. Then, when >60% of the patient's needs are met enterally, PN should be weaned [9].

After defining the timing and the route, the energy/protein goal should be achieved progressively and not before the first 48–72 h to avoid over-nutrition. Indeed, in the early phase of critical illness, which is associated with relevant endogenous energy production, the provision of excessive amounts of nutrients by any route should be avoided. In particular, fully targeted medical nutrition therapy should be prescribed within 3–7 days [6]. ASPEN guidelines suggest that in the early phases of critical illness patients requiring PN in the ICU may benefit from a feeding strategy that is hypocaloric ($\leq$20 kcal/kg/day or no more than 80% of estimated energy needs) but provides adequate protein ($\geq$1.2 g protein/kg/day) [9]. This strategy may optimize the efficacy of PN by reducing the potential for hyperglycemia and insulin resistance. Once the patient stabilizes, PN energy may be increased to meet 100% of estimated energy requirements [9]. As a consequence, EN and PN must be initiated slowly and with strict monitoring, in particular in severely malnourished patients at high risk for "refeeding syndrome" [9].

11.5 Refeeding Syndrome Prevention

The refeeding syndrome describes a constellation of metabolic disturbances potentially fatal that occur as a result of the reinstitution of nutrition to patients who are starved or severely malnourished [30]. It is defined primarily by manifestations of severe hypophosphatemia (including respiratory failure, cardiovascular collapse, rhabdomyolysis, seizures, and delirium), associated with hypokalemia and hypomagnesemia. In order to avoid refeeding syndrome calories may be increased to attempt weight gain once the patient is stable.

This syndrome is due to the sudden increase in insulin levels caused by the transition from a catabolic state in which lipids and proteins are used as a caloric source to a condition in which glucose is reused as an energy source. The increase in insulin level concentrations results in the reduction of thiamine and intracellular input of phosphorus, magnesium, and potassium [11]. Thus, Wernicke's encephalopathy may also occur in these patients. As a consequence, patients with chronic undernourishment should receive supplemental thiamine prior to the initiation of artificial nourishment to prevent Wernicke syndrome.

The main parameter used to make the diagnosis of refeeding syndrome is hypophosphatemia, which appears within 72 h after the start of nutrition (both in EN and PN) [11]. Intensivists should suspect the onset of this syndrome, especially in the presence of a patient with manifest malnutrition, in obese subjects with important recent weight loss, in patients with decompensated diabetes mellitus, in chronic alcoholism, in malabsorption syndromes, and in patients with prolonged intake of diuretics and antacids. In all of these patients, therefore, a nutritional supplement of 50% of the estimated caloric requirement (calculated on body weight at the time of admission) should be initiated. Then, nutrition is susceptible to a gradual and progressive increase until the target goal is reached over the course of about 10 days. In addition, non-nutritional sources of calories (e.g., propofol infusion) should always be considered in the caloric calculation.

Finally in all malnourished patients the following good practice rules should be adopted to prevent refeeding syndrome: (1) adequate thiamine intake should also be provided at the start of artificial nutrition (thiamine 100–200 mg/day i.v. in the first 3 days) associated with daily phosphate monitoring. (2) If hypophosphatemia appears within 3 days after the start of nutrition, caloric intake should always be reduced [11].

11.6 What Is the Best Method for Determining Energy and Protein Needs in Critically Ill Patients?

11.6.1 Energy Requirement

Clinicians should determine energy requirements to establish the goals of nutrition therapy. Energy requirements may be calculated through simple weight-based equation (20–30 kcal/kg/day), published predictive equations, carbon dioxide production (VCO_2), or indirect calorimetry (IC) [6, 9]. Achieving energy balance as guided by IC or VCO_2 measurements compared with predictive equations may lead to more appropriate nutrition intake. However, the applicability of IC and VCO_2 may be limited at most institutions by availability and cost [31]. The predictive equations are associated with significant inaccuracy (up to 60%), leading to over- or under-evaluation of the needs and inducing over- or underfeeding [6]. ASPEN and ESPEN guidelines suggest that IC be used to determine energy requirements when available [6, 9]. If calorimetry is not available, using VCO_2 (carbon dioxide production) will give a better evaluation of REE (REE = $VCO_2 \times 8.19$) than predictive equations [6]. In the absence of IC and VCO_2, these guidelines suggest that a published predictive equation or a simplistic weight-based equation should be used to determine energy requirements [6, 9]. Equations derived from testing hospital patients (Penn State, Ireton-Jones, Swinamer) are no more accurate than equations derived from testing normal volunteers (Harris-Benedict, Mifflin St. Jeor) [9]. The only advantage of using weight-based equations over other predictive equations is simplicity.

Additional energy provided by dextrose-containing fluids and lipid-based medications such as propofol should be accounted for.

Current body weight is used in weight-based equations. However, in critically ill patients following aggressive volume resuscitation or in the presence of edema or anasarca, clinicians should use the usual body weight (i.e., dry body weight) in these equations [9].

For underweight patients (BMI < 18.5 kg/m²), for normal-weight patients (BMI 18.5–24.9 kg/m²), and for overweight patients (BMI 25–29.9 kg/m²), the use of current weight is suggested. In fact, with regard to underweight patients, using the ideal weight would result in excessive caloric intake that could induce the refeeding syndrome [37]. For patients with peripheral edema, in theory, the weight derived from peripheral edema should be subtracted. For obese patients (BMI > 30 kg/m²) the ASPEN guidelines suggest going so far as to administer: (1) 11–14 kcal/kg of current weight in patients with BMI between 30 and 50 kg/m²; (2) 22–25 kcal/kg calculated on ideal weight in patients with BMI > 50 [9].

The required caloric need must be achieved gradually and incrementally in no less than 48 h. The guidelines [6, 9] suggest reaching the estimated caloric goal in 3–7 days for both PN and EN. In particular, they recommend starting both PN and EN with a caloric intake ≤20 kcal/day (or not exceeding 70% of measured REE) and reaching the estimated requirement after 3 days of nutrition. In fact, in the acute phase, critically ill patients have significant endogenous energy production in response to stress. Therefore, both PN and EN should be started slowly to avoid excessive calorie intake. This strategy during PN is also helpful in reducing the risk of hyperglycemia from insulin resistance.

Carbohydrates are believed to be the preferred energy source during this period because fat mobilization is impaired [32] and because of the preference for glucose in organs such as the brain, red blood cells, immune cells, renal medulla, and all the transparent tissues of the eyes [6]. However, in critical illness, insulin resistance and hyperglycemia are common secondary to stress, and excessive glucose-based energy provision is associated with enhanced CO_2 production, enhanced lipogenesis, increased insulin requirements, and no advantage in protein sparing in comparison with a lipid-based energy provision. As a consequence, the amount of glucose (PN) or carbohydrates (EN) administered to ICU patients should not exceed 5 mg/kg/min (i.e., 7.2 g/kg/day) [6]. The caloric contribution of dextrose in medical solutions is 3.4 kcal/g, which differs from dietary carbohydrate (4 kcal/g). The reason for the difference is that water contributes to the weight of the dextrose-hydrate that is used to prepare parenteral nutrition.

The hyperglycemia related to PN enriched in dextrose requires higher doses of insulin. The use of diabetic-specific enteral formula in ICU patients suffering from type 2 diabetes mellitus seems to improve the glucose profile. Citrate use in continuous veno-venous hemo-dia-filtration (CVVH) is also associated with increased carbohydrate load and should be taken into account as a non-nutritional calorie intake.

In 2001, a landmark trial showed that tight glucose control (TGC) (80–110 mg/dL) with intensive insulin therapy (IIT) was associated with reduced sepsis, reduced ICU LOS, and lower hospital mortality compared with conventional insulin therapy (keeping blood glucose levels <200 mg/dL) [33]. However, the NICE-SUGAR study, the largest trial, randomly assigned 6104 patients in 42 hospitals who were primarily fed via the enteral route to a blood glucose target of approximately 80–100 mg/dL (TGC) or <180 mg/dL (MGC). Patients in the TGC group had an increased risk of death at 90 days [34]. There was concern that severe hypoglycemia in this study might exacerbate deficits in the injured brain. As a consequence, ASPEN guidelines recommend a target blood glucose range of 140–180 mg/dL for the general ICU population [9].

For intravenous lipids (including non-nutritional lipid sources) the upper recommendation is 1 g/kg body weight/day with a tolerance up to 1.5 g/kg/day and should be adapted to individual tolerance [6]. The caloric contribution of a typical lipid emulsion is 10 kcal/g. Fat can be administered enterally or parenterally, and as for carbohydrates, the exact amount required is unknown. Fat absorption is impaired in critical illness. Lipid metabolism is modified in critical illness, and low plasma triglyceride levels and high plasma HDL cholesterol levels are associated with improved survival. Special attention should be paid if propofol is administered, since it is a source of fatty acids (FAs). This lipid solution contains 1.1 kcal/mL and can provide a large calorie load over and above nutritional support. Regarding the FA composition of the lipid emulsions, it is clear that the use of intravenous fat emulsions based solely on a soybean oil rich in 18 carbon omega-6 FA should be avoided due to their likely pro-inflammatory effects. Alternative lipid emulsions have become available, including sources that incorporate olive oil, fish oil, and coconut oil in various combinations. Meta-analyses have shown an advantage to lipid emulsions enriched in fish oil or olive oil [35]. Thus, the recent ESPEN recommendations indicate that a blend of FAs should be considered, including medium-chain triglycerides (MCTs), n-9 monounsaturated FAs, and n-3 polyunsaturated FAs [9]. However, the ASPEN recommendations do not acknowledge any advantage to new lipid emulsions [6].

Manipulation of the inflammatory process has been of strong interest in the nutrition support. One meta-analysis of 49 randomized trials reported that omega-3 fatty acid-enriched PN was associated with a 40% lower risk of infection compared with patients receiving standard parenteral nutrition without omega-3 fatty acid enrichment [12]. Hospital and ICU length of stay was also lower in the fatty-acid-enriched group. Parenteral lipid emulsions enriched with EPA + DHA (fish oil dose 0.1–0.2 g/kg/day) can be provided in patients receiving PN [6]. However, large, randomized trials are needed before parenteral nutrition with omega-3 fatty acids should be recommended.

ESPEN meta-analysis found a trend for advantage in oxygenation for enteral formulas enriched with omega-3 FA in pulmonary cardiogenic edema. As a consequence, EN enriched with omega-3 FA within nutritional doses can be administered. However, high-dose omega-3-enriched enteral formulas should not be given on a routine basis [6].

The administration of marked amounts of carbohydrates and lipids can lead to hyperglycemia and liver function test abnormalities, while high-fat administration can lead to lipid overload, and especially unsaturated fat can lead to impaired lung function and immune suppression. Close monitoring of triglycerides and liver function tests may guide the clinician for the best glucose/lipid ratio [6]. Blood triglyceride levels may be monitored at baseline and then generally weekly, particularly in patients with known lipid disorders, pancreatitis, or liver or renal disease, to assess clearance of intravenous fat [1]. Emergent hypertriglyceridemia or worsening of existing hypertriglyceridemia may result from the infusion of lipid emulsion. Cautious initiation of lipid emulsion has been recommended when serum triglycerides exceed 200 mg/dL (e.g., infuse lipid emulsion three times weekly) [36]. Concentrations up to 400 mg/dL are acceptable during therapy without altering the rate of lipids during therapy [36]. Doses of lipid emulsion should be reduced when triglyceride concentrations rise above 400 mg/dL (e.g., once or twice per week). It is also reasonable to attempt decreasing the proportion of calories provided by dextrose. Levels >1000 mg/dL are a contraindication to infusion [36]. Consequently, triglyceride levels should be measured at baseline and at least once each week. In addition, some authors observed improvement in liver enzymes in many patients with parenteral nutrition-related hepatic dysfunction when switching from soy-base to mixed lipid emulsions and when the percentage of fat and total calories is decreased.

11.6.2 Protein Requirement

The basis of protein prescriptions is the hope for mitigation of the breakdown of muscle proteins into amino acids. In the critical care setting, protein appears to be the most important macronutrient for healing wounds, supporting immune function, and maintaining lean body mass.

ESPEN guidelines suggest that 1.3 g/kg protein per day should be delivered progressively [6]. On the other hand, ASPEN guidelines suggest a protein provision of 1.2–2.0 g/kg/day [9]. A high protein intake can be considered in the stable phase of the patient and should be accompanied by the monitoring of azotemia, creatininemia, and excess bases. If metabolic acidosis appears and/or creatininemia increases decreasing protein intake should be considered [11]. For patients undergoing continuous renal replacement therapy (CRRT), a reduction in protein intake is not expected.

For most critically ill patients, protein requirements are not easily met by provision of routine enteral formulations, which have a high nonprotein calorie/nitrogen ratio. Patients with suboptimal EN due to frequent interruptions may benefit from protein supplementation.

The amino acid glutamine (GLN) is a normal component of proteins, representing around 8% of all amino acids. Glutamine is a precursor for nucleotide synthesis and an important fuel source for rapidly dividing cells, such as gastrointestinal epithelia. It is present in standard commercial enteral feeds. GLN for parenteral use is also available. For stability reasons, it was not present in standard PN preparations. Despite evidence that indicates that parenteral glutamine may be beneficial to patients who are receiving PN [14, 38], it is controversial whether or not to use parenteral glutamine.

The efficiency of enteral GLN on infection reduction was suggested in major burns [39] and in major trauma [40]. In other critically ill patients, the MetaPlus trial showed no advantage in terms of infection of a feeding solution containing additional enteral GLN [41]. As a consequence, ESPEN guideline [6] suggest that (1) in ICU patients, except for burn and trauma patients, additional enteral GLN should not be administered; (2) in patients with burns >20% body surface area additional enteral doses of GLN (0.3–0.5 g/kg/day) should be administered for 10–15 days as soon as EN is commenced; (3) in critically ill trauma additional EN doses of GLN (0.2–0.3 g/kg/day) can be administered for the first 5 days with EN. In the case of complicated wound healing it can be administered for a longer period (i.e., 10–15 days). During continuous renal replacement therapy, losses of about 1.2 g GLN/day are observed. These patients might be candidates for enteral complementation.

11.6.3 Micronutrients

Micronutrients consist of trace elements (i.e., Fe, Zn, etc.) and vitamins. They have numerous functions that they generally exert in combination: they are essential for the metabolism of carbohydrates, proteins, and lipids (i.e. nutrition), for immunity and antioxidant defense, for endocrine function, and for DNA synthesis. Providing a full range of trace elements and vitamins is an integral part of nutritional support. PN solutions contain no micronutrients for stability reasons. Thus, PN requires their separate prescription, and they should be provided daily [6]. In contrast, EN bags contain both vitamins and trace elements, and no additional supply is required.

11.7 Parenteral Nutrition (PN)

PN should be prescribed, tailoring the access for PN, the composition, and the infusion rate to the needs of each patient.

11.7.1 PN Venous Access

PN can be given either by peripheral or central vein. However, because of the risk of phlebitis, peripheral-vein parenteral nutrition cannot be highly concentrated (i.e., >600 mOsm/L), and therefore it must be given in a large volume to meet nutrient requirements. Fluid restriction because of renal, hepatic, or cardiac dysfunction often precludes the use of large fluid volumes; thus, peripheral-vein PN is generally not indicated in ICU patients. In these cases, PN must be delivered via a central venous catheter because it tolerates high osmotic load [42].

ASPEN guidelines for adult home PN administration [43] use an arbitrary cutoff of 30 days to distinguish short-term from long-term PN use. Patients in whom short-term administration of PN is desirable, it should be delivered through a peripherally inserted central catheter (PICC). Alternatively, while not preferable, PN may be administered through a subclavian, internal jugular, or femoral central venous catheter if PN is only needed for very short periods (e.g., a few days) or if a PICC is not feasible or reasonable. Tradition teaches that the femoral site is least desirable due to an increased risk of catheter-related bloodstream infections (CRBSIs) and is consequently not preferred.

For long-term administration of PN, ASPEN guidelines indicated a preference for a tunneled central venous catheter (TCVC; e.g., Hickman catheter, Groshong catheter, or implanted infusion port). However, the rationale for this choice is based upon expert opinion and observational studies. On the other hand, one systematic review suggested that CRBSIs rates were no different between PN delivered through a PICC compared with a TCVC [44]. As a consequence, many authors use PICCs preferentially because of the relative ease of removal and insertion compared to TCVC.

If a multiple lumen central venous catheter is used, it should have one port dedicated solely for the infusion of PN. In addition, catheter manipulations should be minimized. These precautions may decrease the infectious complications associated with PN [45, 46]. For patients who have an existing CVC, a new CVC is not typically required unless there has been septicemia during the life of the existing line.

11.7.2 PN Prescription

PN is a mixture of solutions that contain dextrose, amino acids, electrolytes, vitamins, minerals, and trace elements. Lipid emulsion may be infused separately or added to the mixture. However, mixing all three, a so-called total nutrient admixture, or three-in-one parenteral nutrition, is favored by most experts [47]. PN solutions contain approximately 1 kcal/mL.

Dextrose-containing solutions are available in a variety of concentrations, most commonly 40%, 50%, and 70%.

Lipids are provided as an emulsion that may be infused separately or added to the mixture. In Europe, in addition to only soybean oil-based fat emulsions there are also intravenous fish oil, mixtures of olive and soybean oils, medium-chain triglyceride–soybean oil mixtures, and combinations of these oils, all approved for use in PN. Regarding the lipid emulsions, the recent expert recommendations indicated that a blend of fatty acids (FAs) should be considered, including medium-chain triglycerides (MCTs), n-9 monounsaturated FAs, and n-3 polyunsaturated FAs. At this stage, the evidence for n-3 FA-enriched emulsions in non-surgical ICU patients is not sufficient [6].

In view of the fact that egg phospholipid is used to emulsify the triglycerides in intravenous fat emulsions and allergic cross-reactions have been reported, intravenous fat emulsions should be given with care to patients with prior allergy to eggs. However, these reactions are very rare.

Amino acid solutions contain most essential and nonessential amino acids. The exceptions are arginine and glutamine. The caloric contribution of amino acids is approximately 4 kcal/g.

Patients receiving PN must receive adequate *vitamins and minerals* to prevent deficiencies. For most patients, a unit dose of a standard multivitamin and multi-trace element solution will suffice to provide minimum daily requirements. It is advisable that patients with cholestasis do not receive copper or manganese, as these are excreted in bile. A total bilirubin of 2 is often used as a cutoff to restrict these.

11.7.3 Complications

Patients who receive PN are at risk for CRBSIs, complications related to venous access (i.e., bleeding, vascular injury, pneumothorax, venous thrombosis, arrhythmia, and air embolism), and adverse metabolic effects, including hyperglycemia, serum electrolyte alterations, hypertriglyceridemia, refeeding syndrome, Wernicke's encephalopathy, and hepatic dysfunction.

Patients receiving PN are at slightly increased risk of acquiring CRBSIs (bacterial and fungal; approximately one episode per 100 inpatient PN days) [48]. Factors that are independently associated with CRBSIs include poor patient hygiene, insertion of the central venous catheter under emergent circumstances, and, to a lesser extent, the severity of illness and duration of central venous catheterization [49].

11.8 Enteral Nutrition

EN refers to the provision of calories, protein, electrolytes, vitamins, minerals, trace elements, and fluids via an intestinal route. EN is most commonly delivered into the stomach (gastric feeding). However, it can also be administered into more distal parts of the alimentary tract (post-pyloric), particularly in those intolerant of gastric enteral nutrition (e.g., those with delayed gastric emptying or gastric outlet obstruction). There is no evidence that either continuous or bolus (i.e., intermittent) EN is superior to the other. Two randomized trials compared the two approaches and found no differences in mortality, infections, or ICU length of stay [50–52]. Nonetheless, EN is typically administered as a continuous infusion by many experts, particularly in patients at high risk of vomiting, reflux, and aspiration.

11.8.1 Access

Gastric feeding is typically delivered via an orogastric or nasogastric tube. Such tubes are available in two varieties: decompression tubes and feeding tubes.

Decompression tubes are larger and stiffer. They are generally inserted for gastric decompression and then used for short periods to deliver enteral nutrition when gastric decompression is no longer necessary. Concerns about longer-term use include nasal and esophageal erosion and sinusitis.

Feeding tubes are of smaller diameter, more flexible, and often require a stylet for insertion. A feeding tube's position should be confirmed radiographically before it is used because it is frequently misplaced into an airway [53]. Once its position is confirmed, the stylet should be removed and never replaced. Trying to replace the stylet while the tube is in the patient can lead to the stylet protruding from the outlet of the tube and result in inadvertent bowel puncture. Some feeding tubes cannot be used for gastric decompression because the soft walls tend to collapse when suction is applied.

Nasogastric tube is used for short-term EN (expected duration <4 weeks), while percutaneous or surgical access (gastrostomy or jejunostomy) is used when long-term EN is expected (expected duration >4 weeks) [11].

Feeding via tube through percutaneous endoscopic gastrostomy (PEG), percutaneous radiologic gastrostomy, and surgical gastrostomy are alternative approaches to delivering gastric feedings. A surgical gastrostomy tube can be inserted laparoscopically or by an open surgical approach. Post-pyloric tube placement is often challenging and may need to be reserved for patients with documented delayed gastric emptying or gastric outlet obstruction. Several techniques have been described for blind insertion of feeding tubes that terminate beyond the pylorus, usually ending in the first or second part of the duodenum. All are technically difficult and require advanced training. Other alternatives include endoscopically placed nasal tube, percutaneous endoscopic, percutaneous radiological, or surgical feeding enterostomy. Tubes used for post-pyloric feeding may have two ports, a proximal port to drain the stomach and a distal port to deliver EN into the distal duodenum or proximal jejunum.

All feeding tubes should have periodic water flushes to minimize clogging. Only water should be used for flushing.

11.8.2 Formulations

There are many products available for EN. Common differences between formulas include osmolarity, caloric density, and amount of protein per calorie, as well as electrolyte, vitamin, and mineral content. Most are formulated to provide 100% of recommended daily vitamin and mineral dose when a minimum of approximately 1000 or more kilocalories are delivered per day. In addition, there may be differences related to whether they are intact or pre-digested, fiber is present or absent, and disease-specific nutrients are present or absent.

For the majority of patients in an ICU setting, a standard polymeric isotonic or near-isotonic 1- to 1.5-kcal/mL formula is appropriate and will be well tolerated. In addition, no clear benefit to patient outcome has been shown in the literature for the routine use of specialty formulas in a general ICU setting, including those that are designed to be organ specific (pulmonary, renal, hepatic), semi-elemental, elemental, or immune-modulating [9]. In particular the rationale for pulmonary formulas (high fat to carbohydrate to reduce respiratory quotient) has been shown to be erroneous (effect seen only with overfeeding), and their high content of omega-6 fatty acid may drive inflammatory processes [9]. As a consequence, ASPEN guidelines suggest using a standard polymeric formula when initiating EN in the ICU setting and suggest avoiding the routine use of all specialty formulas in critically ill patients, and disease-specific EN is not recommended over the traditional types of enteral nutrition [9]. The exceptions are renal formulas for patients requiring fluid and electrolyte restriction, and glycemic control formulas for diabetic patients.

The following characteristics are typical of *standard enteral nutrition*: (1) isotonic to serum; (2) caloric density of approximately 1 kcal/mL; (3) lactose-free; (4) intact (nonhydrolyzed) protein content of about 40 g/1000 mL (40 g/1000 kcal); (5) mixture of simple and complex carbohydrates and long-chain fatty acids (although some are now including medium-chain and omega-3 fats); and (6) essential vitamins, minerals, and micronutrients. Standard EN delivers 49–53% of calories as carbohydrate and 29–30% of calories as fat. Low-carbohydrate/high-fat and high-carbohydrate/low-fat formulations exist, but neither is recommended for routine enteral nutrition. Standard EN delivers an intact (nonhydrolyzed) protein content of about 40 g/1000 kcal. In contrast, most renal enteral nutrition formulas deliver a protein content of 44 g/1000 kcal. Low-protein enteral nutrition was originally developed for patients with renal disease because of the widespread belief that protein restriction delays the progression of renal disease. However, clinical trials have shown that patients with renal failure can tolerate protein intake as high as 2.5 g/kg/day during critical illness. All feeding products consist of only 70–80% water. As a result, they are unable to meet patients' normal water requirements alone (enteral nutrition providing 25 kcal/kg with a 1 kcal/mL formula provides an average of only 20 mL/kg of water). This may be beneficial for patients who require fluid restriction, but most patients require another source of water. In addition, feeding tubes must be flushed regularly with water to avoid clogging.

Concentrated enteral nutrition may be useful for critically ill patients who require volume restriction (e.g., patients with respiratory failure or volume overload). The standard composition of concentrated EN is similar to that of standard EN, except that it is mildly hyperosmolar to serum and has a caloric density of 1.2, 1.5, or 2.0 kcal/mL. Historically, the hyperosmolality of concentrated EN was thought to predispose patients to diarrhea. However, current adult formulations rarely exceed approximately 750 mOsm/L and are rarely the primary cause of diarrhea.

Fiber-containing formulas are frequently used to correct diarrhea or constipation in patients who are already receiving EN [9]. However, there is no evidence that routine supplementation of EN with fiber can prevent either problem [55–59], and therefore its routine use for prophylaxis of diarrhea or constipation is not recommended [60]. However, based on consensus opinion, switching to a mixed fiber-containing formula is appropriate when there is persistent diarrhea [60].

Renal formulas may be helpful in managing patients who require fluid and/or electrolyte restriction, such as patients with acute renal failure complicated by fluid overload, hyperkalemia, and/or hyperphosphatemia, or those on hemodialysis with difficulties managing electrolytes and volume. Standard feedings, however, are acceptable in patients with renal failure when electrolytes and volume are adequately managed. Continuous renal replacement (CRRT) is highly effective at moving electrolytes such as potassium and phosphate. As a consequence, many authors prefer standard feeds, fluid restricted if necessary, for patients on CRRT.

More recent formulas for patients with renal failure have a high protein content (44 g/1000 kcal) in contrast to older formulations that contained a low-protein intake. In fact, recent studies have shown that these patients when admitted to the ICU, ventilated, and receiving CRRT tolerate up to 2.5 g/kg/day [54]. Such formulations are useful for feeding patients who require low water intake and low electrolyte intake.

Pre-digested EN (previously called semi-elemental, or elemental) differs from standard EN in that the protein is hydrolyzed to short-chain peptides and the carbohydrates are in a less complex form. The total amount of fat may be decreased, with an increased proportion of medium-chain triglycerides, or the triglycerides altered or structured to contain various mixes of fatty acids. The original formulations of pre-digested EN included amino acids instead of peptides or proteins. These formulations are less commonly used today, since they are more hypertonic and may be less well tolerated. Pre-digested EN usually has a caloric density of 1 or 1.5 kcal/mL. It is not recommended as an initial tube feed in critically ill patients [9]. The use of pre-digested EN is weakly supported by data. These have been proposed as potentially beneficial in patients with the following problems: (1) digestive defects (e.g., malabsorptive syndromes that are unresponsive to supplementation of pancreatic enzymes); (2) failure to tolerate standard EN, such as persistent diarrhea; (3) thoracic duct leak, chylothorax, or chylous ascites, since the medium-chain triglycerides do not enter the lymphatic capillaries in the small intestine.

Supplementation of enteral formulas with antioxidants plus omega-3 fatty acids was proposed with the hope it would have an anti-inflammatory effect in the lung. This led to the evaluation of these feeding products in patients with acute lung injury or acute respiratory distress syndrome (ALI/ARDS). Evidence from randomized trials and meta-analyses is conflicting, and data from large, randomized trials and meta-analyses suggest that it is unlikely to be beneficial and may be harmful [61–63]. As a consequence, supplementation of EN with antioxidants plus omega-3 fatty acids is not recommended in critically ill patients.

Enteral formulations enriched with glutamine were proposed because glutamine is a precursor for nucleotide synthesis and an important fuel source for rapidly dividing cells that is rapidly depleted in catabolic patients. Glutamine-enriched EN is not recommended for routine use in most critically ill patients because trials have not found consistent improvement in clinical outcomes [64, 65]. They can be used in patients with severe burns or trauma.

Arginine-enriched enteral formulations have been proposed because arginine is considered conditionally essential during critical illness because it is utilized more quickly. It is required for normal immune function and healing, and it has important roles in nitrogen metabolism, ammonia metabolism, and the generation of nitric oxide. Despite this, arginine-enriched EN is not recommended for routine use in critically ill patients. It has been extensively compared to standard enteral nutrition, with inconsistent results. Whereas one randomized trial found that arginine-enriched EN reduced infections and length of stay in burn patients [62], other studies suggested that it was not beneficial and potentially harmful [66]. Therefore, these formulations are not recommended for routine use in critically ill patients.

Probiotics are nondigestible carbohydrates that are used as enteral nutrition supplements with the hope of promoting the growth of beneficial bacteria in the bowel and of hindering the growth of harmful bacteria. Probiotics (e.g., *Lactobacillus* species) are living microorganisms that could provide a health benefit to the host when ingested. Routine supplementation of enteral nutrition with prebiotics or probiotics is not recommended because the pooled results from randomized trials demonstrate no effect on mortality or infectious complications.

11.8.3 EN Prescription

Determination of the presence of gut contractility is subjective and not an absolute requirement prior to initiation. Early EN (within 48 h of ICU admission) should also be performed during ECMO, in acute severe pancreatitis, during permissive hypercapnia, in the postoperative gastro-enteric surgery, in abdominal trauma (provided gastro-enteric tract continuity is confirmed or restored), in patients with an open abdomen or with controlled gastro-enteric bleeding (in the absence of signs of recurrence), and in patients with diarrhea [6, 10]. Low doses of EN should be prescribed in the following conditions [6, 10]: (1) during therapeutic hypothermia; (2) in patients with abdominal hypertension without compartment syndrome (the dose should be further reduced if EN results in further increase in intra-abdominal pressure); (3) in shock controlled with vasopressors/inotropes, paying special attention to the possibility of intestinal ischemia arising; (4) in patients receiving neuromuscular blocking agents; (5) in patients managed in prone position.

Contraindications to EN are described in Table 11.1 [6, 10, 11]. In all such cases, EN should be deferred.

ESPEN guidelines recommend gastric access should be used as the standard approach to initiate EN [6]. Continuous rather than bolus EN should be used, because ESPEN meta-analysis found a significant reduction in diarrhea with continuous versus bolus administration [6]. The practical approach to EN is described in Table 11.2 and is focused on early recognition/treatment of signs of EN intolerance and prevention of inhalation and other complications.

11.8.4 Complications

The most common complications are aspiration, diarrhea, metabolic abnormalities (including hyperglycemia, micronutrient deficiencies, and refeeding syndrome), and mechanical complications, such as increased abdominal pressure in patients with gastroparesis and/or intestinal paralysis.

Insertion of a nasogastric or nasoenteric tube can cause mechanical complications, such as insertion into the lung. Feeding through such tubes should not begin until its proper position has been confirmed radiographically.

Based on expert consensus, ASPEN guidelines suggest that nursing directives to reduce the risk of aspiration and VAP be employed. In all intubated ICU patients receiving EN, the head of the bed should be elevated 30°–45°, and the use of chlorhexidine mouthwash twice a day should be considered [9].

The measurement of gastric residual volume (GRV) for the assessment of gastrointestinal dysfunction is common and may help to identify intolerance to EN during initiation and progression of EN. Guidelines suggest that enteral feeding should be delayed when GRV is >500 mL/6 h. In this situation, and if examination of the abdomen does not suggest an acute abdominal complication, application of prokinetics should be considered [6]. In critically ill patients with gastric feeding intolerance intravenous erythromycin (usually at dosages of 100–250 mg three times a

Table 11.2 Practical approach to enteral nutrition

- Start within 48 h unless contraindicated (see Table 11.1)
- Start by using the gastric route
- Verify that the tube is correctly positioned before starting (radiological confirmation)
- Maintain the elevated chest position of 35°–40° and use oral cavity rinses with chlorhexidine twice daily
- Infuse the preparation by continuous infusion
- Use standard preparations (except for diabetic patient, patients with renal insufficiency, patients requiring important water restriction)
- Start with low doses and reach the expected caloric load only after 4–7 days
- Combine vitamins as long as EN <1000 kcal/day
- Monitor blood glucose and electrolytes
- Monitor for signs of gastroparesis (increased gastric residual volume, vomiting, abdominal distension, increased intra-abdominal pressure). If present reduce infusion rate or temporary stop and start prokinetics
- Consider increased gastric residual volume if >200 mL/6 h. If it is >500 mL/6 h, EN should be temporarily discontinued
- Monitor for signs of intestinal paralysis (abdominal distension, vomiting, increased gastric residual volume, increased intra-abdominal pressure). If present reduce infusion rate or temporary stop and start prokinetics and laxatives
- Erythromycin is considered the prokinetic of first choice (100–250 mg three times/day). Alternatively, or in combination, metaclopramide iv (10 mg 2–3 times/day) can be used for no more than 5 days while monitoring QT on the ECG (both drugs can prolong QT)
- If a gastric residual volume >500 mL/6 h persists despite the use of prokinetics, after excluding intestinal obstruction, intestinal perforation, and severe abdominal distension, post-pyloric EN should be considered
- If severe diarrhea appears reduce infusion rate, search for cause (rule out infection), discontinue laxatives and prokinetics
- In patients with persistent diarrhea, in whom infectious cause and drug diarrhea have been ruled out, if the patient is not at high risk of intestinal ischemia and severe intestinal dysmotility, consider enteral preparations containing fiber or semi-elemental preparations
- If more than 60% of the caloric and protein target is not achieved with EN within 7–10 days combine PN

day) should be used as a first-line prokinetic therapy. Alternatively, intravenous metoclopramide (at usual doses of 10 mg two to three times a day) or a combination of metoclopramide and erythromycin can be used as a prokinetic therapy [6]. Both agents have been associated with QT prolongation and a predisposition to cardiac arrhythmias. If a large (>500 mL) GRV still persists, the use of post-pyloric feeding should be considered over withholding EN, unless a new abdominal complication (obstruction, perforation, or severe distension) is suspected [9]. Post-pyloric, mainly jejunal feeding should be performed in patients deemed to be at high risk for aspiration.

Diarrhea in ICU patients receiving EN may be a serious complication, as it often results in electrolyte imbalance, dehydration, perianal skin breakdown, and wound contamination. The definitions most commonly used are two to three liquid stools per day or >250 g of liquid stool per day.

The following factors may contribute to acute diarrhea: type and amount of fiber in formula, osmolality of formula (short-chain carbohydrates are highly osmotic), delivery mode, EN contamination, medications (antibiotics, proton-pump inhibitors, prokinetics, glucose-lowering agents, nonsteroidal anti-inflammatory drugs, selective serotonin reuptake inhibitors, laxatives, and sorbitol-containing preparations), infectious etiologies, including *Clostridium difficile*.

If unable to control the diarrhea, clinicians often stop EN, resulting in inadequate nutrition intake. Based on expert consensus, ASPEN guidelines suggest that EN should not be automatically interrupted for diarrhea but rather that feeds be continued while evaluating the etiology of diarrhea in an ICU patient to determine appropriate treatment [9]. Those patients with persistent diarrhea (in whom other sources of diarrhea have been excluded, such as medications and *C. difficile*) may benefit from the use of a mixed fiber-containing formula or a small peptide semi-elemental formula. Commercial fiber-containing formulas are mixed, containing both soluble and insoluble fibers. ASPEN guidelines suggest considering the use of a commercial mixed fiber-containing formulation if there is evidence of persistent diarrhea and suggest avoiding these formulations in patients at high risk for bowel ischemia or severe dysmotility [9]. On the other hand, commercial mixed fiber formulas should not be used routinely in the adult critically ill patient prophylactically to promote bowel regularity or prevent diarrhea [9].

ASPEN guidelines recommend that in patients at either low or high nutrition risk, use of supplemental PN should be considered after 7–10 days if unable to meet >60% of energy and protein requirements by the enteral route alone [6, 9].

11.9 Conclusions

The importance of proper nutrition in ICU patients is increasingly clearly highlighted in the literature, especially in those with a long-term ICU staying. A hands-on approach to nutrition involving both medical and nursing staff is essential in order to ensure the safety and effectiveness of proper nutritional intake.

References

1. Ziegler TR. Parenteral nutrition in the critically ill patient. N Engl J Med. 2009;361:1088–97.
2. Heyland DK, Dhaliwal R, Jiang X, Day AG. Identifying critically ill patients who benefit the most from nutrition therapy: the development and initial validation of a novel risk assessment tool. Crit Care. 2011;15(6):R268.
3. McClave SA, Lowen CC, Kleber MJ, et al. Are patients fed appropriately according to their caloric requirements? JPNE J Parenter Enteral Nutr. 1998;22:375–81.
4. Villet S, Chiolero RL, Bollmann MD, et al. Negative impact of hypocaloric feeding and energy balance on clinical outcome in ICU patients. Clin Nutr. 2005;24:502–9.
5. Zaloga GP. Parenteral nutrition in adult inpatients with functioning gastrointestinal tracts: assessment of outcomes. Lancet. 2006;367:1101–11.
6. Singer P, Blaser AR, Berger MM, Alhazzani W, Calder PC, Casaer MP, Hiesmayr M, Mayer K, Montejo JC, Pichard C, Preiser JC, van Zanten ARH, Oczkowski S, Szczeklik

W, Bischoff SC. ESPEN guideline on clinical nutrition in the intensive care unit. Clin Nutr. 2019;38(1):48–79.

7. Schneider SM, Veyres P, Pivot X, et al. Malnutrition is an independent factor associated with nosocomial infections. Br J Nutr. 2004;92:105–11.

8. Dvir D, Cohen J, Singer P. Computerized energy balance and complications in critically ill patients: an observational study. Clin Nutr. 2006;25:37.

9. McClave SA, Taylor BE, Martindale RG, Warren MM, Johnson DR, Braunschweig C, McCarthy MS, Davanos E, Rice TW, Cresci GA, Gervasio JM, Sacks GS, Roberts PR, Compher C, Society of Critical Care Medicine; American Society for Parenteral and Enteral Nutrition. Guidelines for the provision and assessment of nutrition support therapy in the adult critically ill patient: Society of Critical Care Medicine (SCCM) and American Society for Parenteral and Enteral Nutrition (A.S.P.E.N.). JPEN J Parenter Enteral Nutr. 2016;40(2):159–211.

10. Reintam Blaser A, Starkopf J, Alhazzani W, Berger MM, Casaer MP, Deane AM, Fruhwald S, Hiesmayr M, Ichai C, Jakob SM, Loudet CI, Malbrain ML, Montejo González JC, Paugam-Burtz C, Poeze M, Preiser JC, Singer P, van Zanten AR, De Waele J, Wendon J, Wernerman J, Whitehouse T, Wilmer A, Oudemans-van Straaten HM, ESICM Working Group on Gastrointestinal Function. Early enteral nutrition in critically ill patients: ESICM clinical practice guidelines. Intensive Care Med. 2017;43(3):380–98.

11. Preiser JC, Arabi YM, Berger MM, Casaer M, McClave S, Montejo-González JC, Peake S, Reintam Blaser A, Van den Berghe G, van Zanten A, WerENrman J, Wischmeyer P. A guide to enteral nutrition in intensive care units: 10 expert tips for the daily practice. Crit Care. 2021;25(1):424.

12. Braunschweig CA, Sheean PM, Peterson SJ, et al. Intensive nutrition in acute lung injury: a clinical trial (INTACT). JPEN J Parenter Enteral Nutr. 2015;39:13.

13. Gramlich L, Kichian K, Pinilla J, Rodych NJ, Dhaliwal R, Heyland DK. Does enteral nutrition compared to parenteral nutrition result in better outcomes in critically ill adult patients? A systematic review of the literature. Nutrition. 2004;20(10):843–8.

14. Heyland DK, Dhaliwal R, Drover JW, et al. Canadian clinical practice guidelines for nutrition support in mechanically ventilated, critically ill adult patients. JPEN J Parenter Enteral Nutr. 2003;27:355–73.

15. Tian F, Heighes PT, Allingstrup MJ, Doig GS. Early enteral nutrition provided within 24 hours of ICU admission: a meta-analysis of randomized controlled trials. Crit Care Med. 2018;46:1049.

16. Artinian V, Krayem H, DiGiovine B. Effects of early enteral feeding on the outcome of critically ill mechanically ventilated medical patients. Chest. 2006;129:960.

17. McClave SA, Heyland DK. The physiologic response and associated clinical benefits from provision of early enteral nutrition. Nutr Clin Pract. 2009;24:305.

18. Alverdy JC, Laughlin RS, Wu L. Influence of the critically ill state on host-pathogen interactions within the intestine: gut-derived sepsis redefined. Crit Care Med. 2003;31:598.

19. Casaer MP, Mesotten D, Hermans G, Wouters PJ, Schetz M, Meyfroidt G, Van Cromphaut S, Ingels C, Meersseman P, Muller J, Vlasselaers D, Debaveye Y, Desmet L, Dubois J, Van Assche A, Vanderheyden S, Wilmer A, Van den Berghe G. Early versus late parenteral nutrition in critically ill adults. N Engl J Med. 2011;365(6):506–17.

20. Koretz RL, Lipman TO, Klein S, American Gastroenterological Association. AGA technical review on parenteral nutrition. Gastroenterology. 2001;121:970.

21. Kutsogiannis J, Alberda C, Gramlich L, et al. Early use of supplemental parenteral nutrition in critically ill patients: results of an international multicenter observational study. Crit Care Med. 2011;39:2691.

22. Doig GS, Simpson F, Sweetman EA, et al. Early parenteral nutrition in critically ill patients with short-term relative contraindications to early enteral nutrition: a randomized controlled trial. JAMA. 2013;309:2130.

23. Mukhopadhyay A, Henry J, Ong V, Leong CS, Teh AL, van Dam RM, Kowitlawakul Y. Association of modified NUTRIC score with 28-day mortality in critically ill patients. Clin Nutr. 2017;36(4):1143–8.

24. Bufo AJ, Feldman S, Daniels GA, Lieberman RC. Early postoperative feeding. Dis Colon Rectum. 1994;37:1260.
25. Reissman P, Teoh TA, Cohen SM, et al. Is early oral feeding safe after elective colorectal surgery? A prospective randomized trial. Ann Surg. 1995;222:73.
26. Kaur N, Gupta MK, Minocha VR. Early enteral feeding by nasoenteric tubes in patients with perforation peritonitis. World J Surg. 2005;29:1023.
27. Andersen HK, Lewis SJ, Thomas S. Early enteral nutrition within 24h of colorectal surgery versus later commencement of feeding for postoperative complications. Cochrane Database Syst Rev. 2006;(4):CD004080.
28. Ceydeli A. Early postoperative enteral feeding increases anastomotic strength in a peritonitis model. Am J Surg. 2003;185:605.
29. Koretz RL, Avenell A, Lipman TO, Braunschweig CL, Milne AC. Does enteral nutrition affect clinical outcome? A systematic review of the randomized trials. Am J Gastroenterol. 2007;102(2):412–29.
30. Mehanna HM, Moledina J, Travis J. Refeeding syndrome: what it is, and how to prevent and treat it. BMJ. 2008;336:1495.
31. Schlein KM, Coulter SP. Best practices for determining resting energy expenditure in critically ill adults. Nutr Clin Pract. 2014;29(1):44–55.
32. Nordenström J, Carpentier YA, Askanazi J, et al. Free fatty acid mobilization and oxidation during total parenteral nutrition in trauma and infection. Ann Surg. 1983;198:725.
33. Van den Berghe G, Wouters P, Weekers F, et al. Intensive insulin therapy in critically ill patients. N Engl J Med. 2001;345(19):1359–67.
34. NICE-SUGAR Study Investigators, Finfer S, Chittock DR, Li Y, et al. Intensive versus conventional glucose control in critically ill patients. N Engl J Med. 2009;360(13):1283–97.
35. Manzanares W, Langlois PL, Hardy G. Intravenous lipid emulsions in the critically ill: an update. Curr Opin Crit Care. 2016;22:308–15.
36. Mirtallo JM, Ayers P, Boullata J, et al. ASPEN lipid injectable emulsion safety recommendations, Part 1: Background and adult considerations. Nutr Clin Pract. 2020;35:769.
37. Kraft MD, Btaiche IF, Sacks GS. Review of the refeeding syndrome. Nutr Clin Pract. 2005;20(6):625–33.
38. Grau T, Bonet A, Miñambres E, et al. The effect of L-alanyl-L-glutamine dipeptide supplemented total parenteral nutrition on infectious morbidity and insulin sensitivity in critically ill patients. Crit Care Med. 2011;39:1263.
39. Blass SC, Goost H, Tolba RH, Stoffel-Wagner B, Kabir K, Burger C, et al. Time to wound closure in trauma patients with disorders in wound healing is shortened by supplements containing antioxidant micronutrients and glutamine: a PRCT. Clin Nutr. 2012;31:469–75.
40. Houdijk APJ, Rijnsburger ER, Wesdorp RIC, Weiss JK, McCamish MA, Teerlink T, et al. Randomised trial of glutamine-enriched enteral nutrition on infectious morbidity in patients with multiple trauma. Lancet. 1998;352:772–6.
41. van Zanten AR, Sztark F, Kaisers UX, Zielmann S, Felbinger TW, Sablotzki AR, et al. High-protein enteral nutrition enriched with immune-modulating nutrients vs standard high-protein enteral nutrition and nosocomial infections in the ICU: a randomized clinical trial. JAMA. 2014;312:514–24.
42. Kuwahara T, Asanami S, Tamura T, Kaneda S. Effects of pH and osmolality on phlebitic potential of infusion solutions for peripheral parenteral nutrition. J Toxicol Sci. 1998;23:77.
43. Kovacevich DS, Corrigan M, Ross VM, et al. American Society for Parenteral and Enteral Nutrition guidelines for the selection and care of central venous access devices for Adult Home Parenteral Nutrition Administration. JPEN J Parenter Enteral Nutr. 2019;43:15.
44. Hon K, Bihari S, Holt A, et al. Rate of catheter-related bloodstream infections between tunneled central venous catheters versus peripherally inserted central catheters in adult home parenteral nutrition: a meta-analysis. JPEN J Parenter Enteral Nutr. 2019;43:41.
45. O'Grady PN, Alexander M, Dellinger EP, et al. Guidelines for the prevention of intravascular catheter-related infections. Centers for Disease Control and Prevention. MMWR Recomm Rep. 2002;51:1.

46. Mirtallo J, Canada T, Johnson D, et al. Safe practices for parenteral nutrition. JPEN J Parenter Enteral Nutr. 2004;28:S39.
47. Slattery E, Rumore MM, Douglas JS, Seres DS. 3-in-1 vs 2-in-1 parenteral nutrition in adults: a review. Nutr Clin Pract. 2014;29:631.
48. Fonseca G, Burgermaster M, Larson E, Seres DS. The relationship between parenteral nutrition and central LiEN-associated bloodstream infections. JPEN J Parenter Enteral Nutr. 2017;42:171.
49. Yilmaz G, Koksal I, Aydin K, et al. Risk factors of catheter-related bloodstream infections in parenteral nutrition catheterization. JPEN J Parenter Enteral Nutr. 2007;31:284.
50. Bonten MJ, Gaillard CA, van der Hulst R, et al. Intermittent enteral feeding: the influence on respiratory and digestive tract colonization in mechanically ventilated intensive-care unit patients. Am J Respir Crit Care Med. 1996;154:394.
51. Steevens EC, Lipscomb AF, Poole GV, Sacks GS. Comparison of continuous vs intermittent nasogastric enteral feeding in trauma patients: perceptions and practice. Nutr Clin Pract. 2002;17:118.
52. MacLeod JB, Lefton J, Houghton D, et al. Prospective randomized control trial of intermittent versus continuous gastric feeds for critically ill trauma patients. J Trauma. 2007;63:57.
53. Sorokin R, Gottlieb JE. Enhancing patient safety during feeding-tube insertion: a review of more than 2,000 insertions. JPEN J Parenter Enteral Nutr. 2006;30:440.
54. Scheinkestel CD, Kar L, Marshall K, et al. Prospective randomized trial to assess caloric and protein needs of critically ill, anuric, ventilated patients requiring continuous renal replacement therapy. Nutrition. 2003;19:909.
55. Dobb GJ, Towler SC. Diarrhoea during enteral feeding in the critically ill: a comparison of feeds with and without fiber. Intensive Care Med. 1990;16:252.
56. Heather DJ, Howell L, Montana M, et al. Effect of a bulk-forming cathartic on diarrhea in tube-fed patients. Heart Lung. 1991;20:409.
57. Schultz AA, Ashby-Hughes B, Taylor R, et al. Effects of pectin on diarrhea in critically ill tube-fed patients receiving antibiotics. Am J Crit Care. 2000;9:403.
58. Spapen H, Diltoer M, Van Malderen C, et al. Soluble fiber reduces the incidence of diarrhea in septic patients receiving total enteral nutrition: a prospective, double-blind, randomized, and controlled trial. Clin Nutr. 2001;20:301.
59. Rushdi TA, Pichard C, Khater YH. Control of diarrhea by fiber-enriched diet in ICU patients on enteral nutrition: a prospective randomized controlled trial. Clin Nutr. 2004;23:1344.
60. Taylor BE, McClave SA, Martindale RG, et al. Guidelines for the provision and assessment of nutrition support therapy in the adult critically ill patient: Society of Critical Care Medicine (SCCM) and American Society for Parenteral and Enteral Nutrition (A.S.P.E.N.). Crit Care Med. 2016;44:390.
61. Pradelli L, Mayer K, Klek S, et al. ω-3 Fatty-acid enriched parenteral nutrition in hospitalized patients: systematic review with meta-analysis and trial sequential analysis. JPEN J Parenter Enteral Nutr. 2020;44:44.
62. Singer P, Theilla M, Fisher H, et al. Benefit of an enteral diet enriched with eicosapentaenoic acid and gamma-linolenic acid in ventilated patients with acute lung injury. Crit Care Med. 2006;34:1033.
63. Rice TW, Wheeler AP, Thompson BT, et al. Enteral omega-3 fatty acid, gamma-linolenic acid, and antioxidant supplementation in acute lung injury. JAMA. 2011;306:1574.
64. Tao KM, Li XQ, Yang LQ, et al. Glutamine supplementation for critically ill adults. Cochrane Database Syst Rev. 2014;9:CD010050.
65. Heyland D, Muscedere J, Wischmeyer PE, et al. A randomized trial of glutamine and antioxidants in critically ill patients. N Engl J Med. 2013;368:1489.
66. Heyland DK, Novak F. Immunonutrition in the critically ill patient: more harm than good? JPEN J Parenter Enteral Nutr. 2001;25:S51.

Patient-Ventilator Interaction in the Patient with ARDS

12

Lucia Mirabella and Cesare Gregoretti

12.1 Introduction

In critically ill patients requiring ventilatory support, the primary goal is to allow spontaneous breathing as soon as possible and avoid diaphragmatic dysfunction [1]. With spontaneous breathing, however, it is critically important to ensure optimal patient-ventilator interaction because poor ventilator-patient coordination makes weaning difficult and prolongs days of mechanical ventilation. Optimal patient-ventilator interaction is crucial to ensure patient comfort and improve outcome. However, good optimization is hardly achieved, resulting in asynchronies, defined as a lack of coordination between patient and ventilator due to a mismatch between the patient's neural time and ventilator support during the respiratory cycle, or a mismatch between the support required and provided [1–5].

12.2 Respiratory Physiology and Mechanical Ventilation

The effects of mechanical ventilation on respiratory exchanges, muscle work, and dyspnea depend on the match between respiratory system and ventilator setting. The patient interacts with the ventilator based on three physiological variables: respiratory drive, amount of support, and inspiratory time [6–10]. At the same time,

L. Mirabella
Department of Medical and Surgical Sciences, University of Foggia,
Hospital OO Riuniti di Foggia, Foggia, Italy

C. Gregoretti (✉)
Department of Surgical, Oncological and Oral Science (Di.Chir.On.S.), University of Palermo, 'Giglio' Foundation, Palermo, Italy
e-mail: c.gregoretti@gmail.com

© The Author(s), under exclusive license to Springer Nature Switzerland AG 2024

231

D. Chiumello (ed.), *Practical Trends in Anesthesia and Intensive Care 2022*,
https://doi.org/10.1007/978-3-031-43891-2_12

physiological variables can be influenced by the synchronization system (trigger variables), pressure or volume (control variables), and the mode of transition from inspiratory to expiratory phase (cycling variables). Perfect synchronization is achieved when each individual act required by the patient is assisted by the ventilator in a way that is optimal for the patient.

12.3 Types of Asynchronies

Patient-ventilator interactions have been studied for years; various authors have identified different factors related to ventilation mode, setting, and patient characteristics; identified different types of asynchronies; and suggested strategies to reduce the triggering mechanisms of such asynchronies (Fig. 12.1). However, to date, it remains an open problem and needs the clinician's thorough knowledge of respiratory physiology and interpretation of ventilator curves during different periods of the respiratory cycle.

Longhini et al. classified asynchronies as major (e.g., ineffective trigger, self-trigger, double trigger) and minor (e.g., premature, prolonged, or delayed cycling and delayed trigger). Table 12.1 lists the different types of asynchronies, their definitions, causes, and strategies to resolve each [11].

Inspiratory asynchronies can be defined as poor coordination between the output of the patient's respiratory center and the initiation of assistance by the ventilator. This may depend on the sensitivity of the trigger set; generally modern ventilators use very sensitive pressure or flow triggers, but sometimes the patient spends much of the inspiratory effort to activate the ventilator trigger [12–23]. Consequently, the trigger should be set to minimize patient effort, and although the definition of "best trigger" is controversial, an optimal response time < 100 ms is universally recognized [24].

Control variables result in the onset of asynchronies when the ventilator is unable to appropriately attend to the patient's demands; for example, an increase in flow in the controlled volume mode may result in a reduction in the patient's respiratory drive, or circuit leaks may reduce ventilator performance [1, 25].

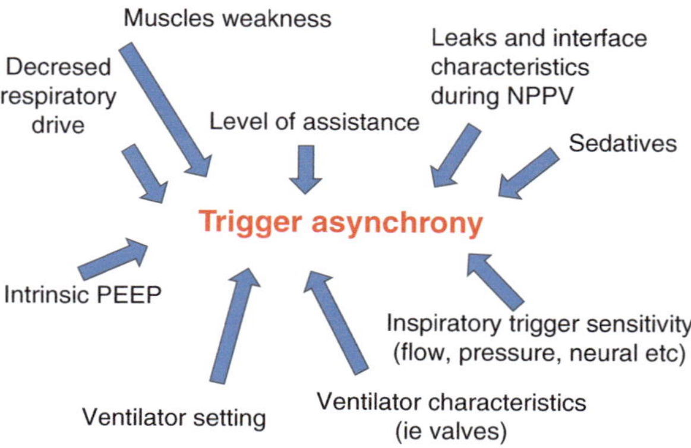

Fig. 12.1 Several factors can cause asynchronies, some depending on patient characteristics and others on the ventilator

Table 12.1 Different types of asynchronies

Asynchrony and its definition	Cause of asynchrony	Solution
Trigger delay *Time lag between onset of effort and onset of ventilator pressurization*	*Respiratory drive—inspiratory trigger asynchrony*	1. Adjust trigger sensitivity 2. Change the type of trigger 3. Remove leaks or switch to a pressure trigger 4. For COPD: increase PEEP to counterbalance PEEPi
Ineffective triggering *Ventilator's incapability to detect the patient's effort despite the presence of an inspiratory effort*	*1. Respiratory drive—inspiratory trigger asynchrony* Less sensitive, *trigger* or insufficient patient effort to initiate a positive pressure breath, *presence of PEEPi, sedatives, metabolic alkalosis* *2. Inspiratory time—ventilator cycling variable asynchrony* *Prolonged cycle due to a longer inspiratory time in a time-cycled mode* or due to a slow expiratory trigger threshold (ETT) in flow-cycled breath(i.e., PSV mode) or due to air leaks causing the hung-up phenomenon *3. Respiratory drive—inspiratory trigger asynchrony and inspiratory time—Vventilator cycling variable asynchrony due to high level of ventilatory assistance causing the respiratory drive depression*	1. Adjust trigger sensitivity 2. Shorten Ti in a time-cycled breath 3. COPD: increase PEEP to counter PEEPi; reduce inspiratory pressure, increase ETT in PSV mode 4. Remove HME, change the endotracheal tube or the interface in NIV 5. Correct metabolic alkalosis 6. Reduce sedation or use drugs with no effect on the respiratory drive
Auto-triggering Mandatory breath not following a patient's inspiratory effort	*Respiratory drive—inspiratory trigger asynchrony ventilatory* Too sensitive inspiratory triggering leaks, random noise into the circuit	1. Adjust trigger sensitivity 2. Reduce noise in the circuit (i.e., condensate) 3. Remove leaks 4. Use appropriate NIV software
Double triggering Two mandatory breaths separated by a very short expiratory time	*1. Inspiratory time—ventilator cycling variable asynchrony* Short cycling as defined as an inspiratory time, less than one-half of the mean inspiratory time *2. Ventilatory need—control variable gas delivery asynchrony Pressure rise time not fast enough to reach the set pressure*	1. Increasing Ti in a time-cycled breath 2. Adjusting the ETT in PSV 3. Optimize pressure rise time in a pressure-controlled time or flow-cycled mode

PEEP positive end-expiratory pressure, *PEEPi* intrinsic positive end-expiratory pressure, *ETT* expiratory trigger threshold, *NIV* noninvasive ventilation, *PSV* pressure support ventilation, *HME* heat and moisture exchanger

Asynchronies generated by cycling variables occur when the inspiratory phase of the respirator does not correspond in duration to the patient's neural inspiratory phase [1, 26–29].

12.4   Triggering Delay

The triggering delay is the "time interval between the onset of patient exertion and the onset of ventilator pressurization." This is typically an asynchrony between respiratory drive and inspiratory trigger, where the phase interval quantifies the delay between the onset of inspiratory muscle activity and the onset of mechanical breathing.

Giuliani et al. reported how the effort performed by the patient during the trigger phase can interfere with the effort performed during the remaining part of the inspiratory phase. Interestingly, at increased inspiratory demand (e.g., high inspiratory drive), the delay in triggering is shorter and the degree of negative pressure curve deflection (P_{aw}) is greater.

In contrast, with lower inspiratory demand (e.g., lower respiratory drive), the trigger delay is greater and the deflection of P_{aw} is lower. In addition, additional load, such as dynamic intrinsic PEEP, may impair the trigger phase.

Finally, ventilator characteristics, such as the location of the flow/pressure sensor (e.g., inside the ventilator or proximal to the patient's airway), a problem related to the valves, the interfaces used (endotracheal tube vs. face mask or helmet), or the high resistances generated by the heat and moisture exchange (HME) filters or the endotracheal tube, are all factors that can influence the trigger delay. Monitoring of esophageal pressure or electrical activity of the diaphragm (EA_{di}) is necessary to detect trigger delay (Fig. 12.2).

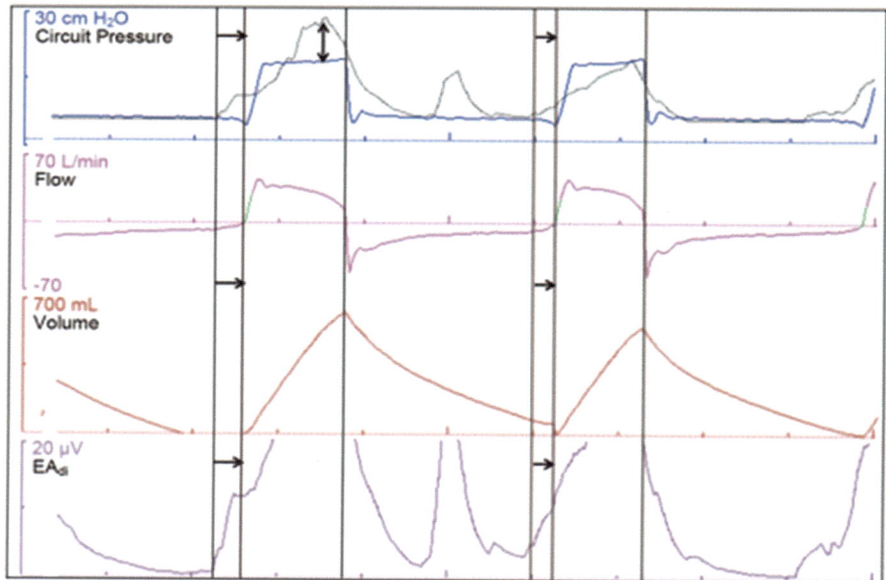

Fig. 12.2 Examples of ventilator-patient asynchronies, (**a**) ineffective trigger, (**b**) trigger delay

12.5   Ineffective Effort

Ineffective effort (Fig. 12.3) is defined as a patient's inspiratory effort that is unable to trigger the ventilator-assisted respiratory act. Ineffective effort represents an asynchrony between the respiratory drive and the inspiratory trigger. From a clinical point of view, ineffective effort can be recognized by analyzing the respiratory rate shown by the ventilator and noting how it is lower than the respiratory rate calculated by observing the patient's rib cage movements. Ineffective effort can also be identified by observing the flow and P_{aw} curves on the ventilator: insufficient patient effort to activate the ventilator output produces a deflection of P_{aw} in conjunction with an increase in flow. There are several causes that can lead to ineffective effort. An insensitive inspiratory trigger may contribute to an ineffective trigger. In patients with obstructive disease, an inspiratory load such as intrinsic PEEP, resulting in air trapping, may cause an ineffective trigger. An external PEEP in spontaneously breathing patients may counterbalance intrinsic PEEP and thus decrease inspiratory effort.

Younes et al. reported how ineffective exertion can also exacerbate dynamic hyperinflation. Metabolic alkalosis can generate ineffective exertion in patients with chronic bicarbonate elevation and hypocapnia by depressing respiratory drive. Sedative drugs may affect the patient's respiratory drive and reduce the ability of respiratory muscles to trigger ventilator; consequently, deep sedation may produce

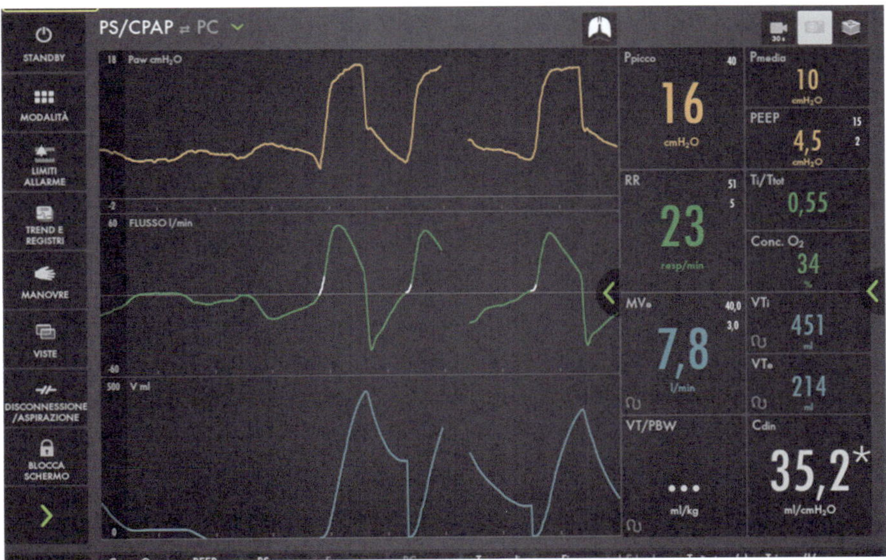

Fig. 12.3 Example of ineffective trigger, patient's inspiratory effort unable to trigger ventilator-assisted breathing act

increased ineffective effort. Several studies have reported how a protocol of minimizing sedation in ICU patients was associated with a reduction in the asynchrony index, as well as a reduction in ventilator days, when compared with a protocol of daily cessation of sedation [30].

De Wit et al. reported how the level of sedation is related to ineffective effort, with a significant increase in the number of ineffective triggers for each increase on the Richmond Agitation-Sedation Scale. Vaschetto et al. showed how, when compared with mild sedation, deep sedation with propofol reduces respiratory drive and respiratory pattern, significantly worsening patient-ventilator interaction [31, 32].

Another cause of ineffective effort may be asynchrony between the neural inspiratory time and the ventilator cycling variable. When the patient's inspiratory time is shorter than the mechanical inspiratory time set on the ventilator, the ventilator continues to insufflate during the neural expiration phase, thus causing hyperinflation. Leung et al. observed that ineffective efforts were more frequent during intermittent mandatory ventilation because of the large tidal volume and prolonged inspiratory time. For these reasons, the use of synchronized intermittent mandatory ventilation (SIMV), especially in patients with COPD, is ineffective in reducing respiratory effort. In contrast, in a flow-cycling mode (e.g., pressure support ventilation [PSV]), the duration of mechanical inspiratory time is determined by the rate of pressure rise and the flow threshold set as the respiratory trigger [6].

Ideally, the ventilator sensor should always detect the patient's flow to ensure synchrony. However, several factors can influence this relationship, such as the patient's respiratory mechanics, ventilator cycling algorithms, and ventilatory parameters. In patients with COPD, increased resistance and compliance generate a slower expiratory time constant. The longer time required for flow to decrease sufficiently to trigger expiration can produce prolonged mechanical inspiration that persists during neural expiration. An appropriate cycling-off setting can reduce the occurrence of ineffective efforts. In addition, the presence of leakage may prevent proper cycling-off during PSV, thus generating prolonged inspiratory time, especially when dedicated NIV software is not used.

Leung et al. reported how a higher level of care can profoundly reduce the patient's respiratory drive, thereby increasing the triggering time (defined by the onset of the patient's inspiratory effort and the onset of the flow increase generated by the ventilator). This causes an extension of mechanical breathing within the patient's expiratory phase, thus going to reduce the time useful for expiration. In patients with COPD, this phenomenon will produce a larger tidal volume that will be associated with a shorter expiratory time, thus possibly causing dynamic hyperinflation and an increase in intrinsic PEEP [6].

12.6 Auto-trigger

Self-trigger is a mechanical breath that is not generated by the patient's inspiratory effort and different from the set acts (e.g., in volume-controlled or pressure-controlled modes). It represents an asynchrony between the respiratory drive and the inspiratory trigger. Self-trigger can be caused by an extremely sensitive inspiratory trigger or by changes in pressure and flow that can be caused by issues in the ventilator circuit (e.g., condensation in the respiratory circuit, leaks, or cardiac oscillations). In particular, an increased systolic output may be able to generate a mechanical act with each cardiac oscillation, especially when the sensitivity of the trigger is too high and the patient's respiratory drive is reduced (e.g., in sedated patients). The potential consequences of self-triggering are respiratory alkalosis, worsening intrinsic PEEP, and cardiac compromise.

12.7 Double Triggering (Double Triggering)

Double triggering, also called double-cycling or breath-stacking, consists of two breaths that may or may not be separated by a very short expiratory time. Double triggering is caused by a very high ventilatory demand combined with a mechanical inspiratory time that is too short compared with the neural time; this generates two inspiratory cycles with a limited expiratory phase.

The double trigger may be due to an asynchrony between the neural inspiratory time and the ventilator cycling variable or an asynchrony between the patient's ventilatory demand and the flow control variable when the ventilator fails to meet the patient's flow demand in either volumetric or pressometric ventilation. This results in prolonged neural effort beyond the ventilator's inspiratory time.

If the patient has a high respiratory drive, additional breathing may or may not be generated accompanied by a very short expiratory time. The double trigger mainly develops when the ventilator delivers a fixed flow or when low tidal volumes are set in the presence of high inspiratory flow demand from the patient.

Double triggering can also occur in the context of a poor match between mechanical inspiratory time and neural time (e.g., asynchrony between the inspiratory neural time and the cycling variable), especially when a high parameter for flow termination is applied to a patient with a restrictive respiratory condition and placed in PSV mode.

In volume-controlled mode, double triggering can be particularly harmful, especially in patients with ARDS on protective ventilation. Double triggering can generate high volumes and cause hyperinflation, thus causing ventilator-induced lung damage and possible increased right ventricular afterload. In contrast, double triggering in the pressure-controlled mode appears to be less dangerous because alveolar pressure increases during inspiration with a concomitant reduction in subsequent breath-driving pressure.

12.8 Reverse-Triggering

Reverse-triggering is a type of asynchrony that occurs when patient exertion takes place after the onset of mechanical breathing (e.g., an act not triggered by the patient).

Usually, reverse-triggering represents a poorly recognized asynchrony in which the ventilator triggers diaphragmatic contraction through activation of the patient's respiratory centers in response to passive insufflation of the lungs. With reverse-triggering, strain frequently begins during insufflation and continues during exhalation.

During pressure-controlled ventilation, patient effort triggered by mechanical breathing is easier to detect the earlier the flow changes within the inspiratory phase. Kaller et al. reported how this type of asynchrony represents a frequent occurrence during protective ventilation. Because the patient's respiratory muscles are still active at the beginning of the expiratory phase, counteracting the elastic return of the respiratory system, the peak expiratory flow is markedly reduced. Reverse-triggering occurs in patients in deep sedation, with or without lung damage, and seems particularly common in the transition from sedation to wakefulness. Interestingly, Haro et al. reported that one-third of double-cycling breaths were due to reverse-triggering, especially in association with deep sedation in patients who did not trigger the ventilator [33, 34].

12.9 Flow Asynchronies

Flow asynchrony is an asynchrony between the ventilatory demand and the gas delivery control variable. Flow asynchrony occurs when the flow output generated by the ventilator does not match the patient's demand. Inadequate gas flow is quite common when too low a flow is set on the ventilator, when the combination of tidal volume and inspiratory time does not generate adequate flow for the injured lung, or when inspiratory flow demand is high and variable from breath to breath. Flow asynchrony seems to be more common with ventilator parameters that generate a fixed flow (e.g., flow-controlled acts) than with flow that varies with effort (e.g., pressure-controlled acts).

12.10 Cyclic Asynchronies

A cycling asynchrony can be defined as an imbalance between the patient's respiratory centers and the ventilator's inspiratory time. If the inspiratory time set on the ventilator is higher than the neural inspiratory time, so-called delayed cycling occurs. A pressure spike in the PSV mode, originating from activation of the expiratory muscles in response to excessive distension, can then be identified. Delayed cycling can also occur due to unintentional leakage that may prevent the ventilator from cycling from the inspiratory to expiratory phase (e.g., so-called inspiratory hang-up). This is most frequently observed during NIV performed with ventilators lacking dedicated software to compensate for leaks or a time criterion for cycling. Delayed cycling, especially in obstructive disease, can cause ineffective triggering. If the inspiratory time set on the ventilator is shorter than the neural inspiratory time, early cycling may occur. A high expiratory time threshold in PSV mode can also generate a short inspiratory time and cause early cycling, especially in patients with low compliance such as those with ARDS. Finally, if the patient's effort (neural inspiratory time) exceeds the inspiratory time of the mechanical act, an additional act (e.g., double trigger) may be generated.

12.11 Clinical Implications

Asynchronies are often hardly recognized, underestimated, and inappropriately treated. The frequency of asynchronies during invasive ventilation varies from 10 to 50%, with a prevalence of ineffective efforts, especially in patients with COPD. The incidence of asynchronies has been defined by the asynchrony index (AI), which is a percentage value of total asynchrony events divided by the sum of total ventilatory cycles plus ineffective efforts. A high incidence of asynchrony is commonly defined by an asynchrony index >10% and may be associated with patient discomfort, increased work of breathing, and prolonged weaning time mainly due to diaphragmatic energy dissipation. Several studies have reported how an asynchrony index >10% can significantly prolong the duration of mechanical ventilation and the risk of tracheostomy, as well as be associated with a higher mortality rate. Further studies are needed to define its prognostic role [2, 31, 35].

12.11.1 Ventilator-Induced Diaphragmatic Dysfunction

Ventilator-induced diaphragmatic dysfunction is a major risk factor leading to poor patient-ventilator interaction and contributing to prolonged ventilator dependence as well as a worse outcome. During partial ventilatory support, asynchronies can have a particularly important impact on respiratory muscle function, particularly during the ineffective efforts that occur during the expiratory phase of the just-completed mechanical act, as the inspiratory muscles contract at a time when they should release while lung volume decreases to residual functional capacity. This results in so-called eccentric or plyometric contraction that causes ultrastructural muscle damage, cytokine release, and reduced muscle strength, resulting in a strength deficit and ineffective weaning.

12.11.2 Weaning Difficulties

Weaning difficulty is closely related to asynchronies. Chao et al. reported how diaphragmatic energy wasted due to ineffective efforts can have negative effects on the weaning process, significantly prolonging the duration of mechanical ventilation in subjects ventilated with an asynchrony index >10% compared with those with a synchrony index <10%. More recently, De Wit et al. demonstrated how an asynchrony index >10% correlated with longer duration of mechanical ventilation and reduced ventilator-free survival, as well as lower discharge rates. A similar trend toward longer duration of mechanical ventilation had already been confirmed by other studies that also noted an association between an asynchrony index >10% and a higher mortality rate [31, 35, 36].

12.11.3 Patient Discomfort and Cognitive Dysfunction

Sleep quality can be strongly influenced by patient-ventilator interaction, and a high percentage of asynchronies seems likely to be responsible for sleep deprivation. An improvement in sleep quality can be achieved by a reduction in ventilatory support, which leads to more stable breathing pattern, fewer missed acts, and periodic breathing. In addition, the type of ventilatory support may play a role in sleep quality by reducing the number of asynchronies. However, the relationship between patient-ventilator interaction and sleep quality is still controversial. Alexopoulou et al. did not observe improvements in sleep quality during proportional assisted ventilation+ (PAV+) when compared with PSV, despite the former being able to improve patient-ventilator interaction. In contrast, neural-controlled assisted ventilation (NAVA) demonstrated efficacy in improving sleep quality compared with PSV [37–40].

12.11.4 Dyspnea

Dyspnea, defined as difficulty breathing, is a common consequence of poor patient-ventilator interaction, and in mechanically ventilated patients, it is closely associated with anxiety. In a proportion of up to one-third of patients, changes in ventilatory parameters were successful in reducing dyspnea and associated anxiety, while failure to reduce dyspnea by changing ventilatory parameters appears to be associated with delayed extubation. The relationship between dyspnea and asynchronies has yet to be studied in depth. Finally, in critically ill patients, asynchronies are associated with persistent neurophysiological alterations. Severe sleep alteration, with a high frequency of awakenings, is related to the acute onset of cognitive dysfunction, visual hallucinations, and delusions.

12.11.5 Monitoring of Asynchronies

Carrying out careful monitoring of asynchronies is crucial to reducing and counteracting their effects even if it is still a challenge in practice.

Visual assessment of the flow/time and pressure/time curves in mechanically ventilated patients can highlight the most frequent forms of asynchrony, such as ineffective triggering or double triggering. Paradoxically, visual identification of asynchronies appears very easy in extreme situations where the patient is misfit from the ventilator rather than in clinical situations where no clinical signs of misfit are evident and the patient's true respiratory rate is not assessed. Specific training is therefore required as demonstrated by Colombo et al., who showed that it was more difficult for less experienced intensivists to visually identify asynchronies [41].

The use of additional signals to study asynchronies such as esophageal pressure is generally suggested. **Esophageal pressure** (weight) allows identification of any patient strain and more reliable information regarding ventilator interactions [42].

The simultaneous observation of P_{aw}, inspiratory flow, expiratory flow, and esophageal pressure thus allows a perfect match between the patient's inspiratory effort and the mechanical act of the respirator. An ineffective triggering, e.g., is identified as a deflection of esophageal pressure not followed by a ventilator-assisted respiratory act. However, even though this monitoring is considered the standard in reality, it is not yet part of everyday use [43, 44].

Diaphragmatic electrical activity (EA_{di}) is monitored with the placement of a modified nasogastric tube that allows the neural respiratory signal to be detected and attended to [45]. Currently only one respirator uses the neural signal to trigger the respiratory act and is not part of routine monitoring.

Diaphragmatic ultrasonography is another effective method for detecting asynchronies; in fact, the measurement of diaphragmatic thickness allows inspiratory effort to be evidenced [46]. Although simple and noninvasive, it is not yet a standardized method that requires synchronization between ultrasound signals and respirator waveforms [47].

The automated real-time method for monitoring asynchronies is a machine learning-based approach. It is a very promising method that aims to identify and quantify asynchronies' acts by filtering out all sorts of interferences, such as the patient's secretions or movements [44, 45]. Several systems are being tested for this purpose. Chen et al., for example, tested a software developed to identify ineffective triggering based on the analysis of airway flow and pressure curves [48]. Mulqueeny et al. developed an algorithm integrated into a ventilation system capable of automatically detecting both ineffective triggering and double triggering in real time. The software applied in both invasive and noninvasive ventilation presented >95% accuracy. Younes et al. developed a new method to monitor and optimize patient-ventilator interactions that uses the signal generated by the equation of motion. Other systems are being studied that automatically detect asynchronies and based on spectral analysis of flow, or comparison of P_{aw} and EA_{di} [49].

12.11.6 Strategies for Improving Patient-Ventilator Interactions (Table 12.2)

Patient-ventilator interactions are influenced by the mode of ventilation as well as by the level of sedation. In conventional ventilation modalities, the trigger plays a key role; in fact, a trigger sensitivity that is too low can increase muscle effort to trigger the mechanical respiratory act, whereas a trigger with high sensitivity can trigger self-trigger, especially in patients who have reduced neuromuscular drive as may occur in polyneuropathy [50–52]. In invasive mechanical ventilation, self-trigger can be triggered by interference in the ventilator circuit (e.g., condensation),

Table 12.2 Strategies to improve patient-ventilator interaction

Conventional ventilation	Solution
Trigger sensitivity setting	1. Adjust trigger sensitivity to avoid auto-trigger or ineffective efforts in weak patients 2. Remove random noise (i.e., cleaning the respiratory circuit) 3. Alternative triggers
Level of support	Use 1. Appropriate PSV level in order to avoid hyperinflation in COPD patients 2. Appropriate rise time in pressure-controlled modes 3. Appropriate inspiratory flow in volume-controlled mode
Too long Ti in PSV or ACV/ AC-PCV mode	Check 1 Proper Ti setting in ACV or APCV mode 2. Proper expiratory threshold in PSV mode according to patient's neural time and respiratory mechanics
Too short Ti in PSV or ACV/ AC-PCV mode	Check 1. Proper Ti setting and rise time in ACV or APCV mode 2. Proper expiratory threshold in PSV mode according to patient's neural time and respiratory mechanics
PEEP	Titrate external PEEP to offset auto-PEEP (i.e., COPD)
Leaks during noninvasive ventilation in PSV	1. Use NIV software or turbine-driven ventilator in intentional leak mode 2. Use a maximum inspiratory time in PSV mode 3. Adjust expiratory trigger sensitivity 4. Use NAVA
Appropriate sedative and sedation level	1. Carefully titrate sedative to obtain the desired sedation level 2. Chose the appropriate drug according to the effects on respiratory drive or timing

NIV Noninvasive ventilation, *PEEP* positive end-expiratory pressure, *COPD* chronic obstructive pulmonary disease, *PSV* pressure support ventilation, *APCV* assisted pressure control ventilation, *NAVA neurally adjusted ventilatory assist*

whereas in noninvasive ventilation, self-trigger is more often generated by leakage [53, 54]. Indeed, it is well known that among the newer algorithms and technologies developed to improve patient-ventilator interactions, neural triggering reduces these asynchronies, including those generated by the presence of intrinsic PEEP and circuit leakage [24, 55].

Too high levels of respiratory support cause harmful effects in ventilated patients, and hyperventilation causes increased ineffective efforts, sleep fragmentation, and apnea. Hyperventilation should be avoided in heart failure patients who are sensitive to apneas and abnormal breathing patterns due to increased chemoreceptor sensitivity. COPD patients, at high levels of support, especially when associated with low expiratory triggers, prolong the inspiratory phase beyond the neural inspiratory time, causing dynamic hyperinflation and ineffective efforts. In such a case, the best strategy is to reduce respiratory support so as to reduce ineffective efforts.

Patient-ventilator interactions also worsen with inadequate inspiratory flow in controlled ventilation modes or from ramp time in pressure support ventilation [12, 56].

Proper setting of inspiratory time is another important point of strategies to improve patient-ventilator interactions. If the mechanical act is too long or too short, it can generate asynchronies due to poor matching between mechanical and neural inspiratory time. This phenomenon occurs in both time-cycled (volume-controlled, pressure-controlled) and flow-cycled (pressure support ventilation) modes of ventilation [57, 58], especially if the expiratory time is also not appropriately set. In noninvasive ventilation, the presence of leaks and the use of respirators that do not have leak compensation in the software increase inspiratory time and consequently asynchronies.

Sedation plays an important role in the quality of patient-ventilator interactions. Profound sedation is known to increase the number of missed efforts [59], while nonsedated patients often exhibit high respiratory rates and double triggering. Vaschetto et al. show how deep sedation with propofol has little effect on patient-ventilator interactions [6]. But dexmedetomidine compared with propofol generates even less without having an influence on respiratory drive [60]. Costa et al. report no effect of remifentanil on respiratory drive with increased neural expiratory time resulting in reduced respiratory rate.

Proportional assist ventilation (PAV) and neurally adjusted ventilatory assist (NAVA) are modes of ventilation that support the respiratory act in a manner proportional to the patient's effort and are effective in reducing asynchronies [61–64]. In comparison with PSV, both reduce hyperinflation, improve neuro-mechanical coupling, improve respiratory pattern, and thus improve patient-ventilator interactions [65, 66]. It has been suggested that these modes of ventilation should be considered in patients with significant asynchronies and if they persist despite optimization of ventilation settings.

Noisy ventilation, a ventilation mode that introduces variability in the respiratory pattern in the same way, turns out to be beneficial in these patients and less harmful than PSV by reducing the number of asynchronies and improving lung function [67]. In addition, noisy ventilation does not require a closed-loop algorithm or the use of probes to assess respiratory curves.

In conclusion, monitoring patient-ventilator interactions is a key aspect of the weaning process and should be mandated for all patients. Understanding the genesis of the various types of asynchrony, regardless of the available technology, improves patient-ventilator interactions and consequently the outcome.

Questions
1. Which of the following statements is false?
   A. NAVA is indicated in the chronic ventilation of patients with neuromuscular diseases
   B. NAVA can improve patient-ventilator synchrony
   C. NAVA can improve patient-ventilator synchrony only in patients with ARDS
   D. None of the above
2. Severe patient-ventilator asynchrony means:
   A. AI > 10%
   B. AI < 10%

   C. AI > 20%

   D. None in the previous

3. Can the control variable affect patient-ventilator synchrony?
    A. Yes
    B. Never
    C. Majorly in volumetric ventilation
    D. None in the previous

4. Double triggering consists of:
    A. Consists of two breaths that may or may not be separated by an expiratory time
    B. Consists of three breaths that may or may not be separated by an expiratory time
    C. Consists of one breath that can least be separated by an expiratory time
    D. None of the above statements are correct

5. Analysis of pressure and flow curves can identify asynchronies:
    A. No never
    B. Yes
    C. Yes but only in COPD
    D. Yes but only in the ARDS

6. In chronic diseases such as COPD patient-ventilator asynchrony may be more due to:
    A. Incorrect expiratory trigger setting in PSV
    B. Intrinsic PEEP not counterbalanced by correct PEEP in PSV
    C. Inspiratory support too high in PSV
    D. All previous

7. In patients with ineffective efforts and AI >10% the prognosis is?
    A. Worst
    B. Unchanged
    C. Change with sedation
    D. None of the above

8. Flow asynchrony is an asynchrony:
    A. Flow asynchrony is an asynchrony between the ventilatory demand and the gas delivery control variable
    B. Flow asynchrony is an asynchrony between the patient trigger and the gas delivery control variable
    C. Flow asynchrony is an asynchrony between the patient's expiratory time and the gas delivery control variable
    D. None of the above

9. Which of these statements is not true:
    A. Reverse-triggering is common in awake nonsedated patients
    B. Reverse-triggering is common in sedated
    C. Reverse-triggering is generated by a contraction of the diaphragm
    D. Reverse-triggering can increase the tidal current volume

10. The EA_{di}:
   A. The EA_{di} can recognize patient-fan asynchronies
   B. The EA_{di} consists of small gastric tube with a series of small electrodes
   C. The EA_{di} measures the electrical activity of the diaphragm
   D. All previous

Answers
 1. B: NAVA can improve patient-ventilator synchrony
 2. A: AI > 10%
 3. C: Majorly in volumetric ventilation
 4. A: Consists of two breaths that may or may not be separated by an expiratory time
 5. B: Yes
 6. D: All previous
 7. A: Worst
 8. A: Flow asynchrony is an asynchrony between the ventilatory demand and the gas delivery control variable
 9. A: Reverse-triggering is common in awake nonsedated patients
10. A: The EA_{di} can recognize patient-fan asynchronies

References

 1. Ranieri VM, Squadrone V, Appendini L, Gregoretti C. Patient-ventilator interaction. In: Vincent J-L, Abraham E, Moore FA, Kochanek PM, Fink MP, editors. Textbook of critical care. 7th ed. Philadelphia: Elsevier; 2017. p. 366–72.
 2. Sassoon CS, Foster GT. Patient-ventilator asynchrony. Curr Opin Crit Care. 2001;7(1):28–33.
 3. Kacmarek RM, Pirrone M, Berra L. Assisted mechanical ventilation: the future is now! BMC Anesthesiol. 2015;15:110.
 4. Tobin MJ, Jubran A, Lakes F. Patient-ventilator interaction. Am J Respir Crit Care Med. 2001;163(5):1059–63.
 5. Garofalo E, Bruni A, Pelaia C, Liparota L, Lombardo N, Longhini F, Navalesi P. Recognizing, quantifying and managing patient-ventilator asynchrony in invasive and noninvasive ventilation. Expert Rev Respir Med. 2018;12(7):557–67.
 6. Leung P, Jubran A, Tobin MJ. Comparison of assisted ventilator modes on triggering, patient effort, and dyspnea. Am J Respir Crit Care Med. 1997;155(6):1940–8.
 7. Dick CR, Sassoon CS. Patient-ventilator interactions. Clin Chest Med. 1996;17(3):423–38.
 8. Mead J. Control of respiratory frequency. J Appl Physiol. 1960;15(3):325–36.
 9. Hubmayr RD, Abel MD, Rehder K. Physiologic approach to mechanical ventilation. Crit Care Med. 1990;18(1):103–13.
10. Whitelaw WA, Derenne JP, Milic-Emili J. Occlusion pressure as a measure of respiratory center output in conscious man. Respir Physiol. 1975;23(2):181–99.
11. Longhini F, Colombo D, Pisani L, Idone F, Chun P, Doorduin J, et al. Efficacy of ventilator waveform observation for detection of patientventilator asynchrony during NIV: a multicentre study. ERJ Open Res. 2017;3(4):00075–2017.
12. Ward ME, Corbeil C, Gibbons W, Newman S, Macklem PT. Optimization of respiratory muscle relaxation during mechanical ventilation. Anesthesiology. 1988;69(1):29–35.

13. Puddy A, Younes M. Effect of inspiratory flow rate on respiratory output in normal subjects. Am Rev Respir Dis. 1992;146(3):787–9.
14. Georgopoulos D, Mitrouska I, Bshouty Z, Anthonisen NR, Younes M. Effects of non-REM sleep on the response of respiratory output to varying inspiratory flow. Am J Respir Crit Care Med. 1996;153(5):1624–30.
15. Lakes F, Karamchandani K, Tobin MJ. Influence of ventilator settings in determining respiratory frequency during mechanical ventilation. Am J Respir Crit Care Med. 1999;160(5):1766–70.
16. Banner MJ, Blanch PB, Gabrielli A. Tracheal pressure control provides automatic and variable inspiratory pressure assist to decrease the imposed resistive work of breathing. Crit Care Med. 2002;30(5):1106–11.
17. MacIntyre NR. Improving patient/ventilator interactions. In: Vincent J-L, editor. Yearbook of intensive care and emergency medicine. Berlin: Springer; 1999. p. 235–43.
18. Ranieri VM, Mascia L, Petruzzelli V, Bruno F, Brienza A, Giuliani R. Inspiratory effort and measurement of dynamic intrinsic PEEP in COPD patients: effects of ventilator triggering systems. Intensive Care Med. 1995;21(11):896–903.
19. Alberti A, Gallo F, Fongaro A, Valenti S, Rossi A. P0.1 is a useful parameter in setting the level of pressure support ventilation. Intensive Care Med. 1995;21(7):547–53.
20. Sassoon CS, Gruer SE. Characteristics of the ventilator pressure- and flow-trigger variables. Intensive Care Med. 1995;21(2):159–68.
21. Fabry B, Haberthür C, Zappe D, Guttmann J, Kuhlen R, Stocker R. Breathing pattern and additional work of breathing in spontaneously breathing patients with different ventilatory demands during inspiratory pressure support and automatic tube compensation. Intensive Care Med. 1997;23(5):545–52.
22. Ranieri VM, Giuliani R, Mascia L, Grasso S, Petruzzelli V, Puntillo N, et al. Patient-ventilator interaction during acute hypercapnia: pressure-support vs. proportional-assist ventilation. J Appl Physiol (1985). 1996;81(1):426–36.
23. Nava S, Bruschi C, Fracchia C, Braschi A, Rubini F. Patient-ventilator interaction and inspiratory effort during pressure support ventilation in patients with different pathologies. Eur Respir J. 1997;10(1):177–83.
24. Sinderby C, Navalesi P, Beck J, Skrobik Y, Comtois N, Friberg S, et al. Neural control of mechanical ventilation in respiratory failure. Nat Med. 1999;5(12):1433–6.
25. Beck J, Sinderby C, Lindström L, Grassino A. Effects of lung volume on diaphragm EMG signal strength during voluntary contractions. J Appl Physiol (1985). 1998;85(3):1123–34.
26. Aslanian P, El Atrous S, Isabey D, Valente E, Corsi D, Harf A, et al. Effects of flow triggering on breathing effort during partial ventilatory support. Am J Respir Crit Care Med. 1998;157(1):135–43.
27. Chatburn RL. Classification of mechanical ventilators. In: Tobin MJ, editor. Principles and practice of mechanical ventilation. 2nd ed. New York: McGraw-Hill; 2006. p. 37–52.
28. Parthasarathy S, Jubran A, Tobin MJ. Cycling of inspiratory and expiratory muscle groups with the ventilator in airflow limitation. Am J Respir Crit Care Med. 1998;158(5 Pt 1):1471–8.
29. Tobin MJ, Yang KL, Jubran A, Lodato RF. Interrelationship of breath components in neighboring breaths of normal eupneic subjects. Am J Respir Crit Care Med. 1995;152(6):1967–76.
30. Javaheri S, Kazemi H. Metabolic alkalosis and hypoventilation in humans. Am Rev Respir Dis. 1987;136(4):1011–6.
31. de Wit M, Miller KB, Green DA, Ostman HE, Gennings C, Epstein SK. Ineffective triggering predicts increased duration of mechanical ventilation. Crit Care Med. 2009;37(10):2740–5.
32. Vaschetto R, Cammarota G, Colombo D, Longhini F, Grossi F, Giovanniello A. Effects of propofol on patient-ventilator synchrony and interaction during pressure support ventilation and neutrally adjusted ventilatory assist. Crit Care Med. 2014;42(1):74–82.
33. Kallet RH, Campbell AR, Dicker RA, Katz JA, Mackersie RC. Work of breathing during lung-protective ventilation in patients with acute lung injury and acute respiratory distress syndrome: a comparison between volume and pressure-regulated breathing modes. Respir Care. 2005;50(12):1623–31.

34. de Haro C, López-Aguilar J, Magrans R, Montanya J, Fernández-Gonzalo S, Turon M, et al. Double cycling during mechanical ventilation: frequency, mechanisms, and physiologic implications. Crit Care Med. 2018;46(9):1385–92.
35. Blanch L, Villagra A, Sales B, Montanya J, Lucangelo U, Luján M, et al. Asynchronies during mechanical ventilation are associated with mortality. Intensive Care Med. 2015;41(4):633–41.
36. Thille AW, Rodriguez P, Cabello B, Lellouche F, Brochard L. Patient-ventilator asynchrony during assisted mechanical ventilation. Intensive Care Med. 2006;32(10):1515–22.
37. Bosma K, Ferreyra G, Ambrogio C, Pasero D, Mirabella L, Braghiroli A, et al. Patient-ventilator interaction and sleep in mechanically ventilated patients: pressure support versus proportional assist ventilation. Crit Care Med. 2007;35(4):1048–54.
38. Parthasarathy S, Tobin MJ. Effect of ventilator mode on sleep quality in critically ill patients. Am J Respir Crit Care Med. 2002;166(11):1423–9.
39. Alexopoulou C, Kondili E, Plataki M, Georgopoulos D. Patient-ventilator synchrony and sleep quality with proportional assist and pressure support ventilation. Intensive Care Med. 2013;39(6):1040–7.
40. Delisle S, Ouellet P, Bellemare P, Tétrault JP, Arsenault P. Sleep quality in mechanically ventilated patients: comparison between NAVA and PSV modes. Ann Intensive Care. 2011;1(1):42.
41. Colombo D, Cammarota G, Alemani M, Carenzo L, Barra FL, Vaschetto R, et al. Efficacy of ventilator waveforms observation in detecting patient-ventilator asynchrony. Crit Care Med. 2011;39(11):2452–7.
42. Brochard L. Measurement of esophageal pressure at bedside: pros and cons. Curr Opin Crit Care. 2014;20(1):39–46.
43. Gogineni VK, Brimeyer R, Modrykamien A. Patterns of patient-ventilator asynchrony as predictors of prolonged mechanical ventilation. Anaesth Intensive Care. 2012;40(6):964–70.
44. Doorduin J, van Hees HW, van der Hoeven JG, Heunks LM. Monitoring of the respiratory muscles in the critically ill. Am J Respir Crit Care Med. 2013;187(1):20–7.
45. Dres M, Rittayamai N, Brochard L. Monitoring patient-ventilator asynchrony. Curr Opin Crit Care. 2016;22(3):246–53.
46. Goligher EC, Lakes F, Detsky ME, Farias P, Murray A, Brace D, et al. Measuring diaphragm thickness with ultrasound in mechanically ventilated patients: feasibility, reproducibility and validity. Intensive Care Med. 2015;41(4):642–9.
47. Matamis D, Soilemezi E, Tsagourias M, Akoumianaki E, Dimassi S, Boroli F, et al. Sonographic evaluation of the diaphragm in critically ill patients: technique and clinical applications. Intensive Care Med. 2013;39(5):801–10.
48. Chen CW, Lin WC, Hsu CH, Cheng KS, Lo CS. Detecting ineffective triggering in the expiratory phase in mechanically ventilated patients based on airway flow and pressure deflection: feasibility of using a computer algorithm. Crit Care Med. 2008;36(2):455–61.
49. Gutierrez G, Ballarino GJ, Turkan H, Abril J, De La Cruz L, Edsall C, et al. Automatic detection of patient-ventilator asynchrony by spectral analysis of airway flow. Crit Care. 2011;15(4):R167.
50. Imanaka H, Nishimura M, Takeuchi M, Kimball WR, Yahagi N, Kumon K. Autotriggering caused by cardiogenic oscillation during flow-triggered mechanical ventilation. Crit Care Med. 2000;28(2):402–7.
51. Levine S, Nguyen T, Taylor N, Friscia ME, Budak MT, Rothenberg P, et al. Rapid disuse atrophy of diaphragm fibers in mechanically ventilated humans. N Engl J Med. 2008;358(13):1327–35.
52. Georgopoulos D, Prinianakis G, Kondili E. Bedside waveforms interpretation as a tool to identify patient-ventilator asynchronies. Intensive Care Med. 2006;32(1):34–47.
53. Fabry B, Guttmann J, Eberhard L, Bauer T, Haberthür C, Wolff G. An analysis of desynchronization between the spontaneously breathing patient and ventilator during inspiratory pressure support. Chest. 1995;107(5):1387–94.
54. Vignaux L, Vargas F, Roeseler J, Tassaux D, Thille AW, Kossowsky MP, et al. Patient-ventilator asynchrony during non-invasive ventilation for acute respiratory failure: a multicenter study. Intensive Care Med. 2009;35(5):840–6.

55. Navalesi P, Costa R. New modes of mechanical ventilation: proportional assist ventilation, neurally adjusted ventilatory assist, and fractal ventilation. Curr Opin Crit Care. 2003;9(1):51–8.
56. Kacmarek RM, Chipman D. Basic principles of ventilator machinery. In: Tobin MJ, editor. Principles and practice of mechanical ventilation. 2nd ed. New York: McGraw-Hill; 2006. p. 53–95.
57. Chiumello D, Polli F, Tallarini F, Chierichetti M, Motta G, Azzari S, et al. Effect of different cycling-off criteria and positive end-expiratory pressure during pressure support ventilation in patients with chronic obstructive pulmonary disease. Crit Care Med. 2007;35(11):2547–52.
58. Branson RD, Blakeman TC, Robinson B. Asynchrony and dyspnea. Respir Care. 2013;58(6):973–89.
59. de Wit M, Pedram S, Best AM, Epstein SK. Observational study of patient-ventilator asynchrony and relationship to sedation level. J Crit Care. 2009;24(1):74–80.
60. Conti G, Ranieri VM, Costa R, Garratt C, Wighton A, Spinazzola G, et al. Effects of dexmedetomidine and propofol on patient-ventilator interaction in difficult-to-wean, mechanically ventilated patients: a prospective, open-label, randomized, multicentre study. Crit Care. 2016;20(1):206.
61. Piquilloud L, Vignaux L, Bialais E, Roeseler J, Sottiaux T, Laterre PF, et al. Neurally adjusted ventilatory assist improves patient-ventilator interaction. Intensive Care Med. 2011;37(2):263–71.
62. de la Oliva P, Schüffelmann C, Gómez-Zamora A, Villar J, Kacmarek R. Asynchrony, neural drive, ventilatory variability and COMFORT: NAVA versus pressure support in pediatric patients. A non-randomized cross-over trial. Intensive Care Med. 2012;38(5):838–46.
63. Costa R, Spinazzola G, Cipriani F, Ferrone G, Festa O, Arcangeli A, et al. A physiologic comparison of proportional assist ventilation with load-adjustable gain factors (PAV+) versus pressure support ventilation (PSV). Intensive Care Med. 2011;37(9):1494–500.
64. Kacmarek RM. Proportional assist ventilation and neurally adjusted ventilatory assist. Respir Care. 2011;56(2):140–8.
65. Schmidt M, Kindler F, Cecchini J, Poitou T, Morawiec E, Persichini R, et al. Neurally adjusted ventilatory assist and proportional assist ventilation both improve patient-ventilator interaction. Crit Care. 2015;25:19–56.
66. Yonis H, Crognier L, Conil JM, Serres I, Rouget A, Virtos M, et al. Patient-ventilator synchrony in neurally adjusted ventilatory assist (NAVA) and pressure support ventilation (PSV): a prospective observational study. BMC Anesthesiol. 2015;15:117.
67. Spieth PM, Güldner A, Huhle R, Beda A, Bluth T, Schreiter D, et al. Short-term effects of noisy pressure support ventilation in patients with acute hypoxemic respiratory failure. Crit Care. 2013;17(5):R261.

End-of-Life in Intensive Care

13

Giacinto Pizzilli, Alessio Dell'Olio,
Maria Della Giovampaola, and Luciana Mascia

13.1 Introduction

When organ dysfunction lead by critical illness is insurmountable and life support is not going to result in outcome coherent with patients values, intensive care unit (ICU) clinicians must guarantee patient dying with dignity [1].

ICU mortality rate is reported between 8 and 19% [2], and a growing number of patients spend their end-of-life (EoL) period in ICU. Increasing life expectancy leads to a growing number of elderly patients admitted to ICU with patients aged 80 or over representing 10–20% of all ICU admissions. ICU mortality of elderly patients aged 80 or over is between 15 and 25% [3]. Consequently end-of-life (EoL) care has become an important topic for intensive care unit (ICU) medical practice.

End-of-life is a period which begins with the diagnosis of a fatal disease and recognizes as the main goal the prevention or relief of suffering as much as possible while respecting the patients' desires [4]. Palliative care (PC) is the instrument to achieve this goal and is defined as *"the prevention and relief of suffering for adult and pediatric patients and their families facing the problems associated with life-threatening illness. These problems include physical, psychological, social and spiritual suffering of both patients and family members"* [5]. The main issues that physicians face during the transition from curative to palliative care are prognostication uncertainty, communication with family members, ethical dilemmas during

G. Pizzilli · A. Dell'Olio · M. Della Giovampaola
Dipartimento di Scienze Mediche e Chirurgiche, Anesthesia and Intensive Care Medicine, Policlinico di Sant'Orsola, Alma Mater Studiorum, Università di Bologna, Bologna, Italy

L. Mascia (✉)
Dipartimento di Scienze Biomediche e Neuromotorie, Anesthesia and Intensive Care Medicine, Alma Mater Studiorum, Università di Bologna, Bologna, Italy
e-mail: luciana.mascia@unibo.it

D. Chiumello (ed.), *Practical Trends in Anesthesia and Intensive Care 2022*,
https://doi.org/10.1007/978-3-031-43891-2_13

withholding (WHLST) or withdrawal (WDLST) of life-sustaining therapies and the need to follow the local laws [6, 7].

This chapter will then discuss EoL care focusing on three main topics: (a) prognostication, (b) decision-making process and communication, and (c) clinical management of EoL.

13.2 Prognostication

Uncertainty about outcome in critically ill patients admitted to the intensive care unit (ICU) is heavy to bear for patients and family. Prediction models may orient physicians in their decision-making and communication. Outcome tools for ICU emphasize acute changes in physiology and organ dysfunction, focusing on short-term mortality and providing quite accurate data about specific organ disease (e.g., Glasgow Coma Scale) or patient populations. Prognostication scores are more accurate in predicting the severity of outcome for conditions such as cardiac arrest and traumatic brain injury providing a high level of certainty, while a larger variability remains for other clinical conditions such as sepsis or acute respiratory distress syndrome. Only recently a growing body of literature focused on post-ICU functional outcomes and long-term quality of life, underscoring that this aspect is relevant for patients as much as survival [8, 9].

13.2.1 Neurological and Neurosurgical Patients

Prognostication is a crucial moment of the neurocritical care. Indeed, several prognostic models have been developed for many different clinical conditions keeping in mind that (1) there are significant gaps in optimal methods of prognostication and that (2) treating clinicians should routinely include medical comorbidities in their evaluation. Common concerns are therefore related to the accuracy of prognostic models and how this information is discussed to ensure patient-centered decision.

In a good prognostication model, clinical examination is mandatory in every patient, and EEG- or sensory-evoked potential recording is necessary if pupillary light reflexes are absent at 72 h to predict poor recovery. EEG has been shown to have higher accuracy than sensory-evoked potential for predicting both poor outcome and good recovery, and it is also useful to identify seizure-associated activity.

After cardiac arrest and, in general, after any kind of brain injury, multimodal assessment, including clinical examination and electrophysiological studies (EEG, evoked potentials, or both), should be carried out after return to normothermia, after discontinuation of sedation, and after the removal of any other confounding factor. Absent pupillary and corneal reflexes, EEG with suppressed or burst suppression background and no reactivity, and absent early somatosensory-evoked potentials do not need additional tests. Biochemical markers and imaging are confirmatory but not mandatory tests for poor prognosis. Interruption of life-sustaining measures should be considered only when poor outcome is predicted by at least two methods with very low false positive results for poor outcome—i.e., clinical examination plus electrophysiology—without any discordant information.

13.2.2 General ICU

Since 1980s much has been achieved in general ICU prognostic assessment. Instruments such as the Acute Physiology and Chronic Health Evaluation (APACHE) and the Simplified Acute Physiology Score (SAPS) were developed. These tools aim to assess severity on admission and predicting hospital mortality relying on a set of physiological variables. Over the years these instruments have been updated due to the change in ICU populations (age, severity of chronic disease), available diagnostic techniques, therapeutic options, and statistical calibration models [10, 11]. Prognostication tools have been developed in large databases, but when applying these tools to different populations in different countries, their calibration may be weaker; therefore, attention should be given to the choice of the reference population in order to avoid misleading results [12–14]. Moreover, none of these tools provides information about long-term mortality, functional outcome, and quality of life (QoL) of ICU survivors, potentially reducing the accuracy of the prognostic information provided to patient and relatives. Indeed patients discharged from ICU have a mortality over the first year between 26 and 63% [15], while survivors frequently suffer physical, cognitive, and mental health impairment persisting up to 5–10 years [16]. This global impairment explain why cumulative QoL after ICU admission is significantly lower than that expected for the general population [17].

Two specific patient populations deserve further consideration: geriatric and hematologic patients. Indeed, their ICU admission has increased over the last decades because of improved therapeutic techniques, and consequently factors influencing either short- or long-term prognosis have been separately identified to overcome the limitations of general prediction models.

Older adults admitted to intensive care units are more frail and much more likely to have preexisting comorbidities [18]. The effect of age per se on short-term prognosis is a matter of debate. ICU short-term mortality is in fact related to the severity of the acute illness, while long-term prognosis is related to the underlying condition and preexisting functional limitations more than the age at admission [19]. Frailty is a clinical state in which there is an increase in individual's vulnerability for developing increased dependency and/or mortality when exposed to a stressor. Frailty can occur as the result of several diseases and medical conditions [20]. The VIP1 study group studied a population of 5021 patients of at least 80 years old with a 43% incidence of frailty at admission reporting a linear relationship between increasing frailty class and short-term mortality [21]. Similarly in another multicenter prospective study higher in-hospital mortality, major adverse events, higher prevalence of hospital readmission, and significantly lower quality of life in the subsequent 12 months were found comparing frail and non-frail patients.

Patients with *hematologic* malignancies have a higher ICU mortality than patients with solid tumors. However during the past decade, development of new efficacious chemotherapy lines with lower toxicity improved outcome and increased life expectancy of hematological patients [22]. Consequently, hematological patients are more likely to be admitted to ICU. As treatments improved, neutropenia and autologous stem cell transplantation are no longer defined as adverse prognostic factors for ICU admission. Conversely age, multiorgan failure, poor performance, and acute respiratory failure (ARF) with first-line intubation remain negative prognostic factors [23–25].

13.3 Decision-Making Process and Communication

In clinical medicine, the 'end of life' can be thought as the period preceding an individual's natural death from a process that is unlikely to be arrested by medical care [26].

Despite most people desire to die at home only one-third or less does [27, 28]. Conversely rate of ICU stay in the last month of life has increased up to 30% in 2009 [29]. Therefore, EoL became an important topic in ICU. During this period critical care and palliative care proceed in parallel, and goals of treatment shift from treating organ dysfunction to guarantee dignity to the dying patient and support to family members. To achieve this goal, decision-making should always be shared and built incorporating scientific evidence and the patient's values and preferences [1] preventing unnecessary suffering related to unwelcome interventions. All clinicians involved in EoL care decisions must quickly recognize the "big picture" in which they are involved, and they should act keeping in mind the ABCD of dignity-conserving care (attitudes, behaviors, compassion, and dialogue) [30]. If confusion arises from different points of view, then patients may receive inappropriate palliative care. This risk has been described by Hillman et al. proposing the "conveyor belt" effect: an *"unstoppable chain of events, resulting in patients experiencing their EoL period in hospital"* [31].

The diagnosis of dying is often delayed, and ICU is the last ring of the chain where the intensivist has to take care of this clinical condition. Uncertainty in prognostication is the main factor moving the "conveyor belt," but several factors contribute to this event: (1) lack of communication, (2) failure of people to have stated their wishes regarding EOL care, and (3) unrealistic societal expectations of modern health care [32]. Uncertainty determines reluctance by doctors to label a person as "dying" until death is nearly certain [33]. Even in the ICU, the decision to continue vital support may not be appropriate since many patients discharged from ICU die within the following 12 months [31]. Decision-making models for the ICU vary internationally. The founding principle of decision-making process in most North American and European countries is the patient autonomy. Since most patients are not able to participate in the decision-making process during their ICU stay a surrogate is designated to participate.

Several challenges and concerns are related to EoL decision-making in the ICU. First there is a wide variability among countries and different ICUs of the same country in the practice of end-of-life care [34, 35], including the attention for living wills and the involvement of surrogates in end-of-life decision-making. In the United States, the priority is preserving patient's autonomy principle, even for those patients lacking decisional capacity. Indeed, the unexpected clinical scenario that the patient potentially faces makes living wills ineffective in many situations. In this case a trusted surrogate is designated. Nevertheless in most of studies after decision is made no reduction in high-intensity treatments has been reported [36, 37]. Second, a correct communication is mandatory for family satisfaction with EOL care. After critical illness, patients and their families communicate with unfamiliar clinicians under stressful situation in an unfamiliar environment where they arrive suddenly. Among the different decision-making models, we can vary from one in which physicians share information but maintains the main responsibility to decide, to the other one in which the patient makes the decision with the advice of the physician. In between stands the most common model of shared decision-making where patient, family, and physician share information and participate jointly to the final decision (Fig. 13.1). When patients are unable to make autonomous decision regarding their care, physicians rely on patients' trusted surrogate (or substitute) decision-makers (SDMs), usually family members. Implementation of this model is associated with shorter ICU stay in dying critically ill patients [38]. SDMs represent a sensitive partner that can be challenged by potential conflict between stakeholders [39]. Indeed misinterpretation of patients' preferences, posttraumatic stress disorder (PTSD), anxiety, and depression have been described for surrogates as well [40–42].

Conflict generated by EoL decisions has been reported between medical staff and family members in almost 50% of the cases [39]. To avoid such conflicts, clinicians should acquire communication skills enabling them to elicit negative emotions in a comprehensive way, reducing the impact of emotional, cognitive, and moral factors that may threaten the health of family members. Setting and sharing achievable goals with clear and honest communication among all stakeholders is one of the core elements for providing effective and comprehensive palliative care. Clinicians should be able to explore and clarify all these issues with families, explaining LST withdrawal with open questions and giving necessary time needed to metabolize the emotional burden. To avoid conflict before and during the withdrawal decision, it is strongly recommended that clinicians (a) provide honest, caring, and cultural sensitive communication with family members; (b) explain to family members what to expect after starting the withdrawal procedure; (c) explain the reason for increasing sedation; (d) personalize the patient's environment; (e) encourage family and patient to express their emotions; and (f) guarantee the presence of a spiritual guide, for unlimited periods if required. Sensitive and honest communication with family member is the best strategy to mitigate critical issues on EoL. The use of trained facilitators may improve communication between family members and medical staff, with a lower incidence of depression (but not PTSD) in family members after the loss of their loved ones; the length of stay of the descendants is reduced as well [43].

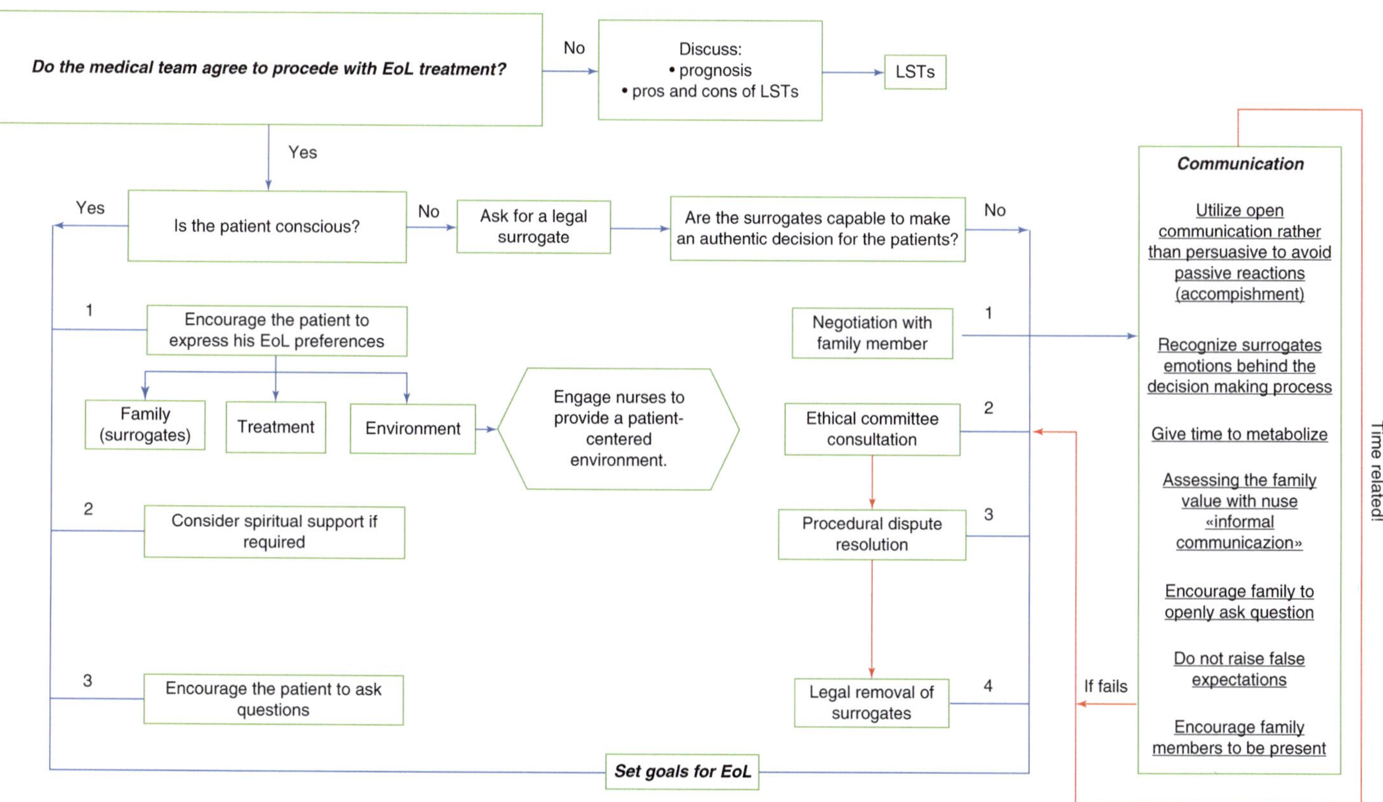

Fig. 13.1 Decision-making process and communication

In conclusion, during critical illness patients and their families communicate with unfamiliar clinicians under stressful situation. When the clinical condition requires the shift from intensive to palliative care, a correct communication is mandatory for family satisfaction.

13.4 End-of-Life Management in the ICU

End-of-life procedures in the ICU include withholding (WHLST) or withdrawal (WDLST) life-sustaining therapies. Withholding treatment is the decision to do not start or increase a life-sustaining intervention. Withdrawing treatment is defined as the decision to actively stop a life-sustaining intervention presently being given. WHLST and WDLST incidence is reported to be between 6 and 14% of patients admitted to ICU [44]. Although most author agree that there is no ethical difference between WHLST and WDLST, a big debate is still occurring about this topic [45, 46].

The first consensus guidelines approaching EoL analgesia and sedation in ICU were published in 2002 [6]. Despite the growing number of scientific recommendations on this topic, the clinical approach to EoL care remains vague, and several studies emphasized the non-uniformity of clinicians in assuming responsibility for EoL decisions. A significant discrepancy about drug management and withdrawal of procedures persists in clinical practice [46, 47]. Inconsistence in clinical decisions may breed serious anger and frustration within family members, as well as other medical team members. Main recommendations are related to (1) pain relief and sedation, and (2) respiratory support.

13.4.1 Pain Relief and Sedation Management

To titrate the correct dose of sedative and analgesic drug, it is crucial to assess patient's distress, severity of pain and agitation, and the potential presence of delirium. In general, ICU patients may not be able to communicate or show any sign of distress, and therefore assessment may be difficult. For this reason, it is fundamental for terminal patients to use the validated scales routinely applied in the ICU general population [48]. Pain is one of the main components afflicting patients in the EoL period; it is defined by the International Association for the Study of Pain as "an unpleasant sensory and emotional experience associated with, or resembling that associated with, actual or potential tissue damage" [49].

Although the ability to assess pain is essential, yet this skill is poorly taught and managed by few clinicians. Moreover, in ICU the assessment of pain may be masked by the patient's condition. In conscious patients, a numeric rating scale (NRS) should be used [50]. If the patient is not able to self-report their condition, validated scales with behavioral and physiologic indicators should be used, such as the Behavioral Pain Scale (BPS) and the Critical Care Pain Observation Tool (CPOT) [51].

As for pain, the assessment of agitation and delirium in ICU terminal patients can be challenging. In this perspective, it is important to understand the definitions of both terms. Agitation is defined by the *Diagnostic and Statistical Manual of Mental Disorders,* Fourth Edition (DSM-V), as an excessive motor activity associated with a feeling of inner tension [52]. On the other hand, delirium can be defined as a syndrome characterized by the acute onset of cerebral dysfunction with a change or fluctuation in baseline mental status, inattention, and either disorganized thinking or an altered level of consciousness [48]. Both for delirium and agitation, guidelines recommend the use of scales validated in critically ill patients, such as the Richmond Agitation and Sedation Scale (RASS) [53] for the detection and quantification of agitation and the Confusion Assessment Method for the Intensive Care Unit (CAM-ICU) [54] and the Intensive Care Delirium Screening Checklist (ICDSC) [55] for the detection of delirium. Assessment of pain and agitation allows the clinician to individualize palliative care, tailoring the correct dose of sedatives and analgesics. These two classes of drugs combined together guarantee better relief from pain and suffering than either class of drug alone.

As stated by the ACCM guidelines, the initial dose of sedation and analgesic drug depends on (1) previous exposure to narcotics, (2) age, (3) previous alcohol and drug use/abuse, (4) underlying organ dysfunction, (5) patient's previous level of sedation and consciousness, (6) available psychological and spiritual support, and (7) patient's wishes.

After the beginning of infusion drug, it is important to frequently re-assess patient's condition with previously mentioned scales to titrate the dose. It is fundamental to underline that, regarding palliation, the dose of drugs needed by the patient can exceed the usual one since there is not a "maximal dose" of drug in relieving pain and suffering.

According to guidelines of the British Medical Council, although the dosage of narcotic/sedative to palliate the dying patients may hypothetically accelerate the death process (the double effect), clinicians should prescribe the maximum achievable dosage to relief patient symptoms, but not for euthanasia. Indeed it is recognized that terminal sedation is fundamentally different from euthanasia [6]. Terminal sedation is different in the intentions and is defined as *bringing the patient into deep sedation while forgoing artificial nutrition or hydration.* Although today there is no maximum dosage for terminal sedation, it must be recognized that without a national legal endorsement for euthanasia, the "maximum dosage" should always be reached by increments.

Another issue to consider about palliative sedation is that clinicians should provide the best achievable interaction between patients and family members. Guidelines for the withdrawal of life-sustaining measures have been proposed by the Canadian Critical Care Society [7].

13.4.2 Respiratory Support

One of the main issues related to the quality of dying in ICU is the control of dyspnea defined by the American Thoracic Society as a "subjective experience of breathing discomfort that consists of qualitatively distinct sensations that vary in intensity" [56, 57]. In a prospective study investigating the quality perception of family members, resident physicians, attending physicians, and nurses, dyspnea was reported as the second main concern related to patient EoL. Furthermore, two-thirds of family members stated that their loved one was breathing uncomfortably for most of the time.

Because of its nature, clinical measures such as peripheral oxygen saturation, arterial blood gas (ABG) analysis, and respiratory rate may not be good tools for its assessment. For this reason, literature recommends the use of numeric or descriptive scales like the Visual Analog Scale (VAS) or the Borg Dyspnea Scale rate for the intensity of the symptoms, or the effect of dyspnea on daily activity or health-related quality of life (HRQoL) [58]. An effective measure to counteract dyspnea in terminal patients can be non-invasive ventilation (NIV). In 2004, a feasibility study in a population of oncological end-stage patients found that the use of NIV as a measure to treat concomitant acute respiratory failure (ARF) is feasible and effective in improving both dyspnea and clinical variables, such as ABG [59]. The efficacy of NIV in reducing dyspnea was confirmed also by Nava et al., who described a reduction of the Borg scales in end-of-life patients with solid tumors after the use of NIV for dyspnea relief, as well as a reduction in the use of opioids [60]. One of the most debated factors concerning the use of NIV for palliation is whether it could worsen symptoms like anxiety and preclude communication with relatives in the final moments of life. A prospective observational cohort study demonstrated that in patients with a "do not intubate order," NIV did not worsen the prevalence of anxiety, depression, and PTSD-related symptoms both in patients and in their relatives. In this context, it is important to underline that the use of NIV, as well as all the other medical treatments, requires the patients and their loved ones to be informed about what to expect about the procedure [61].

13.5   Conclusions

End-of-life is a period which begins with the diagnosis of a fatal disease. When organ dysfunction of critical illness is insurmountable, ICU clinicians must guarantee patient dying with dignity avoiding the "conveyor belt" effect. In the transition from curative to palliative care, the best strategy to mitigate critical issues is prognostication certainty, adequate communication with family members, ethical dilemmas, and legal issue resolution. The main goals of EoL are prevention or relief of suffering, respecting patients and family wishes.

References

1. Cook D, Rocker G. Dying with dignity in the intensive care unit. N Engl J Med. 2014;370(26):2506–14. https://doi.org/10.1056/NEJMra1208795.
2. ICU outcomes. Philip R. Lee Institute for Health Policy Studies. https://healthpolicy.ucsf.edu/icu-outcomes. Accessed 7 Apr 2022.
3. Leblanc G, Boumendil A, Guidet B. Ten things to know about critically ill elderly patients. Intensive Care Med. 2017;43(2):217–9. https://doi.org/10.1007/s00134-016-4477-2.
4. Akdeniz M, Yardımcı B, Kavukcu E. Ethical considerations at the end-of-life care. SAGE Open Med. 2021;9:20503121211000920. https://doi.org/10.1177/20503121211000918.
5. Palliative care. https://www.who.int/health-topics/palliative-care. Accessed 7 Apr 2022.
6. Hawryluck LA, Harvey WR, Lemieux-Charles L, Singer PA. Consensus guidelines on analgesia and sedation in dying intensive care unit patients. BMC Med Ethics. 2002;3(1):3. https://doi.org/10.1186/1472-6939-3-3.
7. Downar J, Delaney JW, Hawryluck L, Kenny L. Guidelines for the withdrawal of life-sustaining measures. Intensive Care Med. 2016;42(6):1003–17. https://doi.org/10.1007/s00134-016-4330-7.
8. Oeyen S, Vermeulen K, Benoit D, Annemans L, Decruyenaere J. Development of a prediction model for long-term quality of life in critically ill patients. J Crit Care. 2018;43:133–8. https://doi.org/10.1016/j.jcrc.2017.09.006.
9. Flaatten H, Oeyen S, deLange DW. Predicting outcomes in very old ICU patients: time to focus on the past? Intensive Care Med. 2018;44(8):1344–5. https://doi.org/10.1007/s00134-018-5262-1.
10. Vincent JL, Moreno R. Clinical review: scoring systems in the critically ill. Crit Care. 2010;14(2):207. https://doi.org/10.1186/cc8204.
11. Moreno RP. Outcome prediction in intensive care: why we need to reinvent the wheel. Curr Opin Crit Care. 2008;14(5):483–4. https://doi.org/10.1097/MCC.0b013e328310dc7d.
12. Poole D, Rossi C, Anghileri A, et al. External validation of the simplified acute physiology score (SAPS) 3 in a cohort of 28,357 patients from 147 Italian intensive care units. Intensive Care Med. 2009;35(11):1916–24. https://doi.org/10.1007/s00134-009-1615-0.
13. On behalf of the ASDI Study Group, Metnitz B, Schaden E, et al. Austrian validation and customization of the SAPS 3 admission score. Intensive Care Med. 2009;35(4):616–22. https://doi.org/10.1007/s00134-008-1286-2.
14. Moreno R, Afonso S. Ethical, legal and organizational issues in the ICU: prediction of outcome. Curr Opin Crit Care. 2006;12(6):619–23. https://doi.org/10.1097/MCC.0b013e328010c800.
15. Williams TA, Dobb GJ, Finn JC, Webb SAR. Long-term survival from intensive care: a review. Intensive Care Med. 2005;31(10):1306–15. https://doi.org/10.1007/s00134-005-2744-8.
16. Desai SV, Law TJ, Needham DM. Long-term complications of critical care. Crit Care Med. 2011;39(2):371–9. https://doi.org/10.1097/CCM.0b013e3181fd66e5.
17. Cuthbertson BH, Roughton S, Jenkinson D, MacLennan G, Vale L. Quality of life in the five years after intensive care: a cohort study. Crit Care. 2010;14(1):R6. https://doi.org/10.1186/cc8848.
18. Ferrante LE, Pisani MA, Murphy TE, Gahbauer EA, Leo-Summers LS, Gill TM. Functional trajectories among older persons before and after critical illness. JAMA Intern Med. 2015;175(4):523–9. https://doi.org/10.1001/jamainternmed.2014.7889.
19. Boumendil A, Maury E, Reinhard I, Luquel L, Offenstadt G, Guidet B. Prognosis of patients aged 80 years and over admitted in medical intensive care unit. Intensive Care Med. 2004;30(4):647–54. https://doi.org/10.1007/s00134-003-2150-z.
20. Morley JE, Vellas B, Abellan van Kan G, et al. Frailty consensus: a call to action. J Am Med Dir Assoc. 2013;14(6):392–7. https://doi.org/10.1016/j.jamda.2013.03.022.
21. Flaatten H, De Lange DW, et al. The impact of frailty on ICU and 30-day mortality and the level of care in very elderly patients (≥80 years). Intensive Care Med. 2017;43(12):1820–8. https://doi.org/10.1007/s00134-017-4940-8.

22. Azoulay E, Pène F, Darmon M, et al. Managing critically ill hematology patients: time to think differently. Blood Rev. 2015;29(6):359–67. https://doi.org/10.1016/j.blre.2015.04.002.
23. Ñamendys-Silva SA, González-Herrera MO, García-Guillén FJ, Texcocano-Becerra J, Herrera-Gómez A. Outcome of critically ill patients with hematological malignancies. Ann Hematol. 2013;92(5):699–705. https://doi.org/10.1007/s00277-013-1675-7.
24. Algrin C, Faguer S, Lemiale V, et al. Outcomes after intensive care unit admission of patients with newly diagnosed lymphoma. Leuk Lymphoma. 2015;56(5):1240–5. https://doi.org/10.3109/10428194.2014.922181.
25. Azoulay E, Pickkers P, et al. Acute hypoxemic respiratory failure in immunocompromised patients: the Efraim multinational prospective cohort study. Intensive Care Med. 2017;43(12):1808–19. https://doi.org/10.1007/s00134-017-4947-1.
26. Lamont EB. A demographic and prognostic approach to defining the end of life. J Palliat Med. 2005;8(Suppl 1):S12–21. https://doi.org/10.1089/jpm.2005.8.s-12.
27. Rothman DJ. Where we die. N Engl J Med. 2014;370(26):2457–60. https://doi.org/10.1056/NEJMp1404427.
28. Sneesby L. Home is where I want to die: Kelly's journey. Contemp Nurse. 2014;46(2):251–3. https://doi.org/10.5172/conu.2014.46.2.251.
29. Teno JM, Gozalo PL, Bynum JPW, et al. Change in end-of-life care for medicare beneficiaries. JAMA. 2013;309(5):470–7. https://doi.org/10.1001/jama.2012.207624.
30. Chochinov HM. Dignity and the essence of medicine: the A, B, C, and D of dignity conserving care. BMJ. 2007;335(7612):184–7. https://doi.org/10.1136/bmj.39244.650926.47. PMID: 17656543; PMCID: PMC1934489.
31. Hillman KM, Rubenfeld GD, Braithwaite J. Time to shut down the acute care conveyor belt? Med J Aust. 2015;203(11):429–30. https://doi.org/10.5694/mja14.01432.
32. Hillman K. Dying safely. Int J Qual Health Care. 2010;22(5):339–40. https://doi.org/10.1093/intqhc/mzq045.
33. Lynn J, Schall MW, Milne C, Nolan KM, Kabcenell A. Quality improvements in end of life care: insights from two collaboratives. Jt Comm J Qual Improv. 2000;26(5):254–67. https://doi.org/10.1016/S1070-3241(00)26020-3.
34. McLean RF, Tarshis J, Mazer CD, Szalai JP. Death in two Canadian intensive care units: institutional difference and changes over time. Crit Care Med. 2000;28(1):100–3. https://doi.org/10.1097/00003246-200001000-00016.
35. Vincent JL. Forgoing life support in western European intensive care units: the results of an ethical questionnaire. Crit Care Med. 1999;27(8):1626–33. https://doi.org/10.1097/00003246-199908000-00042.
36. Johnson SB, Butow PN, Bell ML, et al. A randomised controlled trial of an advance care planning intervention for patients with incurable cancer. Br J Cancer. 2018;119(10):1182–90. https://doi.org/10.1038/s41416-018-0303-7.
37. Mitchell SL, Volandes AE, Gutman R, et al. Advance care planning video intervention among long-stay nursing home residents: a pragmatic cluster randomized clinical trial. JAMA Intern Med. 2020;180(8):1070–8. https://doi.org/10.1001/jamainternmed.2020.2366.
38. Bibas L, Peretz-Larochelle M, Adhikari NK, et al. Association of surrogate decision-making interventions for critically ill adults with patient, family, and resource use outcomes: a systematic review and meta-analysis. JAMA Netw Open. 2019;2(7):e197229. https://doi.org/10.1001/jamanetworkopen.2019.7229.
39. Breen CM, Abernethy AP, Abbott KH, Tulsky JA. Conflict associated with decisions to limit life-sustaining treatment in intensive care units. J Gen Intern Med. 2001;16(5):283–9. https://doi.org/10.1046/j.1525-1497.2001.00419.x.
40. Azoulay E, Pochard F, Kentish-Barnes N, et al. Risk of post-traumatic stress symptoms in family members of intensive care unit patients. Am J Respir Crit Care Med. 2005;171(9):987–94. https://doi.org/10.1164/rccm.200409-1295OC.
41. Pochard F, Darmon M, Fassier T, et al. Symptoms of anxiety and depression in family members of intensive care unit patients before discharge or death. A prospective multicenter study. J Crit Care. 2005;20(1):90–6. https://doi.org/10.1016/j.jcrc.2004.11.004.

42. Shalowitz DI, Garrett-Mayer E, Wendler D. The accuracy of surrogate decision makers: a systematic review. Arch Intern Med. 2006;166(5):493–7. https://doi.org/10.1001/archinte.166.5.493.

43. Curtis JR, Treece PD, Nielsen EL, et al. Randomized trial of communication facilitators to reduce family distress and intensity of end-of-life care. Am J Respir Crit Care Med. 2016;193(2):154–62. https://doi.org/10.1164/rccm.201505-0900OC.

44. Sprung CL, Cohen SL, Sjokvist P, et al. End-of-life practices in European intensive care units: the Ethicus study. JAMA. 2003;290(6):790. https://doi.org/10.1001/jama.290.6.790.

45. Melltorp G, Nilstun T. The difference between withholding and withdrawing life-sustaining treatment. Intensive Care Med. 1997;23(12):1264–7. https://doi.org/10.1007/s001340050496.

46. Mark NM, Rayner SG, Lee NJ, Curtis JR. Global variability in withholding and withdrawal of life-sustaining treatment in the intensive care unit: a systematic review. Intensive Care Med. 2015;41(9):1572–85. https://doi.org/10.1007/s00134-015-3810-5.

47. Sprung CL, et al. End-of-life practices in European intensive care units.pdf. 2003.

48. Barr J, Fraser GL, Puntillo K, et al. Clinical practice guidelines for the management of pain, agitation, and delirium in adult patients in the intensive care unit. Crit Care Med. 2013;41(1):263–306. https://doi.org/10.1097/CCM.0b013e3182783b72.

49. Raja SN, Carr DB, Cohen M, et al. The revised International Association for the Study of Pain definition of pain: concepts, challenges, and compromises. Pain. 2020;161(9):1976–82. https://doi.org/10.1097/j.pain.0000000000001939.

50. Chanques G, Viel E, Constantin JM, et al. The measurement of pain in intensive care unit: comparison of 5 self-report intensity scales. Pain. 2010;151(3):711–21. https://doi.org/10.1016/j.pain.2010.08.039.

51. Use of a Behavioural Pain Scale to assess pain in ventilated, unconscious and/or sedated patients— PubMed. https://pubmed.ncbi.nlm.nih.gov/16198570/. Accessed 13 Apr 2022.

52. American Psychiatric Association. Diagnostic and statistical manual of mental disorders, vol. 3. Washington, DC: American Psychiatric Association; 1980.

53. Ely EW, Truman B, Shintani A, et al. Monitoring sedation status over time in ICU patients: reliability and validity of the Richmond agitation-sedation scale (RASS). JAMA. 2003;289(22):2983–91. https://doi.org/10.1001/jama.289.22.2983.

54. Guenther U, Popp J, Koecher L, et al. Validity and reliability of the CAM-ICU flowsheet to diagnose delirium in surgical ICU patients. J Crit Care. 2010;25(1):144–51. https://doi.org/10.1016/j.jcrc.2009.08.005.

55. Bergeron N, Dubois MJ, Dumont M, Dial S, Skrobik Y. Intensive care delirium screening checklist: evaluation of a new screening tool. Intensive Care Med. 2001;27(5):859–64. https://doi.org/10.1007/s001340100909.

56. Dyspnea. Mechanisms, assessment, and management: a consensus statement. American Thoracic Society. Am J Respir Crit Care Med 1999;159(1):321–340. doi:https://doi.org/10.1164/ajrccm.159.1.ats898.

57. An official American Thoracic Society statement: update on the mechanisms, assessment, and management of dyspnea—PubMed. https://pubmed.ncbi.nlm.nih.gov/22336677/. Accessed 13 Apr 2022.

58. A review of quality of care evaluation for the palliation of dyspnea. Am J Respir Crit Care Med. https://www.atsjournals.org/doi/full/10.1164/rccm.200903-0462PP. Accessed 13 Apr 2022.

59. Cuomo A, Delmastro M, Ceriana P, et al. Noninvasive mechanical ventilation as a palliative treatment of acute respiratory failure in patients with end-stage solid cancer. Palliat Med. 2004;18(7):602–10. https://doi.org/10.1191/0269216304pm933oa.

60. Nava S, Ferrer M, Esquinas A, et al. Palliative use of non-invasive ventilation in end-of-life patients with solid tumours: a randomised feasibility trial. Lancet Oncol. 2013;14(3):219. https://doi.org/10.1016/S1470-2045(13)70009-3.

61. Azoulay E, Kouatchet A, Jaber S, et al. Noninvasive mechanical ventilation in patients having declined tracheal intubation. Intensive Care Med. 2013;39(2):292–301. https://doi.org/10.1007/s00134-012-2746-2.

Point-of-Care Ultrasound (POCUS) in Pediatric Age: Update

14

Giovanna Chidini

14.1 Introduction

The implementation of point-of-care ultrasound (POCUS) has been a profound transformation in clinical practice, especially in the areas of emergency medicine and intensive care. It has emerged in recent years, particularly by borrowing in the pediatric setting the experience gained in the adult setting. POCUS ultrasound used at the patient's bedside is useful both for diagnosing some common pathologies and for performing therapeutic procedures (chest drainage, central and peripheral vascular cannulation). The use of POCUS ultrasonography by pediatric intensivists has increased significantly and equally, both in Western countries (high-cost, high-tech intensive care providers) and in poorer countries in which the costs of intensive care are not fully supported by state budgets. Particularly in the pediatric age, this technology has found wide application in the diagnosis and monitoring of respiratory infections and in the monitoring of chronic and acute pulmonary pathology, allowing less radiological exposure to growing children and thus reducing oncological risks. A number of national and international societies have therefore been engaged in discussions in order to draft shared guidelines on both clinical application and regulation of operator training [1–7]. However, no unified guidelines are currently available for the pediatric and neonatal part, as it is at present for the adult part. The first POCUS application in neonatal and pediatric settings was goal-directed echocardiography. An expert statement was published in 2011, followed by the UK consensus statement on neonatologist-performed echocardiography and recommendations for European training [8–10]. The Australian Clinician Performed Ultrasound (CPU) program represents a well-established academic curriculum

G. Chidini (✉)
Pediatric Intensive Care Unit, Dipartimento Di Emergenza Urgenza, Fondazione IRCCS Cà
Granda Ospedale Maggiore Policlinico, Milan, Italy
e-mail: giovanna.chidini@policlinico.mi.it

D. Chiumello (ed.), *Practical Trends in Anesthesia and Intensive Care 2022*,
https://doi.org/10.1007/978-3-031-43891-2_14

developed to train neonatologists limited to cerebral and cardiac assessment [10, 11]. Recently ESPNIC (European Society for Paediatric and Neonatal Intensive Care) published evidence-based guidelines drafted by an international panelist to define the use and applications of POCUS ultrasound in the pediatric setting, applicable by any professional who is involved in routine or urgent work with the critical child.

This chapter will discuss the following key points:

1. Indications for chest ultrasound in neonatal/pediatric age
2. Modalities of performing bedside chest and cardiac ultrasound in children
3. POCUS: the lung and mechanical ventilation: Lung Ultrasound Score (LUS), neonatal RDS and surfactant, bronchiolitis, pneumonia, pneumothorax and drainage, POCUS and mechanical ventilation, POCUS and intubation

14.2 Indications for Chest Ultrasound in Neonatal/ Pediatric Age

The main indications for lung and chest wall ultrasound in the pediatric population include:

– Diagnosis and follow-up of pediatric pulmonary infectious diseases (especially bronchiolitis and pneumonia) and pulmonary complications (such as pneumothorax, pleural effusion, and lung abscess)
– Diagnosis and follow-up of neonatal lung disease
– Confirmation of prenatal diagnosis of lung malformations
– Diagnosis of chest trauma and early detection of signs of child abuse
– Diaphragmatic echography

14.3 Modalities of Performing Bedside Chest and Cardiac Ultrasound in Children

Thoracic ultrasonography has also been widely used in clinical practice because of the ease of performance and the "opportunity to acquire high-definition" images given the excellent acoustic window of the infant and child.

A high-frequency (10 MHz or higher) linear probe should be used for its best resolution, although other probes can be used if linear probes are not available (e.g., convex or microconvex probe). The high-frequency probe allows scanning of surface structures with good resolution. The probe should be placed perpendicular to the chest and moved perpendicular to the direction from the ribs. The examination must follow a systematic procedure: each hemithorax is divided into three areas: anterior, lateral, and posterior, bounded by the parasternal line, anterior axillary line, and posterior axillary line [12, 13]. In this way, about 70% of the lung surface can be ultrasound screened. The apex of the lung can be adequately seen suprasternally with supraclavicular or infraclavicular approach. Dorsal examination is mandatory, as most pediatric lung pathology is localized to the posterior retrocardiac areas. The examination can be performed when the patient is in a sitting position or in a prone decubitus position or often in mother's arms. Similar to the anterior chest examination, the lung is investigated in the axillary, medial, and posterior paravertebral lines to obtain sagittal and sometimes coronal images.

The scan should reach the diaphragm to confirm complete exploration of the lung and differentiate between intra-abdominal and intrathoracic pathology (e.g., pleural or abdominal effusions).

A 7.5 mHz microconvex probe can be used in cases where the patient has a higher thoracic impedance, high amounts of pleural effusion, in the examination of major consolidations, or for the evaluation of B-line frequencies. For simplification purposes, it is proposed to use a linear probe for the ultrasound examination of the newborn and to reserve a microconvex probe for the examination of the infant and child.

14.4 Ultrasonographic Features in the Healthy Lung

Ultrasonography of the healthy lung consists of artifact detection due to the presence of air and the "air/liquid interface" that is generated from the pleural line. Therefore, when performing an ultrasound examination of the lung, it is critical to identify the pleural line.

The pleural line, a horizontal hyperechogenic reflex formed by the difference in acoustic impedance between the soft tissues of the chest wall and the aerated lung parenchyma, is visible between the acoustic shadows relative to the ribs (bat sign). It appears as a regular and relatively straight hyperechogenic line within which the two pleural leaflets and their relative sliding can be distinguished [13, 14]. The normal pleural line is generally regular, thin, and smooth. Its theoretical width is less than 0.5 mm [15, 16]. Its thickness is rarely measured in clinical practice. In fact, there is no consensus regarding the normal thickness of the pleural line, although it may be useful to detect its appearance, interruption, and granulations.

Pleural sliding is the sliding motion of the visceral pleura over the parietal pleura generated by a respiratory act. The absence of pleural sliding should be carefully evaluated as it may be related to pathology such as pneumothorax (in the absence of A-lines), hypoventilation, reduced respiratory system compliance, failure to intubate, or selective intubation.

Physiological artifacts (A-lines) are visible below the pleural line due to the presence of liquid/air interface originating from the pleural line (less than three/field). Applying M-Mode, a mixed image is produced: in which the pleural line separates an overlying part (air artifact) from an underlying part characterized by a granular pattern generated by pleural sliding (seashore pattern).

A-lines are horizontal, hyperechogenic, and equidistant lines below the pleural line. A-lines constitute the reverberation artifact of the pleural line, and the distance between A-lines is constant. The presence of A-lines and lung glide in an area of the lung guarantees the absence of pathology in that area [17].

B-lines are vertical hyperechogenic lines starting perpendicularly from the pleural line [18].

Their presence is related to the expansion of interlobular septa and the accumulation of fluid in the lung.

B-lines are nonspecific and not useful per se for differentiating lung disease [19, 20]. However, as has been described in adults, based on the distance between two B-lines at the pleural margin, certain pathologies may be more likely: a distance of 3 mm correlates with ground-glass subpleural lesions and a distance of 7 mm with thickened subpleural interlobular septa [21].

14.5 Ultrasound in the Diseased Lung

The main indications for using ultrasonography in lung pathology are the diagnosis of effusion, pneumothorax, interstitial syndrome, atelectasis, and consolidation.

14.5.1 Pleural Effusion

Lung ultrasonography is useful for assessing the presence, volume, and characteristics of thoracic effusions [22]. The procedure of examining the patient does not vary similar to the standard examination. In particular, one must remember to carefully explore the declivous areas in the intubated and supine patient. Ultrasonography provides information on the location of effusions, the type of material, the presence of concameration, and the presence of septa. In addition, LUS is useful in deciding the optimal place to perform thoracentesis or placement of a drain [23, 24]. LUS can detect effusions less than 10 mL. In contrast, chest radiography detects only larger effusions (200 mL). Collection of free fluid is not always anechoic. The presence of multiple mobile echoes in the effusion (the "plankton" sign) can be observed in patients with hemothorax, chylothorax, and pleurisy [25]. The "jellyfish" sign may be present in major effusions. This sign represents the beating of the lung in the effusion. The "sinusoid" sign is specific to pleural effusions. It is obtained with M-mode imaging and indicates variation in pleural during the respiratory cycle.

14.5.2 Pneumothorax

The use of LUS for the diagnosis of pneumothorax dates back to 1995. Since then, pulmonary ultrasound has been used more and more, complementing conventional radiology both in the medical setting and in the management of the polytrauma patient. The sensitivity of radiography for pneumothorax is low because of air that tends to accumulate in the anteromedial and apical areas of the chest. In contrast, ultrasound examination of the chest has high sensitivity and specificity in diagnosing pneumothorax in the intubated and supine patient.

The parietal and visceral pleura are not in contact. In the conventional mode, there is no lung glide or B-lines. The only image obtained is the glare of the A-lines. The presence of B-lines is excluded pneumothorax (100% negative predictive value). The M-mode image will reveal the "stratosphere" sign instead of the "seashore" sign of the normal lung. The "stratosphere" sign has a sensitivity and specificity greater than 90% with 100% negative predictive value [26]. The "lung point" defines the point where the transition between normal lung (with lung sliding and A-lines) and pneumothorax (A-lines only) occurs. Its presence has a 100% specificity for pneumothorax [27–30]. It can be assessed using conventional and M-mode.

Pathognomonic signs of pneumothorax consist of the disappearance of pleural sliding and the presence of the lung point, which represents the exact transition point between the presence and absence of sliding. In pediatric and neonatal age, the ultrasound pattern exactly reproduces that of the adult without any particular specificity [31].

14.5.3 Consolidation (Atelectasis/Pneumonia)

The consolidation pattern is defined as a hypoechogenic area with poorly defined edges and posterior reinforcing B-lines in adjacent areas. The lower edges may be more hyperechogenic and irregular in some cases [32]. Lung parenchyma resembles liver tissue and is called "pulmonary hepatization." Pulmonary flow may be absent. Air sonograms are depicted as branched echogenic structures present in the consolidated area. Even with LUS, it is still difficult to distinguish between pneumonia and atelectasis. In addition, the consolidation pattern can also be seen in pulmonary thromboembolisms and pulmonary contusions. Several recent publications have studied LUS differentiation between pneumonia and atelectasis, and the results are not definitive [32–40]. Two meta-analyses suggested excellent sensitivity and specificity of LUS for the diagnosis of pneumonia [41, 42]. In any case, the current pediatric recommendation is to correlate clinical and LUS findings [43–45]. In pneumonia, consolidation may show a dynamic tree-like air bronchogram that is not always visible. Blood flow may be present, visible by echo-Doppler modality. Of note, perihilar consolidations that do not reach the pleural line may be missed by LUS [46].

Atelectasis presents as consolidations with linear static air bronchograms and generally clear borders. Blood flow is absent.

14.6   Lung Ultrasound Score in the Infant and Child

Children can be scanned in standing, supine, or lateral decubitus positions; in addition, to achieve greater compliance in uncooperative children, the examination can be performed with a heated gel and the child sitting on the caregiver's lap while breastfeeding or using age-appropriate distraction techniques in order to minimize anxiety.

A 10 MHz linear probe is the most commonly used transducer for the LUS examination. This type of transducer, given the use of high frequencies, is optimal for investigating up to about 4 cm depth of the chest and thus accurately visualizing particularly the pleural line and its possible changes. In contrast, the use of low-frequency probes (such as the curvilinear transducer (1–5 MHz) or the phased-array transducer (1–3 MHz) is useful for securing a higher and wider penetration, which is useful for a general assessment of the lung or in suspicion of diffuse disease with a lower resolution than high-frequency linear probes.

Each hemithorax is divided into three areas: (a) anterior area, bounded by parasternal and anterior axillary lines; (b) lateral area, within the anterior and posterior axillary lines; and (c) posterior area beyond the posterior axillary line. Each area is divided into upper and lower halves.

The probe is placed vertically, obliquely, and horizontally relative to the ribs in the anterior, lateral, and posterior thorax and moves from intercostal space to intercostal space in a caudal direction from the apices to the costophrenic angles so as to cover the entire lung surface. To date, several scoring systems have been proposed to assess the degree of lung involvement in a specific disease process.

These systems divide the chest into a different number of zones and score based on the distribution of B-lines in the different explored areas during the scan. Of these, the most widely used in intensive care settings are the 4-zone, 6-zone, and 8-zone systems.

Ultrasound examination of the newborn is performed with a linear neonatal probe, dividing each hemithorax into six zones and assigning each lung zone a severity score describing the loss of lung ventilation. Each lung zone is assigned an incremental severity score (Figs. 14.1 and 14.2).

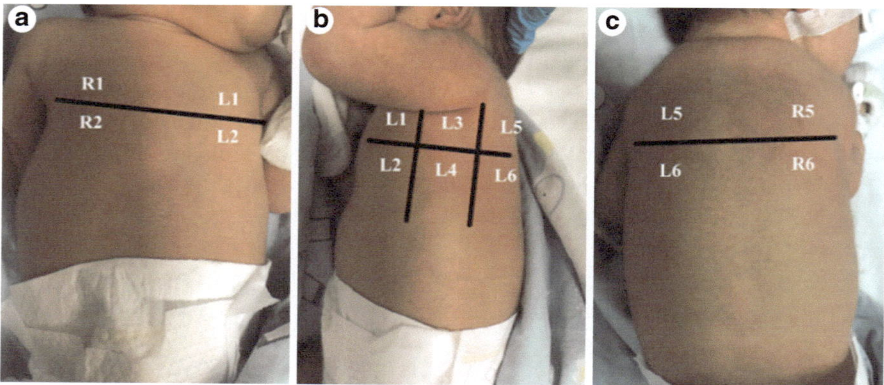

Fig. 14.1 Ultrasound mapping of the infant's chest. (**a**) anterior chest mapping (**b**) lateral chest mapping (**c**) posterior chest mapping

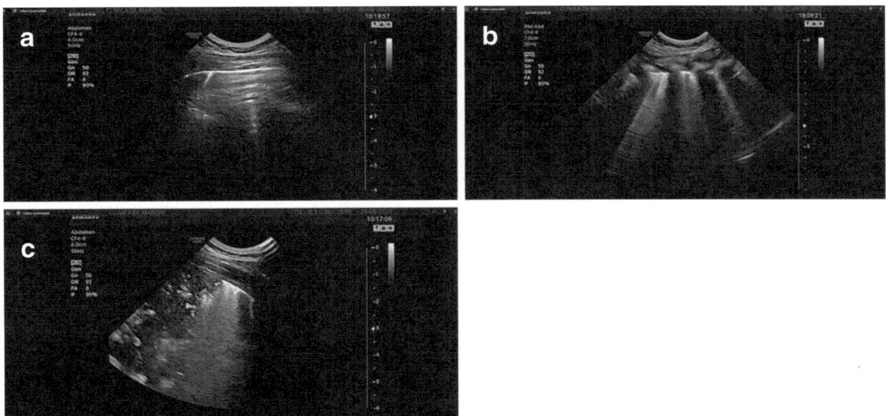

Fig. 14.2 Pediatric Lung Ultrasound Score: definition and ultrasound equivalent. (**a**) Grade 0-Normal Aeration; (**b**) LUS Grade 1: less than 3 B Lines per field; (**c**) LUS Grade 2 (coalescent B lines) and 3 (subpleural consolidation)

14.6.1 LUS POCUS: Bronchiolitis

Bronchiolitis is a viral infection of the lower respiratory tract that affects children younger than 24 months of age and is the leading cause of hospitalization in children. The main pathogen responsible is respiratory syncytial virus (RSV), with infections typically occurring as recurrent seasonal epidemics. Treatment is mainly supportive, and no specific etiologic therapy is routinely used to limit viral infection and reduce the severity of the clinical picture. According to the most recent American Academy of Pediatrics, the diagnosis of bronchiolitis is eminently clinical (presence of respiratory distress, wheezing), and chest radiography should be reserved for more severe cases in which signs of infectious or mechanical complications are present (e.g., bacterial coinfection or pneumothorax). With this in mind, in recent years there has been great interest in using chest ultrasound to differentiate bacterial pneumonia from viral infections [47, 48]. In this sense, LUS may be the definitive tool to diagnose or rule out bacterial pneumonia in children with clinical bronchiolitis and to identify patients who might benefit from initiating antibiotic therapy. In particular, a recent study by Biagi et al. investigated the reliability of LUS in discriminating against children with uncomplicated bronchiolitis from those with concomitant bacterial pneumonia. The results of this study showed a high correlation between chest radiography and POCUS in the diagnosis of complicated bronchiolitis ($r = 0$–64). Table 14.1 and Figure 14.3 show ultrasound and radiology findings related to the discussed pathology. In addition, chest ultrasonography in bronchiolitis helps to identify those patients who need escalation in ventilatory support in high-flow or noninvasive ventilation (see Table 14.1 for Definitions)

Table 14.1 Definition of bronchiolitis severity based on LUS ultrasound pattern [47]

A   Normal or near normal defined as normal lung flow without B-lines or With a limited number of focal B-lines
B1   Moderate interstitial pattern (focal B-lines involving <8 intercostal spaces and/or confluent B-lines involving three intercostal spaces) small subpleural consolidation (depth < 10 mm (a)   Moderate interstitial pattern without consolidation (b)   Moderate interstitial pattern with consolidation
B2   Severe interstitial pattern (generalized focal B-lines and/or confluent B-lines involving four intercostal spaces) lung consolidation with depth 10 mm (a)   Severe interstitial pattern without consolidation (b)   Severe interstitial pattern with consolidation
C   Isolated consolidation (a)   Depth < 10 mm (b)   Depth 10 mm

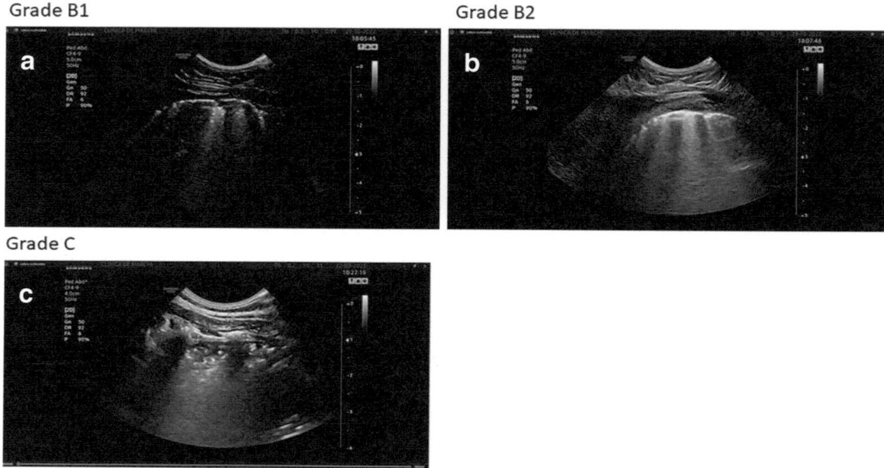

Fig. 14.3 Lung ultrasonography in a patient with bronchiolitis complicated by pneumonia

14.6.2 LUS POCUS and SARS-COV2 Infection

In recent years, lung ultrasound has emerged as a useful bedside tool to identify and monitor many respiratory conditions, especially in pediatric intensive care units. The outbreak of the SARS-COV2 pandemic in December 2019 in China has raised the issue of diagnostics and patient transport to the radiology area for CT diagnostics, which is considered elective [49]. Reports regarding the pediatric population actually later confirmed that in children, SARS-COV2 lung infection was correlated with a milder clinical picture than in adult patients, which is why the use of tomographic diagnostics did not find convincing clinical indications, while chest radiography proved to be a method with low sensitivity and specificity [50, 51]. For these reasons, chest ultrasonography has found wide use in both infants and children for both diagnostic purposes and monitoring of SARS-COV2 respiratory infections [31, 52].

In a recent Chinese study, LUS POCUS showed that the ultrasound, CT, and clinical picture were concordant in describing the severity of the disease.

Both CT and LUS also presented high sensitivity to diagnose COVID-19 pneumonia. In those cases with hemodynamic and respiratory instability or high probability of infection, LUS might be the best option because of its easy accessibility at the bedside.

To date, the sonographic appearance of SARS-COV2 infection has been best described in adult patients. In adults, COVID-19 LUS pneumonia shows bilateral lung involvement with the typical pattern of interstitial syndrome characterized by coalescing isolates/multiples or B-lines, sometimes separated by spared areas, a thinned pleural line with some irregularities, and sometimes pleural effusion and subpleural consolidations. B-lines, whose number increases as the air content in the lung decreases, are considered to be a typical sign of interstitial syndrome, and their distribution seems to correlate with the severity of the clinical picture.

The ultrasound findings described in SARS-COV2 infection are similar to those widely described in patients with other types of pneumonia, including various forms of B-lines, pleural line irregularities or fragmentation, subpleural consolidations, pleural effusion, and absence of lung sliding [31]. In pediatric and neonatal patients with COVID-19, LUS POCUS showed mainly multiform vertical artifacts and separate, coalescing B-lines. Subpleural consolidations <1 cm were found to be the most predominant pattern, and alveolar consolidation was described in some cases. These findings and patterns were equally defined in adults (Fig. 14.4). However, consolidations are less common in our pediatric patients than typically described in adults [31]. The cited studies conclude that LUS has shown great utility for the management of children with COVID-19 because of its easy access, safety, and low cost.

14.6.3 LUS POCUS: Diagnosis and Follow-Up of Neonatal Lung Disease

Many lung diseases, such as respiratory distress syndrome (RDS), transient tachypnea, pneumonia, atelectasis, and pneumothorax, can cause respiratory distress in infants, especially among premature infants. Differential diagnosis of these diseases is often difficult, but LUS can help discriminate these diseases [53–55].

Neonatal respiratory distress syndrome (RDS) is characterized by functional and structural immaturity of the lung, resulting in respiratory distress at birth. Ultrasonographic findings consist of the presence of coalescent, diffuse, and symmetrically distributed B-lines in both lungs (Fig. 14.5).

These lines are due to the presence of fluid in the interstitial or alveolar compartment, and in general, their number correlates the severity of the disease, up to "white lung" in severe cases. The pleural line appears irregular, ill defined, and thickened. In addition, small areas of subpleural hypoechogenic nodularity are present especially at the declivous areas.

The 2019 European consensus guidelines on the management of RDS state that lung ultrasound could be a useful tool for clinical decision making, and it seems to be able to differentiate RDS from other common respiratory disorders of the newborn, reducing exposure to ionizing radiation [56]. In addition, some recent studies have shown how it emphasized that chest ultrasonography performed in the first 12 h of life may be useful in early identification of patients who are more likely to require surfactant therapy or CPAP regardless of oxygenation criteria [57].

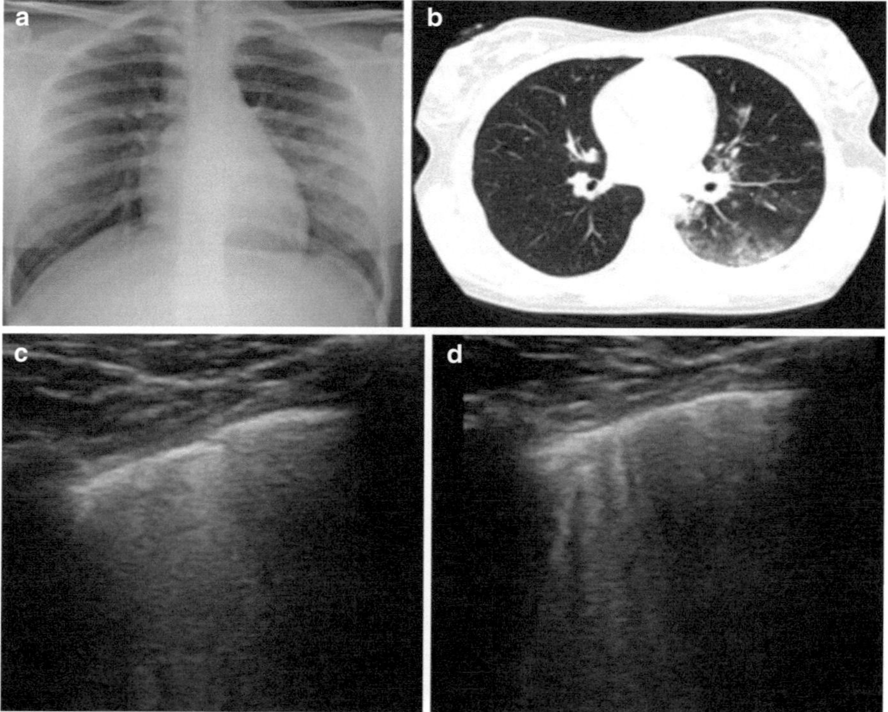

Fig. 14.4 SARS-COV2 infection in adult patient. (**a**) Chest X-ray; (**b**) Chest CT; (**c, d**) LUS POCUS. Adapted from [31]

Fig. 14.5 Neonatal respiratory distress syndrome (RDS). Coalescent B-lines, irregularity of the pleural line, and subpleural consolidation are visible. Adapted from [55]

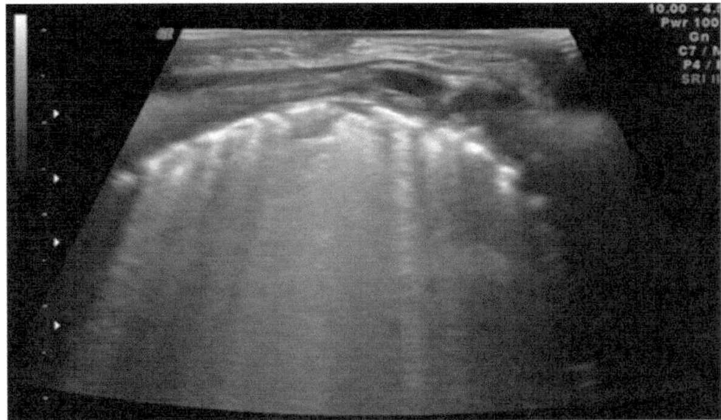

Fig. 14.6 Transient tachypnea of the newborn. Dashed line shows the ultrasound demarcation line between the upper and lower lung fields: double lung point (white arrow). Adapeted from [59]

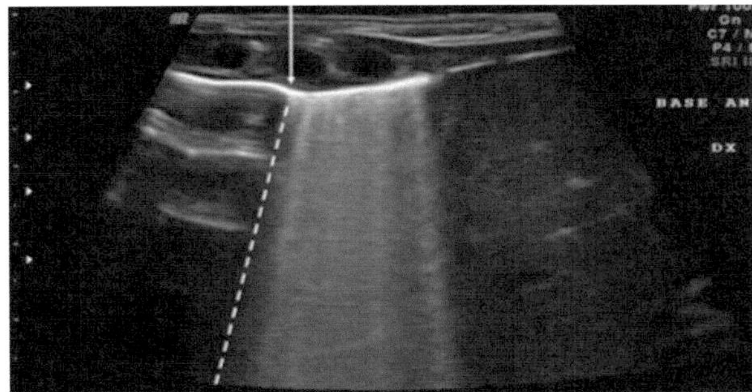

Transient tachypnea of the newborn (TTN), also known as "wet lung," is caused by failure of lymphatic reabsorption and clearance from the fetal lung.

It is a typical picture in the term newborn or in the newborn in cases of rapid delivery or cesarean section [23]. Infants with TTN have compact B-lines in the lower lung fields and increasingly less compact B-lines at the top in one or both lungs.

In TTN, chest ultrasonography demonstrates a clear sonographic demarcation line between the upper and lower lung fields of both lungs (Fig. 14.6) [58]. The pleural line is regular, with normal echogenicity and motion; no subpleural consolidations are observed. Due to these typical ultrasonographic findings, lung ultrasonography may be useful in the early diagnosis of TTN and differentiate TTN from NRDS as early as the first hours of life [59].

Meconium aspiration syndrome (MAS) refers to a multitude of respiratory symptoms caused by the aspiration of meconium during delivery. It is more common in post-term infants.

The ultrasound findings of MAS are as follows: coalescent or noncoalescent B-line pattern.

Several subpleural consolidations spread asymmetrically over both lung fields (white lung).

14.7 Congenital Pulmonary Airway Malformation (CPAM)

Congenital pulmonary airway malformation (CPAM), formerly known as congenital cystic adenomatoid malformation (CCAM), is a congenital disease of the lung similar to bronchopulmonary sequestration. In CPAM, usually an entire lung lobe is replaced by a nonfunctioning cystic piece of abnormal lung tissue. This abnormal tissue will never function as normal lung tissue.

In most cases, the outcome of a fetus with CPAM is very good. In rare cases, the cystic mass becomes so large that it restricts the growth of the surrounding lung and causes pressure against the heart. In these situations, CPAM can be life-threatening for the fetus.

Malformation (CPAM) or congenital diaphragmatic hernia is usually diagnosed by ultrasonography and prenatal MRI. Recently, lung ultrasonography has been proposed as an aid in the evaluation of an infant with respiratory distress in whom CPAM is suspected or to confirm a prenatal suspicion of CPAM [60–62].

The typical sonographic appearance of CPAM is not yet well defined or unambiguous, but a large single hypoechogenic cystic lesion, small communicating cystic lesions, and consolidations similar to those seen in other lung diseases have been described in several patients (Fig. 14.7).

To date, the gold standard for postnatal diagnosis of these malformations remains a CT scan of the chest, but ultrasound may, in the future, be a useful test to confirm an uncertain diagnosis or follow the patient over time.

Fig. 14.7 CPAM, prenatal morphologic ultrasound 29 weeks. Adapted from [60]

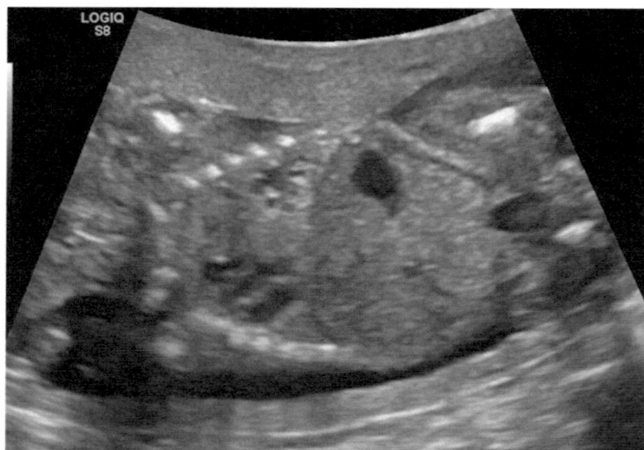

14.7.1 Congenital Malformations of the Lung or Chest Wall

14.8 Chest Trauma and Detection of Signs of Child Abuse

Ultrasound plays a primary role in the management of the polytrauma patient. As in the adult patient, so too in pediatric trauma management, FAST extended ultrasound (chest, heart, abdomen) remains essential for emergency department management in primary assessment [63, 64].

With progressively better defined semeiotics of the healthy and pathologic lung, ultrasonography is now an irreplaceable tool in the emergency department with greater sensitivity for pneumothorax and hemothorax than chest X-ray [65].

In addition, recent evidence has shown that ultrasound can be a useful tool for the detection of bone fractures, particularly rib and skull theca fractures, indicative of child abuse [80]. A rib fracture is diagnosed when a discontinuity in cortical alignment is observed as a clear interruption of the anterior echogenic margin of the rib (Fig. 14.8). Also, in the case of previous fractures, it is possible to observe on ultrasonography the bony callus, which results in an irregular cortical profile different from that of the adjacent ribs.

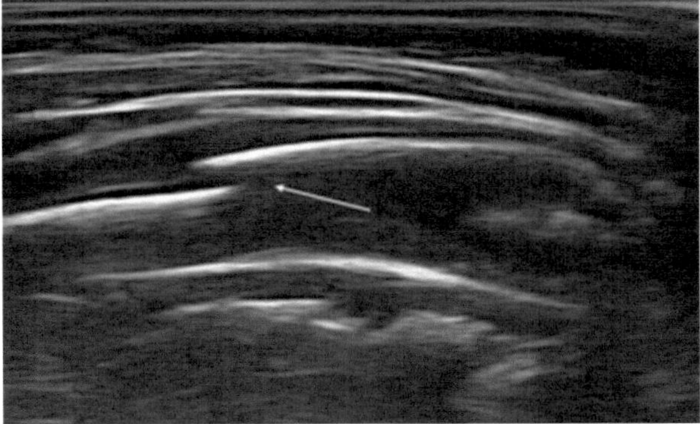

Fig. 14.8 Rib fracture in transverse scan along the major axis of the rib (white arrow). Adapted from [63]

14.9 Ultrasound of the Diaphragm

Ultrasonography can be useful in assessing diaphragmatic function in terms of diagnosis and monitoring of diaphragmatic paralysis, neuromuscular disorders, guidance for needle electromyography, evaluation in chronic diseases, traumatic rupture of the diaphragm, detection of postoperative complications, difficult weaning, estimation of respiratory work, and titration of ventilatory support [66].

Several publications on the subject have highlighted the predictive value of diaphragmatic ultrasound for monitoring respiratory weaning. In particular, some authors have studied the predictive value of diaphragmatic thickening fraction and diaphragm excursion.

In addition, an interesting application is that described by Buonsenso et al., who demonstrated the correlation between ultrasound parameters of the diaphragm and (diaphragm excursion, inspiratory excursion, thickness at the end of inspiration) and clinical outcomes [67, 68].

14.9.1 LUS POCUS and Intubation

Although capnography is the gold standard for confirmation of tracheal intubation in adult and pediatric patients, it has some technical limitations in neonates due to physiological peculiarities of the neonatal lungs and technical characteristics of the capnometers themselves.

First, gas exchange differs between small and adult lungs because of the greater impact of small airway gas exchange, the greater impact of ventilation circuit dead space, and the presence of airway leaks in infants intubated with non-cuffed tubes. In addition, the high respiratory rate and low tidal volume typical of infants, particularly those with rigid lungs, require mainstream sensors with fast response times, minimal dead space, and reduced suction flow.

If these technical requirements are not met, the $ETCO_2$ value that should reflect the end-expiration measurement could be misleading.

Recent studies have suggested that POCUS ultrasound can be used to confirm tracheal tube placement.

In a recent review and meta-analysis analyzing the sensitivity and specificity of ultrasonography to confirm endotracheal tube placement, it is shown that estimated sensitivity and specificity of ultrasonography for confirming endotracheal tube position was 0.98 (95% CI: 0.98–0.99) and 0.94 (95% CI 0.91–0.96).

The conclusion of this meta-analysis reports that ultrasound has high diagnostic accuracy and can be used as a tool for confirmation of endotracheal tube placement especially in critically ill patients or when capnography is not available or its result is equivocal [69].

The examination is performed with a linear probe placed in a mid-cervical anterior transverse plane. Trachea and esophagus are thus visualized. The examination can be conducted in intra- and extra-hospital settings.

The placement of the tracheal tube in the esophagus makes the pathognomonic sign of double trachea.

14.9.2 Point-of-Care Ultrasound: ESPNIC Guidelines

The use of POCUS by intensive care providers has increased significantly in recent years, and in adult emergency management, structured guidelines for POCUS implementation and training of medical and nursing staff have been published [1–7]. However, unified guidelines on the use of POCUS and training do not yet exist for pediatric and neonatal self-critical care. Therefore, the European Society of Pediatrics and the Neonatal Intensive Care Unit (ESPNIC) has published a consensus document on the use of POCUS in the infant and child. The feature of this panel is to include in the indications not only ultrasound and chest, but also the use of POCUS for the determination of cardiac, pulmonary, cerebral, and vascular function.

The directions are given below, highlighting the recommendations with strong agreement (SA) and referring the remainder to reading the literature ref.

1. POCUS should not be used as a screening tool for the diagnosis of congenital heart disease in infants and children unless pediatric neonatologists/intensivists have received advanced echocardiographic training specifically for this purpose (SA).
2. POCUS may be useful for assessing cardiac filling (preload assessment) and intravascular volume status in infants and children (SA).
3. POCUS may be useful for assessing fluid responsiveness in infants and children (SA).
4. POCUS may be useful for qualitative assessment of cardiac function at visual inspection in infants and infants (SA).
5. POCUS is useful for semiquantitative assessment of cardiac function in infants and children [however, detailed functional assessment should be performed by a person with advanced echocardiographic training].
6. POCUS is useful for evaluation of pulmonary artery systolic pressure in pulmonary hypertension in infants and infants (SA).
7. POCUS is useful for semiquantitative assessment of pulmonary hypertension in infants and children (SA).
8. POCUS is useful for diagnosing pericardial effusion in infants and children (SA).
9. POCUS is useful for guiding pericardiocentesis in infants and children (SA).
10. POCUS should be used to assess ductus arteriosus patency in infants and children (SA).
11. POCUS can be used to detect vegetation to make or exclude the diagnosis of endocarditis [however, a diagnosis requires detailed evaluation by a pediatric cardiologist].
12. POCUS is useful to distinguish between respiratory distress syndrome (RDS) and transient tachypnea of the newborn (TTN).

13. POCUS is useful for detecting pneumonia in infants and children.
14. POCUS is useful for semiquantitatively assessing lung ventilation and aiding the management of respiratory intervention in acute respiratory distress syndrome (ARDS) in infants and children.
15. POCUS is useful for recognizing meconium aspiration syndrome (MAS).
16. POCUS is useful for descriptive purposes in viral bronchiolitis but cannot provide a differential etiologic diagnosis (SA).
17. POCUS is useful for accurately detecting pneumothorax in infants and children (SA).
18. POCUS is useful for placing chest drainage (SA).
19. POCUS is useful for detecting pleural effusions in infants and children (SA).
20. POCUS is useful for guiding thoracentesis in infants and children (SA).
21. POCUS is useful for assessing pulmonary edema in infants and children.
22. POCUS is useful for detecting anesthesia-induced atelectasis in infants and children.
23. POCUS-guided technique should be used for internal jugular vein (IJV) line placement in infants and children (SA).
24. POCUS-guided technique is useful for anonymous vein line placement in infants and children (SA).
25. POCUS-guided technique is useful for femoral line placement in infants and children (SA).
26. The POCUS-guided technique is useful for arterial catheter placement in children.
27. POCUS-guided technique is useful for peripherally inserted central catheters in children.
28. POCUS is useful for locating catheter tip position in infants and children (SA).
29. POCUS is useful for detecting changes in cerebral blood flow secondary to vasospasm in patients with traumatic brain injury and nontraumatic intracranial hemorrhage.
30. POCUS is useful to detect changes in optic nerve sheath diameter (ONSD) indicative of ICP with fused skull bones.
31. POCUS is useful for detecting cerebral midline shift in infants and children.
32. POCUS is useful for the detection of free intra-abdominal fluid in infants and children (SA).
33. POCUS can detect parenchymal changes in abdominal organs in infants and children [although as a definitive diagnosis a detailed evaluation should be performed by a pediatric radiologist].
34. POCUS can detect obstructive uropathy in infants and children [although for a definitive diagnosis an evaluation should be performed by a pediatric radiologist].
35. POCUS can recognize hypertrophic pyloric stenosis [although for a definitive diagnosis a detailed evaluation should be performed by a pediatric radiologist].
36. POCUS can guide peritoneal drainage or aspiration of peritoneal fluid in infants and children (SA).

14.10 Conclusions

In recent years, due to increasing evidence and greater knowledge of ultrasound semeiotics of the healthy and pathological lung, the use of lung ultrasound is increasingly used in the pediatric setting, especially in the diagnosis, clinical management, and follow-up of lung disease in children and infants.

Speed, repeatability, low cost, and the possibility of being performed at the patient's bedside represent the strengths of this method, which, if wisely applied, could result in many benefits, contributing to a better use of the health system's economic resources and a reduction, in the pediatric population, of exposure to ionizing radiation.

References

1. Ma IWY, Arishenkoff S, Wiseman J, Desy J, Ailon J, et al.; On behalf of The Canadian Internal Medicine Ultrasound (CIMUS) Group*. Internal medicine point-of-care ultrasound curriculum: consensus recommendations from the Canadian Internal Medicine Ultrasound (CIMUS) Group. J Gen Intern Med. 2017;32:1052–7.
2. Expert Round Table on Ultrasound in ICU. International expert statement on training standards for critical care ultrasonography. Intensive Care Med. 2011;37:1077–83.
3. Frankel HL, Kirkpatrick AW, Elbarbary M, Blaivas M, Desai H, Evans D, et al. Guidelines for the appropriate use of bedside general and cardiac ultrasonography in the evaluation of critically ill patients-part I: general ultrasonography. Crit Care Med. 2015;43:2479–502.
4. Moore CL, Copel JA. Point-of-care ultrasonography. N Engl J Med. 2011;364:749–57.
5. Evans N, Gournay V, Cabanas F, Kluckow M, Leone T, Groves A, et al. Point of-care ultrasound in the neonatal intensive care unit: international perspectives. Semin Fetal Neonatal Med. 2011;16:61–8.
6. Longjohn M, Wan J, Joshi V, Pershad J. Point-of-care echocardiography by pediatric emergency physicians. Pediatr Emerg Care. 2011;27:693–6.
7. Vignon P, Dugard A, Abraham J, Belcour D, Gondran G, Pepino F, et al. Focused training for goal-oriented hand-held echocardiography performed by noncardiologist residents in the intensive care unit. Intensive Care Med. 2007;33:1795–9.
8. Mertens L, Seri I, Marek J, Arlettaz R, Barker P, McNamara P, et al. Targeted neonatal echocardiography in the neonatal intensive care unit: practice guidelines and recommendations for training. J Am Soc Echocardiogr. 2011;24:1057–78.
9. Singh Y, Gupta S, Groves AM, Gandhi A, Thomson J, Qureshi S, et al. Expert consensus statement neonatologist-performed echocardiography (NoPE)-training and accreditation in the UK. Eur J Pediatr. 2016;175:281–7.
10. de Boode WP, Singh Y, Gupta S, Austin T, Bohlin K, Dempsey E, et al. Recommendations for neonatologist performed echocardiography in Europe: consensus statement endorsed by European Society for Paediatric Research (ESPR) and European Society for Neonatology (ESN). Pediatr Res. 2016;80:465–71.
11. Australasian Society for Ultrasound Medicine. Proficiency and appropriate use statement [Internet]. https://www.asum.com.au/files/public/SoP/Current/Paediatrics_and_Neo-Natal/Proficiency-and-Appropriate-UseStatement-for-Neonatal-Ultrasound-G1.pdf.
12. Volpicelli G, Elbarbary M, Blaivas M, Lichtenstein DA, Mathis G, Kirkpatrick AW, et al. International evidence-based recommendations for point-of-care lung ultrasound. Intensive Care Med. 2012;38(4):577–91.
13. Cattarossi L. Lung ultrasound: its role in neonatology and pediatrics. Early Hum Dev [Internet]. 2013;89(Suppl 1):S17–9. https://doi.org/10.1016/S0378-3782(13)70006-9.

14. Lichtenstein DA. Ultrasound examination of the lungs in the intensive care unit. Pediatr Crit Care Med. 2009;10(6):693.
15. Lichtenstein DA, Mezière G, Lascols N, Biderman P, Courret JP, Gepner A, et al. Ultrasound diagnosis of occult pneumothorax. Crit Care Med. 2005;33(6):1231–8.
16. Copetti R, Cattarossi L, Macagno F, Violino M, Furlan R. Lung ultrasound in respiratory distress syndrome: a useful tool for early diagnosis. Neonatology. 2008;94(1):52–9.
17. Sharma D, Farahbakhsh N. Role of chest ultrasound in neonatal lung disease: a review of current evidences. J Matern Neonatal Med [Internet]. 2017:1–7. https://www.tandfonline.com/doi/full/10.1080/14767058.2017.1376317.
18. Lichtenstein D. Fluid administration limited by lung sonography: the place of lung ultrasound in assessment of acute circulatory failure (the FALLS-protocol). Expert Rev Respir Med. 2012;6(2):155–62.
19. Tomà P, Owens CM. Chest ultrasound in children: critical appraisal. Pediatr Radiol. 2013;43(11):1427–34.
20. Martelius L, Heldt H, Lauerma K. B-lines on pediatric lung sonography: comparison with computed tomography. J Ultrasound Med. 2016;35(1):153–7.
21. Lichtenstein DA, Mezière G, Lagoueyte J-F, Biderman P, Goldstein I, Gepner A. A-lines and B lines. Lung ultrasound as a bedside tool for predicting pulmonary artery occlusion pressure in the critically ill. Chest. 2009;136:1014–20.
22. Brogi E, Gargani L, Bignami E, Barbariol F, Marra A, Forfori F, et al. Thoracic ultrasound for pleural effusion in the intensive care unit: a narrative review from diagnosis to treatment. Crit Care. 2017;21(135):1–11.
23. Gryminski J, Krakowka P, Lypacewicz G. The diagnosis of pleural effusion by ultrasonic and radiologic techniques. Chest. 1976;70(1):33–7.
24. Lichtenstein D, Mauriat P. Lung ultrasound in the critically ill neonate. Curr Pediatr Rev [Internet]. 2012;8(3):217–223.
25. Salamonsen M, Lo A, Ng A, Bashirzadeh F, Wang W, DIK F. Novel use of pleural ultrasound can identify malignant entrapped lung prior to effusion drainage. Chest [Internet]. 2014;146(5):1286–1293. https://doi.org/10.1378/chest.13-2876.
26. Volpicelli G, Boero E, Sverzellati N, Cardinale L, Busso M, Boccuzzi F, et al. Semiquantification of pneumothorax volume by lung ultrasound. Intensive Care Med. 2014;40(10):1460–7.
27. Raimondi F, Rodriguez Fanjul J, Aversa S, Chirico G, Yousef N, De Luca D, et al. Lung ultrasound for diagnosing pneumothorax in the critically ill neonate. J Pediatr. 2015;175:74.
28. Moreno-Aguilar G, Lichtenstein D. Lung ultrasound in the critically ill (LUCI) and the lung point: a sign specific to pneumothorax which cannot be mimicked. Crit Care [Internet]. 2015;19(1):19–20. https://doi.org/10.1186/s13054-015-1030-6.
29. Cattarossi L, Copetti R, Brusa G, Pintaldi S. Lung ultrasound diagnostic accuracy in neonatal pneumothorax. Can Respir J. 2016;2016:6515069.
30. Frankel H, Kirkpatrick A, Elbarbary M, Blaivas M, Desai H, Evans D, et al. Guidelines for the appropriate use of bedside general and cardiac ultrasonography in the evaluation of critically ill patients—part I: general ultrasonography. Crit Care Med. 2015;43(11):2479–502.
31. Peng QY, Wang XT, Zhang LN. Findings of lung ultrasonography of novel corona virus pneumonia during the 2019-2020 epidemic. Intensive Care Med. 2020;46(5):849–50. https://doi.org/10.1007/s00134-020-05996-6.
32. Stadler JAM, Andronikou S, Zar HJ. Lung ultrasound for the diagnosis of community-acquired pneumonia in children. Pediatr Radiol. 2017;47:1412–9.
33. Claes AS, Clapuyt P, Menten R, Michoux N, Dumitriu D. Performance of chest ultrasound in pediatric pneumonia. Eur J Radiol [Internet]. 2017;88:82–87. https://doi.org/10.1016/j.ejrad.2016.12.032.
34. Ibrahim M, Omran A, Ibrahim M, Bioumy N, El-Sharkawy S. Lung ultrasound in early diagnosis of neonatal ventilator associated pneumonia before any radiographic or laboratory changes. Case Rep Pediatr [Internet]. 2016;2016:1–4. https://www.hindawi.com/journals/cripe/2016/4168592/.

35. Mongodi S, Via G, Girard M, Rouquette I, Misset B, Braschi A, et al. Lung ultrasound for early diagnosis of ventilator-associated pneumonia. Chest [Internet]. 2016;149(4):969–980. https://doi.org/10.1016/j.chest.2015.12.012.
36. Guerra M, Crichiutti G, Pecile P, Romanello C, Busolini E, Valent F, et al. Ultrasound detection of pneumonia in febrile children with respiratory distress: a prospective study. Eur J Pediatr. 2016;175(2):163–70.
37. Jones BP, Tay ET, Elikashvili I, Sanders JE, Paul AZ, Nelson BP, et al. Feasibility and safety of substituting lung ultrasonography for chest radiography when diagnosing pneumonia in children: a randomized controlled trial. Chest [Internet]. 2016;150(1):131–138. https://doi.org/10.1016/j.chest.2016.02.643.
38. Ambroggio L, Clohessy C, Shah SS, Ambroggio L, Sucharew H, Macaluso M, et al. Lung ultrasonography: a viable alternative to chest radiography in children with suspected 13 pneumonia? J Pediatr [Internet]. 2016;176:93–98.e7. https://doi.org/10.1016/j.jpeds.2016.05.033.
39. Esposito S, Papa SS, Borzani I, Pinzani R, Giannitto C, Consonni D, et al. Performance of lung ultrasonography in children with community-acquired pneumonia. Ital J Pediatr. 2014;40(1):1–6.
40. Shah VP, Tunik MG, Tsung JW. Prospective evaluation of point-of-care ultrasonography for the diagnosis of pneumonia in children and young adults. JAMA Pediatr. 2013;167(2):119–25.
41. Caiulo VA, Gargani L, Caiulo S, Fisicaro A, Moramarco F, Latini G, et al. Lung ultrasound characteristics of community-acquired pneumonia in hospitalized children. Pediatr Pulmonol. 2013;48(3):280–7.
42. Xin H, Li J, Hu HY. Is lung ultrasound useful for diagnosing pneumonia in children?: a meta-analysis and systematic review. Ultrasound Q. 2018;34(1):3–10.
43. Balk DS, Lee C, Schafer J, Welwarth J, Hardin J, Novack V, et al. Lung ultrasound compared to chest X-ray for diagnosis of pediatric pneumonia: a meta-analysis. Pediatr Pulmonol. 2018;53(8):1130–9.
44. Liu J, Chen SW, Liu F, Li QP, Kong XY, Feng ZC. The diagnosis of neonatal pulmonary atelectasis using lung ultrasonography. Chest. 2015;147(4):1013–9.
45. Kurepa D, Zaghloul N, Watkins L, Liu J. Neonatal lung ultrasound examination guidelines. J Perinatol [Internet]. 2018;38(1):11–22. https://doi.org/10.1038/jp.2017.140.
46. Urbankowska E, Krenke K, Drobczyński Ł, Korczyński P, Urbankowski T, Krawiec M, et al. Lung ultrasound in the diagnosis and monitoring of community acquired pneumonia in children. Respir Med. 2015;109(9):1207–12.
47. San Sebastian Ruiz N, Rodríguez Albarrán I, Gorostiza I, Galletebeitia Laka I, Delgado Lejonagoitia C, Samson F. Point-of-care lung ultrasound in children with bronchiolitis in a pediatric emergency department. Arch Pediatr. 2021;28(1):64–8. https://doi.org/10.1016/j.arcped.2020.10.003. 0929-693X/Published by Elsevier Masson SAS on behalf of French Society of Pediatrics.
48. Soldati G, Smargiassi A, Inchingolo R, Buonsenso D, Perrone T, Briganti DF, Perlini S, Torri E, Mariani A, Mossolani EE, Tursi F, Mento F, Demi L. Proposal for international standardization of the use of lung ultrasound for COVID-19 patients; a simple, quantitative, reproducible method. J Ultrasound Med. 2020;39:1–7. https://doi.org/10.1002/jum.15285.
49. Lepri G, Orlandi M, Lazzeri C, et al. The emerging role of lung ultrasound in COVID-19 pneumonia. Eur J Rheumatol. 2020;7:S129–33. https://doi.org/10.5152/eurjrheum.2020.2063.
50. Pan F, Ye T, Sun P, Gui S, Liang B, Li L, Zheng D, Wang J, Hesketh RL, Yang L, Zheng C. Time course of lung changes on chest CT during recovery from 2019 novel coronavirus (COVID-19) pneumonia. Radiology. 2020;295:200370–721. https://doi.org/10.1148/radiol.2020200370.
51. Ong JSM, Tosoni A, Kim YJ, Kissoon N, Murthy S. Coronavirus disease 2019 in critically ill children: a narrative review of the literature. Pediatr Crit Care Med. 2020;21(7):662–6. https://doi.org/10.1097/PCC.00000000002376.
52. Soldati G, Smargiassi A, Inchingolo R, Buonsenso D, Perrone T, Briganti DF, Perlini S, Torri E, Mariani A, Mossolani EE, Tursi F, Mento F, Demi L. Is there a role for lung ultrasound during the COVID-19 pandemic? J Ultrasound Med. 2020;39:1–4. https://doi.org/10.1002/jum.15284.

53. Lichtenstein D, Mauriat P. Lung ultrasound in the critically ill neonate. Curr Pediatr Rev. 2012;8:217–23. [CrossRef].
54. Sharma D, Farahbakhsh N. Role of chest ultrasound in neonatal lung disease: A review of current evidences. J Matern Fetal Neonatal Med. 2019;32:310–6. [CrossRef].
55. Copetti R, Cattarossi L, Macagno F, Violino M, Furlan R. Lung ultrasound in respiratory distress syndrome: a useful tool for early diagnosis. Neonatology. 2008;94:52–9. [CrossRef].
56. Sweet DG, Carnielli V, Greisen G, Hallman M, Ozek E, Pas AT, Plavka R, Roehr CC, Saugstad OD, Simeoni U, et al. European consensus guidelines on the management of respiratory distress syndrome—2019 update. Neonatology. 2019;115:432–50. [CrossRef] [PubMed].
57. Gregorio-Hernández R, Arriaga-Redondo M, Pérez-Pérez A, Ramos-Navarro C, Sánchez-Luna M. Lung ultrasound in preterm infants with respiratory distress: experience in a neonatal intensive care unit. Eur J Pediatr. 2020;179:81–9. [CrossRef].
58. Reuter S, Moser C, Baack M. Respiratory distress in the newborn. Pediatr Rev. 2014;35:417–28. [CrossRef] [PubMed].
59. Liu J, Wang Y, Fu W, Yang CS, Huang JJ. Diagnosis of neonatal transient tachypnea and its differentiation from respiratory distress syndrome using lung ultrasound. Medicine. 2014;93:e197. [CrossRef].
60. David M, Lamas-Pinheiro R, Henriques-Coelho T. Prenatal and postnatal management of congenital pulmonary airway malformation. Neonatology. 2016;110:101–15. [CrossRef].
61. Farrugia M, Raza S, Gould S, Lakhoo K. Congenital lung lesions: classification and concordance of radiological appearance and surgical pathology. Pediatr Surg Int. 2008;24:987–99. [CrossRef].
62. Yousef N, Mokhtari M, Durand P, Raimondi F, Migliaro F, Letourneau A, Tissières P, De Luca D. Lung ultrasound findings in congenital pulmonary airway malformation. Am J Perinatol. 2018;35:1222–7.
63. Wongwaisayawan S, Suwannanon R, Prachanukool T, Sricharoen P, Saksobhavivat N, Kaewlai R. Trauma ultrasound. Ultrasound Med Biol. 2015;41:2543–61. [CrossRef].
64. Flato U, Guimarães H, Lopes RD, Valiatti JL, Flato EM, Lorenzo RG. Usefulness of extended-FAST (EFAST-extended focused assessment with sonography for trauma) in critical care setting. Rev Bras Ter Intensiva. 2010;22:291–9. [CrossRef].
65. Staub L, Biscaro R, Kaszubowski E, Maurici R. Chest ultrasonography for the emergency diagnosis of traumatic pneumothorax and haemothorax: a systematic review and meta-analysis. Injury. 2018;49:457–66. [CrossRef].
66. Sferrazza Papa G, Pellegrino G, Di Marco F, Imeri G, Brochard L, Goligher E, Centanni S. A review of the ultrasound assessment of diaphragmatic function in clinical practice. Respiration. 2016;91:403–11. [CrossRef] [PubMed].
67. Xue Y, Zhang Z, Sheng C-Q, Li Y-M, Jia F-Y. The predictive value of diaphragm ultrasound for weaning outcomes in critically ill children. BMC Pulm Med. 2019;19:270. [CrossRef].
68. Buonsenso D, Supino MC, Giglioni E. Point of care diaphragm ultrasound in infants with bronchiolitis: a prospective study. Pediatr Pulmonol. 2018;53:778–86. [CrossRef].
69. Farrokhi M, Yarmohammadi B, et al. Screening performance characteristics of ultrasonography in confirmation of endotracheal intubation; a systematic review and meta-analysis. Arch Acad Emerg Med. 2021;9(1):e68. https://doi.org/10.22037/aaem.v9i1.1360.

Prehospital and Early Intrahospital Management of Trauma

15

Luca Bolgiaghi, Fabrizio Sammartano, and Davide Chiumello

To date, trauma represents one of the leading causes of death worldwide. Approximately 9% of annual deaths, or more than five million people, die as a result of trauma, whether deliberate or intentional; no less important is the impact, in both social and economic terms, represented by trauma survivors and the care they receive [1]. In the United States, a country that has historically delved into the issue of trauma in both civilian and military settings, it is estimated that just under $900 billion is spent annually on the management of the trauma patient, to which must be added another $450 billion or so, representing economic losses resulting from lost wages and lost productivity.

15.1 Prehospital Management

Prehospital rescue and all those involved in carrying it out therefore play a crucial role in reducing the social cost derived from trauma; from this consideration comes the importance of knowing how to recognize major trauma and potential rapidly developing injuries and knowing how to implement actions to reduce the damage [2].

L. Bolgiaghi (✉)
Department of Anesthesia and Resuscitation, ASST Santi Paolo e Carlo, San Paolo University Hospital, Milan, Italy
e-mail: luca.bolgiaghi@hotmail.it

F. Sammartano
San Carlo Borromeo Trauma Center, ASST Santi Paolo e Carlo, San Carlo University Hospital, Milan, Italy

D. Chiumello
Department of Anesthesia and Resuscitation, ASST Santi Paolo e Carlo, San Paolo University Hospital, Milan, Italy

Department of Health Sciences, University of Milan, Milan, Italy

D. Chiumello (ed.), *Practical Trends in Anesthesia and Intensive Care 2022*, https://doi.org/10.1007/978-3-031-43891-2_15

Traumatic injuries have a typical bimodal distribution, with a primary injury occurring at the very moment of the trauma, on which preventive systems can possibly be put in place, such as the correct use of personal protective equipment, but on which there is no possibility of direct action by the rescuer; and a secondary injury, which has its onset minutes or hours after the trauma and is the main cause of the worsening of the primary injury: our attention should focus on this second type of injury. In fact, the goal of the rescuer's work is precisely to prevent the onset or minimize the consequences of the secondary injury, thus improving the patient's prognosis and being able to reduce the social and economic costs resulting from the traumatic event [3]. Following this temporal distinction, trauma mortality can be divided into three moments:

- Immediate (minutes): which can vary only by the application of education and prevention
- Early (hours-days): dependent on the timeliness and appropriateness of prehospital care
- Late (weeks): dependent on proper patient allocation and hospital care

Golden principles of prehospital trauma care
• Scene safety assessment
• Scene assessment and determination of need for additional resources
• Recognize dynamics and kinematics of trauma
• Carry out primary assessment and identify immediately life-threatening injuries of the patient
• Proper airway management and manual stabilization of the cervical spine
• Support ventilation with target SpO_2 of at least 94%
• Early recognition and control of massive hemorrhage
• Immobilize musculoskeletal injuries that may result in hemodynamic instability, maintain body temperature
• Maintain manual spinal stabilization until definitive immobilization
• Infusion of warm intravenous fluids if necessary
• Collect medical history and perform secondary evaluation as soon as life-threatening problems are excluded or treated
• Managing pain appropriately
• Provide accurate communication with receiving facility

Clinical Case Sunday, 10 a.m.: activation of advanced rescue vehicle for traffic accident, bystanders report unconscious woman found with altered consciousness inside vehicle. Fire department and traffic police on the way

From the moment the *dispatch is* received, the leader of the advanced rescue vehicle must inform the rest of the crew of the event and, as far as possible with the information available, divide the roles and share the material to be brought to the scene; the event preparation phase is carried out on the way between stationing and the event site.

Upon arrival at the scene, even before they have left the rescue vehicle, the team members, in a phase that is referred to as a *glimpse*, can get an initial idea about the type of event they will have to deal with: number of vehicles/persons involved, environmental situation, macroscopic hazards evident, e.g., open flames [4]. The phase of assessing the safety of the scene and the possible need to alert additional resources begins at this time and then continues outside the rescue vehicle [5].

Clinical Case High-clearance provincial road, no emergency vehicles yet on scene, evidence of two cars involved in head-on collision, no open flames and no obvious fluid leaks from vehicles. two conscious people sitting on the ground about 5 m from the vehicles. Head-on impact with obvious deformation of the passenger compartment of one of the two vehicles, inside which a female patient is sitting, eyes closed.

With the information gathered through a look at the scene they are facing, the team can already get an idea of the event. In this case we are dealing with an event that involved multiple people, at least three from an initial estimate. The incident occurred on a high traffic road, so the speed and energies involved could be high: this assumption is supported by the appearance of the vehicles. The leader, in order to allow an optimal management of the service, therefore has the task of giving an initial report to the emergency system so as to activate the number and type of res-cue vehicles congruous for the situation (possibly also figures different from the medical, such as FF.O. or V V.F.): the disproportion between victims and rescuers, in fact, would not allow the correct assessment and the right treatment for each patient. The association between high kinetic energy, the number of people involved, and the patient still in the vehicle likely with altered consciousness leads to the decision by the rescue system to activate a second vehicle on a rotary wing.

Confirmation of the presence of normal consciousness and the absence of mas-sive hemorrhage in the two involved seated shifts the team's attention to the patient still in the vehicle; it will be the leader's task, upon the arrival of additional means of managing and directing them as needed. Special attention should be applied to the identification of the following conditions:

(a) Conditions that immediately put the patient's life at risk
(b) Conditions that may result in the loss of a limb
(c) Conditions that are not life-threatening or do not result in serious harm in the short term

In the trauma patient with multi-system injuries, involving more than one system or more than one area of the body, e.g., patient with head injury, splenic injury resulting in shock, and lower extremity fracture, the priority of treatment is recogni-tion and management of the immediately life-threatening condition.

Clinical Case Unconscious patient inside deformed cockpit, door opened by bystanders, cockpit motor intrusion with patient's lower limbs incarcerated under steering wheel and dashboard. Patient unresponsive to call, radial pulse undetectable, bilateral chest excursion but evident tachypnea, lip cyanosis.

The team identifies the patient as extremely critical and likely rapidly evolving; therefore, the patient would be extricated with rapid maneuvering and taken out of the vehicle and laid down on the ground where primary assessment can be undertaken, which should be done quickly and in a logical order. In analogy to ACLS, in which the priorities changed from ABD to CAB, primary trauma assessment also currently emphasizes control of severe external bleeding as the first step in the sequence. While in teaching the various steps of primary assessment are illustrated sequentially, many of these steps can, and should, be performed simultaneously. The steps can be memorized using the X-ABCDE sequence:

- X: control of massive external hemorrhage
- A (AIRWAYS): airway assessment and management and cervical spine stabilization
- B (BREATHING): assessment and management of ventilation and oxygenation
- C (CIRCULATION): assessment of circulation and perfusion
- D (DISABILITY): neurological framework assessment
- E (EXPOSURE): patient exposure and assessment

In the primary evaluation of a polytrauma patient, massive external hemorrhages should be immediately identified and treated [6]; when present, these should be treated prior to, or concurrently, if the number and skillfulness of rescuers dictate, airway evaluation and spinal immobilization. The best treatment of massive bleeding of an extremity is *tourniquet* placement; other measures include direct pressure or the use of hemostatic dressings and compression bandages—the latter should be used only in cases of nonarterial bleeding. Severe bleeding in junctional areas, i.e., areas of transition between two anatomic districts, e.g., the groin or axillary cavity, can be managed by placing gauze with hemostatic products combining dressing and compression bandaging.

The airway of the polytrauma patient must be rapidly assessed to ensure that it is patched; unconsciousness immediately identifies a nonpervious airway. If airway patency is compromised, the airway should first be opened manually, foreign bodies in the oral cavity should be removed if necessary, and then, if the situation, rescuers' skills and availability of devices, permits, a definitive airway should be established; the choice of which device to use is beyond the scope of this chapter [7]. In any patient victim of trauma with high kinetic energy, the presence of a spinal cord injury should be suspected until its possible exclusion: this translates into the need to keep the patient's cervical spine protected from unnecessary movement; this can be ensured especially in the initial stages of rescue, until at least the pre-transport phase, with manual stabilization of the spine with the aid or without the cervical collar; manual stabilization will end when the patient is properly immobilized on the most suitable presidium (scoop, spinal board, or vacuum mattress).

Respiratory function ensures the proper supply of oxygen to the patient's lungs in order to maintain normal cellular aerobic metabolism and ensures the proper clearance of CO_2, so that basic acid balance is maintained in the normal range. Hypoxia can set in as a result of various types of damage, not necessarily to the airways, lung parenchyma, or thorax, but it results in reduced blood oxygenation in any case, which inevitably leads, if untreated, to cellular hypoxia. Respiratory function can be improved rapidly but just as effectively by applying the acronym OPACS:

- O: Observes thoracic expansion, presence, extent, and symmetry
- P: Palpate the chest looking for crackles (subcutaneous emphysema), rushes, and irregularities (rib fractures)
- A: Auscultation of respiratory noises
- C: Breathing rate counts
- S: Saturimetry

In the patient with impaired ventilation who complains of dyspnea or whose dynamics of trauma lead one to suspect chest trauma, the chest should be exposed and palpated rapidly; just as rapidly, auscultation is continued in order to identify respiratory sounds and any alterations. The main injuries that can impede ventilation include pneumothorax, hypertensive pneumothorax (which is **an emergency** that can rapidly result in the patient's death), rib *volet*, and extra-thoracic injuries, such as head trauma or spinal cord injuries [8]. The injuries reported here must be suspected and identified during the primary evaluation and require the immediate establishment of respiratory support; the modes of support and available devices are beyond the scope of this chapter.

The next step in the treatment of the trauma patient is the assessment of impairment or possible failure of the circulatory system. In the primary assessment, the rescuer needs to quickly recognize the presence of alterations in the patient's peripheral perfusion that may endanger the patient. The assessment of the peripheral pulse, its presence/absence, amplitude and frequency, skin temperature and coloration, and the presence of sweating are easy-to-find information that, although with limitations (external temperatures, patient's age, pathologies in history), can give us important information about peripheral perfusion. Combining the parameters just described with the measurement of arterial pressure and the measurement of capillary refill time (assessed by compressing the nail bed and releasing the pressure, the normal value of which is <2 s) allows us to have a good assessment of circulatory adequacy and allows, on the ground, to make choices regarding the treatment to be implemented. As is well known, in trauma patients, the most frequent cause of shock is hemorrhage; as soon as altered perfusion is recognized, it will be necessary to hypothesize the most likely site of hemorrhage, if not already recognized (X-ABCDE) [9]. Potential sites of hemorrhage in the polytrauma patient include the thorax (hemothorax), the peritoneum (hemoperitoneum), the pelvis in case of pelvic fractures, and fractures of long bones, particularly the femur. If hemorrhage is suspected at any of these sites, the thorax, abdomen, pelvis, and lower extremities should be carefully examined for signs of injury; in the prehospital setting, however, control of hemorrhage at these sites is not easy to obtain: certainly the use of a pelvic belt in suspected pelvic injuries can be instrumental in ensuring hemodynamic

Table 15.1 Target pressures in the polytrauma patient

Trauma	Target pressure	Physiological objective
Penetrating trauma	PAS 70 mmHg	Ensure organ perfusion by preventing rebleeding
Closed trauma	PAS 80–90 mmHg	Ensuring organ perfusion No "pop the clot"
Hemorrhagic head trauma	PAS 100 mmHg	Compromise between cerebral perfusion and bleeding
Closed-head trauma	PAS 110 mmHg	Ensuring cerebral perfusion

stability of the patient (particularly in open-book fractures). In the remaining cases, the main goal for these patients remains rapid transport to the most appropriate facility, represented by the Trauma Center. Depending on the type of injury one is faced with, the vital parameters collected in the primary evaluation, and the assessment of the presence of signs of shock (altered consciousness, tachy-bradypnea, hypoperfusion at the periphery), there are indications regarding the fluidic treatment to be carried out in the territory (Table 15.1), to reduce the risk of hypoperfusion and tissue damage on the one hand and to avoid the increase of blood loss on the other.

Once alterations leading to alterations in oxygen transport to the lung parenchyma and the rest of the body have been recognized and corrected, the next step is to assess brain function, which is an indirect measure of central nervous system (CNS) perfusion. Alterations in the level of consciousness should direct the rescuer to the following alterations:

- Decreased cerebral oxygenation or severe hypoventilation
- CNS injuries
- Exposure to toxic substances (alcohol, drugs, or substances of abuse)
- Metabolic alterations

The Glasgow Coma Scale (GCS) is a simple, objective, and rapid tool for determining the presence of brain dysfunction and is predictive, especially in its motor component, of the severity of the impairment and the patient's prognosis; it allows easy handoffs in what concerns brain function and provides a baseline assessment in anticipation of future reevaluations [10]. As shown in Table 15.2, the GCS is divided into three sections: eye opening, verbal response, and motor response.

An early step that allows for careful primary assessment is to remove the patient's clothing: this allows all injuries to be detected and thus ensures the patient receives the best level of care. Although it is important to complete the primary assessment of the trauma patient by exposure, it should not be forgotten that hypothermia is a serious problem in trauma management, which can exacerbate the clinical picture by leading to alterations in the patient's acid base balance and coagulative pattern. It is therefore important to remember to expose only the external parts to the external environment and, as soon as possible, proceed to cover the patient to prevent further heat loss.

Table 15.2 Glasgow Coma Scale and related scores (Min 3–Max 15)

	Eyes	Verbal	Motor
1	Absence of opening	No response	No response
2	Opens to pain	Incomprehensible words	Extension to pain
3	Opens to the call	Inappropriate words	Flexion to pain
4	Spontaneous opening	Confused	Retraction from pain
5		Oriented	Stimulus localization
6			Executes simple orders

Case Report Patient extracted with rapid extrication maneuver, no evidence of massive hemorrhage in place; subluxation of mandible in order to ensure airway patency and ventilation with AMBU self-expanding balloon; normo-expandable chest no flails or emphysema; confirmed no peripheral pulse, carotid pulse 155 bpm, pale periphery, PA undetectable; found 16G large-caliber peripheral venous access, infused bolus of crystalloids 250 mL. Abdominal defense reaction, evidence of deformity to pelvis and femurs bilaterally, exposed decomposed fracture of legs bilaterally. GCS 4 (M2V1E1)

Definitive airway secured by orotracheal intubation. Lower-extremity immobilization and pelvic belt placement; definitive immobilization of patient on spinal board. Contact with emergency medical emergency system operations center in order to centralize the patient.

The choice of definitive treatment site for a critically ill polytrauma patient assumes the same importance as any other treatment delivered at the scene and is based on knowledge and evaluation of key centralization criteria. It is important to balance the risk of overestimation (*overtriage*) and underestimation (*undertriage*) of injuries and clinical conditions. The use of *scores* is very common in medicine and certainly helps in patient categorization, but it is not practical in the emergency system; the Injury Severity Score (ISS), for example, is a score used to define and categorize the patient with major trauma, but in order to be calculated, it requires that the patient has performed all the necessary diagnostic-therapeutic steps. It seems clear therefore how it is unusable during primary rescue; the usefulness of these scores is instead greater for data collection and subsequent analysis.

International literature and guidelines from major scientific societies dealing with major trauma have identified three main criteria to be used in the evaluation of a patient with major trauma.

Physio-pathological criteria (consider alteration of vital parameters):

- Altered consciousness with GCS < 9
- GCS > 9 but persistent agitation or other neurological signs
- Persistent PAS < 90 mmHg after crystalloid infusion
- Tachypnea >29 or Bradypnea <10 acts/min after analgesia

Anatomical criteria (take into consideration the body district affected by the trauma):

- Exposed skull fracture—skull theca sinking—suspected skull base fracture (periorbital hematoma, rhino-liquor)
- Smashing of the facial massif
- Spinal trauma with motor and/or sensory deficits
- Penetrating wounds at head—neck—trunk—limb root level
- Amputation, subamputation, or limb crushing
- Pelvic fractures with hemodynamic instability
- Chest trauma with respiratory distress signs, rib *volet*, multiple rib fractures with subcutaneous emphysema

Event dynamics criteria (they basically consider kinetic energy)

- Fall from height >3 m
- Distance projection >3 m or ejection from the cockpit
- Projection from the motorcycle
- Intrusions of part of the vehicle into the passenger compartment
- Rolling
- Presence of another deceased patient

In addition to these criteria, which can be called the main ones, there are also special considerations not to be forgotten that can mislead the rescuer in the primary assessment of the patient:

- Extremes of ages
- Taking anticoagulated drugs
- Pregnancy
- Presence of burns and their degree and extent

Clinical Case Patient was transported by helicopter, during transport administered additional crystalloids (total 750 mL) without ever obtaining a detectable PA value. In shock room performed echo-fast with finding bilateral pleural sliding, intraperitoneal free effusion, and pubic symphysis diastasis. The patient was then transferred to the operating room for continuation of treatment.

In conclusion, the likelihood of survival for a polytrauma patient depends on the immediate identification and correction or mitigation of conditions that interfere with tissue perfusion: these conditions are identified only by using a systematic approach with defined priorities and consequent actions; this constitutes the patient assessment, which begins with the assessment of the scene and its safety and continues by using the X-ABCDE sequence so as to gather information that, when analyzed, forms the basis for immediate care and for the choice on whether to centralize the patient. Despite the sequential presentation, these assessments and actions are often performed simultaneously; immediate hazards must be quickly corrected as soon as they are recognized. Once massive hemorrhage has been controlled, airways managed if necessary, breathing and hemodynamics optimized, and the event and the victim's condition clearly and accurately communicated to the operations center, the patient should be transported without wasting additional valuable time at the scene. Primary and possibly secondary assessment should be repeated many times, including during transport, so that any changes in the patient's condition or the emergence of new problems requiring rapid intervention can be identified.

15.2 Early Intrahospital Management

The *trauma team* represents a group of medical professionals, nurses, and support staff whose task is to ensure the management of the major trauma patient in a coordinated and multidisciplinary manner. The numerosity and composition of the trauma team depend on the resources available and influence the type of approach to the patient (vertical vs. cross-cutting). The vertical approach, in which a single figure handles the entire assessment from head to toe, is reserved for facilities with few resources. In contrast, in centers dedicated to trauma care, the approach is transversal, with multiple professional figures simultaneously, in a coordinated manner and under the supervision of a team leader, performing maneuvers on the patient.

The team leader, regardless of specialty, represents the figure within the group with the most experience and cultural background in trauma. He or she should be a physician not directly involved in the various procedures, but with exclusive supervisory duties, such as:

– Activation and team composition in the imminence of patient arrival
– Preparation of the shock room with all the necessary equipment
– Information exchange with prehospital personnel
– Selection of diagnosis and treatment priorities with communication of strategies to other team members
– Performing or supervising primary, secondary assessment, and life-saving maneuvers
– Involvement of specialists and coordination of various procedures, until the final admission of the patient
– Supervision of the accuracy of clinical documentation
– Communication with the patient if conscious, family members, and the media

The professionals who make up the trauma team within an emergency department aimed at delivering definitive care to major trauma are (Table 15.2) the following.

1. **Medical airway expert**: Within the trauma team, the medical airway expert (MVA) is usually an anesthesiologist-resuscitation (AR) or emergency physician (MURG). He or she positions himself or herself at the patient's head and serves the function of checking cervical spine protection, acquiring the airway by intubation if necessary, performing the puncture for pleural decompression, funneling the central venous tract, placing the gastric tube (SNG), and perform-

ing E-FAST ultrasound (if no 24/7 radiologist available and if not surgeon *expertise*). If the airway physician is an anesthesiologist, he or she is responsible for intra-operative management of the patient. Otherwise, provision should be made for an anesthesiologist to join the team at the time the patient enters the operating room.

2. **Trauma surgeon**: Since there is no specific professional figure in Italy, this role is usually filled by a general surgeon (CHIR) who assumes special expertise in performing emergency procedures during the initial management of major trauma. He or she initially positions himself or herself at one side of the patient and provides when necessary surgical acquisition of airway and infusion routes, thoracostomy drainage and decompressive thoracotomy, temporary control of external bleeding, fracture reduction and *splinting*, and bladder catheter placement. He also performs E-FAST if more experienced in this procedure than the airway physician (if no 24/7 radiologist available). The team surgeon obviously performs emergency surgeries, expertise being required to perform life-saving surgical maneuvers in all body districts.

3. **Trauma Nurse 1**: This is the nurse (IP1) who complements and assists the airway expert physician and performs some procedures (e.g., SNG placement) on his or her delegation to expedite operations.

4. **Trauma Nurse 2**: This is the nurse (IP2) who supports and assists the trauma surgeon in all procedures by performing some of them by proxy (e.g., bladder catheterization, acquisition of peripheral venous pathways, dressing of bleeding wounds, placement of *splints*).

5. **Radiology Technician**: It is essential to have a radiology technician (TRSM) in the shock room who is responsible for setting up the ultrasound equipment and performing the initial (or first-level) radiological investigations in the emergency room on the instructions of the team leader.

6. **Auxiliary staff**: One or two auxiliaries (AUs) are needed to provide the team with materials that may not be in the shock room, dispatch blood requests, preserve the patient's personal belongings, assist medical and nursing staff with procedures, help with transfers, accompany family members to the interview rooms, and provide psychological support to them.

7. **Physician who records procedures**: This is usually a physician-in-training (SPEC) whose function is not only to work alongside one of the physicians on the team to become familiar with the various procedures, but also to record on paper or computer the primary and secondary assessment data, medical history, parameters, and procedures performed. In his absence, this role is performed by the airway physician or surgeon.

   Three other medical figures who are often indispensable from the earliest stages of major trauma management:

8. **Radiologist**: The radiologist (RAD) can perform E-FAST in the shock room themselves, which then takes on a higher diagnostic value and subsequently decides in consultation with the team leader on the choice and sequence of the most appropriate second-level investigation techniques to arrive at a definitive lesion assessment.

9. **Orthopedist**: The presence of the orthopedist (ORTO) in the shock room is necessary from the earliest stages after patient arrival in cases of severe pelvic fractures, as he or she can provide temporary pelvic stabilization to reduce retroperitoneal bleeding. In addition, the orthopedic surgeon can oversee the maneuvers of reduction and temporary immobilization of extremity fractures as well as indicate the diagnostic findings necessary for their definition.

10. **Neurosurgeon**: In case of worsening of consciousness or appearance of side signs and in the presence of para-tetraplegia, neurosurgical intervention may be immediately necessary. Therefore, it is critical that once the breathing and circulation issues have been managed in the suspected CNS injury, the neurosurgeon (NCH) views the patient and decides in consultation with the team leader on subsequent diagnostic and therapeutic procedures.

Other surgical area specialists who may be needed in special cases within the trauma team include the thoracic surgeon, vascular surgeon, cardiac surgeon, obstetrician-gynecologist, plastic-reconstructive surgeon, maxillofacial surgeon, otolaryngologist, ophthalmologist, and pediatric surgeon. The availability of these specialists should be ensured on call within the same hospital or through appropriate protocols of agreement.

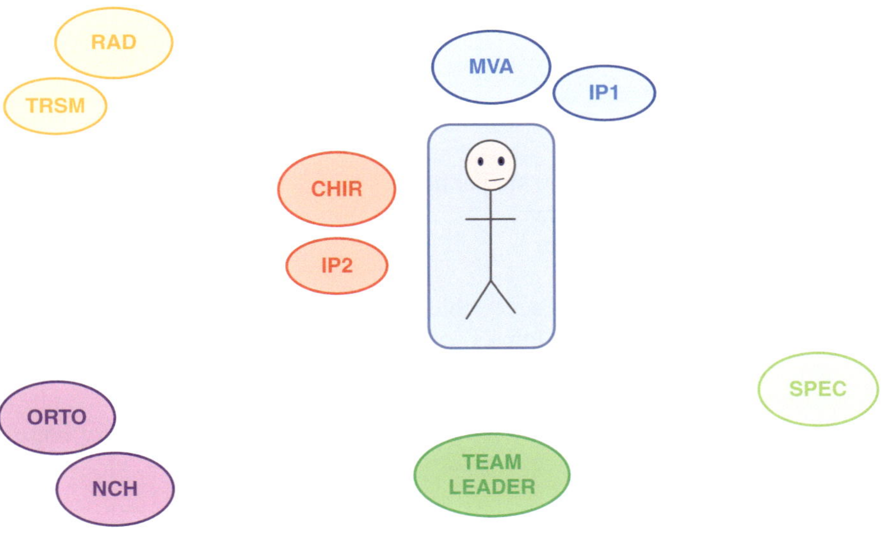

15.3   The Activation of the Trauma Team

It is necessary for the trauma team to be activated correctly, based on specific criteria, usually characterizing red or yellow triage codes. The following are those criteria:

15.3.1 Code Red

Vital Parameters
- GCS < 14 or neurological deterioration
- PAS < 90 mmHg (at least one detection in the prehospital)
- FR <10 or >29 or impaired respiratory mechanics or need for prehospital intubation

Anatomy of the Lesion
- Penetrating wound of head, neck, chest, abdomen, proximal extremities at elbow or knee
- Combination of trauma and burn of second or third
- Clinical suspicion of pelvic fracture
- Clinical suspicion of fracture of two or more proximal long bones (femur or humerus)
- Paralysis of one or more limbs
- Complete or incomplete proximal amputation at the wrist or ankle

15.3.2 Code Yellow

Dynamics of Trauma
- Violent impact
- Ejection from vehicle
- Vehicle speed greater than 60 km per hour
- External deformation >50 cm
- Sheet metal intrusion >30 cm
- Rolling of the vehicle
- Death of an occupant of the same vehicle
- Car/pedestrian or car/cyclist impact with speed >10 km/h
- Car/pedestrian or car/cyclist impact with projection or rolling up of the victim
- Motorcyclist fell at speeds >40 km/h
- Fallen motorcyclist with separation from the vehicle and/or secondary impact and/or rolling over
- Fall from height >6 m
- Extrication >20 min

Clinical Conditions of Increased Risk
- Age <12 years or >70 years
- Known or presumed pregnancy
- Serious known chronic diseases
- Anticoagulant therapy

15.4   First-Level Diagnostics

15.4.1 Extended Focused Assessment Sonography for Trauma (E-FAST)

This term refers to ultrasound scanning for free effusion to be performed with the following scans:

- Right hypochondrium (Morrison's pouch) and left (spleno-renal recess)
- Pelvic excavation
- Pericardium
- Costophrenic breakthroughs bilaterally
- Parasternal scans with a linear probe to visualize the sliding of pleural leaflets during respiratory acts

The absence of sliding (sliding) is indicative of pneumothorax; this condition, as well as the finding of hemothorax, may be indicative of the need for thoracostomy drainage.

A free abdominal effusion associated with a hemodynamic unstable condition is an indication for emergency laparotomy.

The advantages of E-FAST are rapid performance, high sensitivity (90%) and specificity (95.6%), and the ability to be repeated frequently. However, it is an operator-dependent examination, which does not allow identification of hollow viscera lesions and evaluation of the retroperitoneum.

The widespread use of E-FAST has almost completely replaced the practice of diagnostic peritoneal lavage (DPL) in the emergency evaluation of the abdomen of the trauma patient.

15.4.2 Chest X-Ray

To be performed with patient supine, in antero-posterior projection.

The chest X-ray reading should consider:

- Soft tissue and bone components: presence of fractures of skeletal components (ribs, clavicles, scapulae), presence of swelling or air in soft tissue, indicative for pneumothorax
- Airway and mediastinum: position of the trachea and main bronchi (a deviation of the trachea is indicative of hypertensive pneumothorax), correct positioning of the endotracheal tube if present, widening of the mediastinum
- Lung fields: assessment of lung field expansion, presence of contusions (if associated with rib volet may be the cause of marked hypoxia with a need for mechanical ventilation), pneumothorax or hemothorax

– Cardiac image and aortic profile: assessment of heart size and contours, regularity of aortic profile
– Diaphragm: integrity of hemidiaphragms (evidence of gastric bubble or SNG in chest is indicative of diaphragmatic injury), occupation of costophrenic sphincters
– Additional devices: correct positioning of pipes and lines
– Identification of thoracic injuries on standard radiography indicates, in major trauma, the need for CT with contrast medium.

15.4.3 X-Ray of the Pelvis

To be performed in antero-posterior projection.

It allows identification of pelvic girdle fractures, potentially causing hemodynamic instability, and planning of subsequent diagnostic-therapeutic choices.

In interpreting the X-ray of the pelvis, one must evaluate:

– Presence of any disruption of the pelvic ring bordering the small pelvis
– Presence of fracture rhymes at the different bony components of the pelvis, acetabulum bilaterally, and L5
– Enlargement of pelvic volume by diastasis of the pubic symphysis (>2.5 cm) or sacroiliac joints posteriorly
– The rise of a hemipelvi relative to the contralateral

15.5 Second-Level Diagnostics

They are performed after secondary evaluation or at the end of any emergency surgery for hemorrhagic injuries.

15.5.1 X-Ray of the Spine

The study of the spine is deferred after the resolution of any emergencies identified by previous assessments, thus also after emergency surgeries. In that case, cervical immobilization by collar and dorso-lumbar immobilization by spine board or rigid mattress if available should be maintained until the spine can be investigated. The spine should be fully investigated in the case of trauma patients with altered sensory (coma, sedation, alcohol, or drug use). In the awake, cooperating patient, the spine is investigated on the basis of clinical assessment if there is tenderness, neurological deficit, or mechanism of trauma at risk.

For the dorso-lumbosacral spine, two projections should be performed (anterolateral and latero-lateral); the projections, if adequate, should visualize all metameres included in the investigated spine tract. For the cervical spine and the cervico-dorsal hinge, it is preferable to perform a CT scan of the spine in order to have a better diagnostic definition; in fact, the interposition of the shoulders does not allow a proper evaluation of the spine with X-rays alone, and at the same time, the trans-oral projection for the evaluation of the epistropheus tooth is not executable in the trauma patient.

15.5.2 X-Rays of the Limbs

To be performed in cases of obvious or suspected long bone fractures.

As in the case of the spine, such investigations should be performed only after stabilization of the patient's vital functions. They do, however, possess the character of urgency in the presence of exposed fractures and fractures associated with vascular lesions, as these problems require the earliest possible surgical treatment in order to save the limb.

TC:

Is performed as an in-depth diagnostic in all cases in which clinical evaluation or first-level investigations have shown or placed suspicion of injury to various body districts.

Because patient transport is required in an environment that does not often allow for adequate vital function supports, the patient must be stable. If not, the patient must first undergo all stabilization procedures (intubation, drainage of hypertensive pneumothorax, surgical control of a hemorrhage, etc.) before undergoing the examination.

CT should be performed by the following method:

- Without infusion of intravenous contrast medium for study of the encephalon or for targeted study of vertebral metameres.
- After contrast medium injection (cmdc) for the study of the thorax of the abdomen and pelvis; it allows the study of parenchyma and the identification of vascular lesions (contrast medium extravasation or *blushing*) that can benefit from angiography. Visualization of air by appropriate windowing allows evaluation in the thorax for the presence of small flaps of pneumothorax and in the abdomen for the presence of free air as an indirect sign of perforation of a hollow viscera.
- After administration of endoluminal contrast agent: administration of water-soluble contrast agent via SNG or rectal probe is indicated in the evaluation of the integrity of hollow viscera in cases of penetrating trauma.

15.5.3 Angiography

Allows the study of the arterial vascular tree and the treatment of lesions amenable to embolization or placement of endoprostheses (*stents*). The indication for angiography is the visualization on CT of bleeding from the vessels of the various parenchyma and pelvis in cases of pelvic fracture. In the patient with stable hemodynamics, endovascular treatment, if effective, can avoid surgical intervention, particularly in cases of pelvic, liver, spleen, and kidney injuries. Another indication for angiography is the absence of an arterial pulse distal to a fracture focus in a limb. The angiographic study is necessary to place the indication for a revascularization procedure.

15.5.4 Nuclear Magnetic Resonance Imaging (RMN)

Is used as a second-level investigation in the patient with head trauma in cases of discrepancy between CT images and neurological objectivity (e.g., in cases of diffuse axonal damage and in the presence of suspected brainstem injury). In the patient with vertebrospinal cord injury, it allows definition of the extent of spinal cord damage. MRI should be performed urgently in the presence of incomplete spinal cord injury or progressive worsening of neurological damage as it may indicate the need for emergency neurosurgical intervention. The use of cholangio MRI in traumatic liver injury for the diagnosis of biliary complications is emerging.

It is possible that a patient initially classified as stable and started to a nonintensive care observation post in the emergency department or in radiology, such as in the CT room, will show a sudden deterioration of the hemodynamic picture. In such an eventuality, the patient should be immediately returned to the emergency room (where supplies and equipment for life support are available), and the steps of the ABC sequence should be repeated. The team leader should follow the patient as he or she moves along with at least three other team members and is responsible for the continuation of any life support and monitoring of parameters.

The diagnostic and therapeutic *process* is decided by the team leader with the support of the other members of the trauma team and any consultants involved.

References

1. Gunst M, Ghaemmaghami V, Urban J, et al. Changing epidemiology of trauma deaths leads to a bimodal distribution. Proc (Bayl Univ Med Cent). 2010;23(4):349–54.
2. Sobrino J, Shafi S. Timing and causes of death after injuries. Proc (Bayl Univ Med Cent). 2013;26(2):120–3.
3. Centers for Disease Control and Prevention. Leading causes of death. https://www.cdc.gov/injury/wisquars/index.html. Updated Apr 2017.
4. Reichard A, Marsh S, Moore P. Fatal and nonfatal injuries among emergency medical technicians and paramedics. Prehosp Emerg Care. 2011;15(4):511–7.
5. Brown JB, Rosengart MR, Forsythe RM, et al. Not all prehospital time is equal: influence of scene time on mortality. J Trauma Acute Care Surg. 2016;81:93–100.
6. Bulger EM, Snyder D, Schoelles K, et al. An evidence-based prehospital guideline for external hemorrhage control: American College of Surgeons Committee on Trauma. Prehosp Emerg Care. 2014;18(2):163–73.
7. Stockinger ZT, McSwain NE Jr. Prehospital endotracheal intubation for trauma does not improve survival over bag-mask ventilation. J Trauma. 2004;56(3):531.
8. Jones KM, Reed RL, Luchette FA. The ribs or not the ribs: which influences mortality? Am J Surg. 2001;202(5):598–604.
9. Brown JB, Choen MJ, Minei JP, et al. Goal directed resuscitation in the prehospital setting: a propensity adjusted analysis. J Trauma Acute Care Surg. 2013;74(4):295–300.
10. Kerby JD, Maclennan PA, Burton JN, et al. Agreement between prehospital and emergency department Glasgow Coma Scores. J Trauma. 2007;63(5):1026–31.